Making Sense of IBS

Making Sense of IBS

*A Physician Answers
Your Questions about
Irritable Bowel Syndrome*

SECOND EDITION

Brian E. Lacy, Ph.D., M.D.

Johns Hopkins University Press
Baltimore

Note to the reader: This book is not meant to substitute for medical care, and treatment should not be based solely on its contents. Instead, treatment must be developed in a dialogue between you and your doctor. It is especially important to discuss the use of any medications with your doctor.

© 2006, 2013 Johns Hopkins University Press
All rights reserved. Published 2013
Printed in the United States of America on acid-free paper
9 8 7 6 5 4 3 2 1

Johns Hopkins University Press
2715 North Charles Street
Baltimore, Maryland 21218-4363
www.press.jhu.edu

Library of Congress Cataloging-in-Publication Data

Lacy, Brian E.
    Making sense of IBS : a physician answers your questions about irritable bowel syndrome / Brian E. Lacy, Ph.D., M.D. — Second edition.
        pages   cm. — (A Johns Hopkins Press health book)
    Includes bibliographical references and index.
    ISBN-13: 978-1-4214-1115-6 (pbk. : alk. paper)
    ISBN-10: 1-4214-1115-6 (pbk. : alk. paper)
    ISBN-13: 978-1-4214-1116-3 (electronic)
    ISBN-10: 1-4214-1116-4 (electronic)
    1. Irritable colon. I. Title. II. Title: Making sense of irritable bowel syndrome.
    RC862.I77L33 2013
    616.3′42—dc23   2013006074

A catalog record for this book is available from the British Library.

All illustrations except Figure 11.1 are by Jacqueline Schaffer.

Special discounts are available for bulk purchases of this book. For more information, please contact Special Sales at 410-516-6936 or specialsales@press.jhu.edu.

Johns Hopkins University Press uses environmentally friendly book materials, including recycled text paper that is composed of at least 30 percent post-consumer waste, whenever possible.

Contents

Preface

If you've picked up this book, then it is quite likely that you or a friend, a coworker, or someone in your family has irritable bowel syndrome (IBS). I can safely make that statement because 1 in 6 to 1 in 7 adult Americans suffers from this problem. Although the condition is quite common, people who have IBS have often found it difficult to get help for their symptoms or answers to their questions. Fortunately, over the past 10 years, significant advances have been made in our understanding of IBS. We now have a much clearer picture of why IBS develops, and we also better understand the very complex interactions that occur between the brain and the gut in patients who have IBS. In addition, researchers, scientists, and physicians have made significant contributions to our ability to manage the multiple symptoms of this often frustrating disorder.

Because education of patients and health care providers about IBS has been limited, I wanted to write this book to share this wealth of new information with more people. The book has several goals:

- to convey what we currently understand about IBS
- to clear up the many misconceptions and misperceptions that surround IBS
- to help you recognize the symptoms of IBS
- to describe tests that may be used during the evaluation of IBS symptoms
- to discuss the many treatment options available for the diverse symptoms of IBS

- to provide information that will allow people who have IBS to better understand their symptoms, institute changes, and improve their quality of life.

To accomplish these goals, I have divided this book into four parts. Part 1 provides a general introduction to the disorder. Part 2 focuses on the evaluation and diagnosis of a patient who has symptoms of IBS. Part 3 focuses on the treatment of IBS, and Part 4 discusses children who have IBS and the future for IBS treatments and education. Terms used in the book are defined in a glossary at the back, and at the front of the book is a list of abbreviations. There is also a short appendix about the design and importance of clinical studies.

I hope that this book will answer your many questions about IBS and allow you to make sense of this common disorder.

Acknowledgments

The process of writing, editing, and publishing a book is a significant undertaking that represents the collective efforts of many people. Unfortunately, and unfairly, the cover of a book lists only the author's name and does not credit the many others so intimately involved in this lengthy process. Although it is not possible to properly thank everyone who contributed to this project, I would like to acknowledge some of them.

First, I want to thank all of the patients who have IBS whom I have seen over the past fifteen years. I appreciate their willingness to describe their symptoms and share how IBS affects their lives. I hope that this book will provide them with new ideas and information that will enable them to better understand this complex disorder and ameliorate their symptoms.

Thanks also go to Executive Editor Jacqueline Wehmueller and to Sara Cleary, both of the Johns Hopkins University Press, for their cogent thoughts, continued encouragement, and tireless efforts in editing and revising the manuscript. In addition, I owe great thanks to all of my friends and colleagues at Dartmouth for their wonderful suggestions, advice, and support.

Finally, I dedicate this book to the memory of my father, who taught me to be patient and understanding, and to Elaine, for her unwavering patience, support, and selflessness.

Abbreviations

Abbreviations will usually be defined where they first appear in the text. This list is provided for convenient reference.

ANS   autonomic nervous system
CBC   complete blood count
CBT   cognitive behavioral therapy
CFS   chronic fatigue syndrome
CMV   cytomegalovirus
CNS   central nervous system
CPP   chronic pelvic pain
CRF   corticotropin releasing factor
CRP   C-reactive protein
CT   computed tomography
DNA   deoxyribonucleic acid
EGD   esophagogastroduodenoscopy
ENS   enteric nervous system
ESR   erythrocyte sedimentation rate
FDA   Food and Drug Administration
5-HT   5-hydroxytryptamine, also called serotonin
GERD   gastroesophageal reflux disease

GI	gastrointestinal
gm	gram(s)
Hct	hematocrit
Hgb	hemoglobin
HIV	human immunodeficiency virus
IBD	inflammatory bowel disease
IC	interstitial cystitis
LES	lower esophageal sphincter
LFTs	liver function tests
mg	milligram(s)
ml	milliliter(s)
MRI	magnetic resonance imaging
MSG	monosodium glutamate
OAB	overactive bladder
O&P	ova and parasites
OTC	over-the-counter
PEG	polyethylene glycol
PET	positron emission tomography
PMR	polymyalgia rheumatica
p.r.n.	*pro re nata* (as needed)
RAP	recurrent abdominal pain
SLE	systemic lupus erythematosus
SSRI	selective serotonin reuptake inhibitor
TCA	tricyclic antidepressant
TIA	transient ischemic attack
TMJ	temporomandibular joint
TSH	thyroid stimulating hormone
US	ultrasound
UTI	urinary tract infection
WBC	white blood cell

PART I

Irritable Bowel Syndrome: The Basics

CHAPTER 1

Overview of IBS

Irritable bowel syndrome is one of the most common disorders seen in medical practice today. During a typical week, the average family practitioner or internist will see more patients who have irritable bowel syndrome (IBS) than patients who have asthma, diabetes, hypertension, or cardiovascular disease. To help put this into perspective, consider that approximately 15 percent of adult Americans have symptoms of IBS, which translates to approximately 45 million adult Americans having recurring symptoms of abdominal pain, discomfort, bloating, distention, and either constipation or diarrhea (or both). This helps to explain why the aisles in your local pharmacy or drugstore are packed with over-the-counter medications designed to treat digestive problems.

Although IBS is common, the condition remains poorly understood. Lack of understanding of this prevalent, complex disorder is pervasive among family members and coworkers of people who have IBS as well as insurers, health care plans, the public at large, and even some physicians. People misunderstand IBS on many different levels. For example, some people believe that IBS is an uncommon disorder and that the attention paid to it occurs only because of the actions of a very small but vocal group of people who have IBS. On the contrary, multiple large population-based research studies have shown that up to 15 percent of adult Americans have IBS.

Another common misconception is that IBS affects only young women. In fact, nothing could be further from the truth. Irritable bowel syndrome is an equal opportunity disorder. It does not discriminate based on age, sex, race, or nationality. Some insurance companies and health care providers believe that IBS is nothing more than an annoyance and that it should not even be considered a medical problem. It is well documented, however, that from a patient's perspective, this common disorder significantly affects patients' quality of life on a daily basis.

Finally, some people mistakenly argue that IBS is a new problem that has appeared in response to the stresses of an industrialized society or that it is a problem manufactured by pharmaceutical companies solely to improve their revenue. But multiple studies have clearly shown that IBS is found throughout the world and is not just limited to Western societies. Irritable bowel syndrome exists in rural areas, underpopulated areas, and nonindustrialized societies. Irritable bowel syndrome is not new; it likely has been present for thousands of years, if not longer. In this book, I address these common misconceptions and provide answers to common questions about IBS using the most recent data from scientific studies performed around the world.

Although irritable bowel syndrome is now a relatively familiar term, the disease was given a number of different names in the past. Some of these are colorful (spastic colitis), while others are somewhat pejorative (nervous colitis), and still others are simply misnomers (mucus colitis, unstable colitis, and inflammatory colitis). These terms are misleading, confusing, and often distressing to people who have IBS. People who receive a diagnosis using one of these old-fashioned terms may be worried that they are receiving a different diagnosis of a more severe disorder rather than IBS. For example, the term "mucus colitis" may lead someone to think that they have ulcerative colitis or Crohn's disease, both of which are inflammatory bowel diseases (see Chapters 7, 8, and 12). For these reasons, such older labels should not be used, and anyone who is diagnosed with one of these labels should ask his or her doctor for a different diagnosis.

Despite the variety of names and labels for IBS, the disease has remained the same over the years. Noted English physician W. Cumming published a description of IBS more than 150 years ago that seems remarkably similar to our current description. In an 1849 passage taken from the *London Gazette*, he described IBS in the following manner: "The bowels are at one time constipated, at another time lax, in the same person. How the disease has two such different symptoms I do not profess to explain."

There is significant confusion over this common medical problem, and a host of unanswered questions remain. What, then, is IBS? Irritable bowel syndrome is a common, chronic (meaning that it continues for a long time or recurs frequently) disorder of the gastrointestinal tract. Characteristic symptoms include abdominal pain or discomfort, in association with disordered bowel habits consisting of either constipation or diarrhea (or alternating symptoms of both, in many cases). Other common symptoms include bloating, gassiness, abdominal distention, passage of mucus with a bowel movement, significant straining during a bowel movement, or the very urgent need to have a bowel movement. Although these symptoms are well recognized, they are not specific to IBS; other medical conditions can cause these or similar symptoms, too. The following story of a young woman referred for the evaluation of chronic gastrointestinal symptoms illustrates the misconceptions and misperceptions that surround this common medical problem.

Meredith is a 29-year-old woman referred by her family practitioner for a second opinion. She explained that her problems first began in college. Every several months she would have several days of lower abdominal cramps and diarrhea. The diarrhea was loose and watery but never bloody. It seemed to be associated with significant bloating and distention of her abdomen. Her friends often joked that during these episodes she looked six months pregnant. She attributed these episodes to a viral illness on one occasion, food poisoning on another, and overly rich food on a third occasion.

After college she worked for a consulting firm. This was a stressful job and she had little free time for exercise or relaxing social activities. Several times a month, she would have three to four days of lower abdominal cramps and pain. The pain would generally start shortly before an episode of diarrhea, and she noted that she would often have to run to the bathroom because the urge to have a bowel movement was so strong and forceful. The cramps and lower abdominal discomfort would eventually subside, but each episode left her feeling exhausted. Her friends suggested that she might be lactose intolerant (unable to break down and digest the major sugar in milk products; see Chapter 10). However, even after she eliminated milk and cottage cheese from her diet, her symptoms continued. Meredith mentioned her symptoms to her gynecologist at her next routine office visit. After examining her, he told her he could find nothing wrong and that it was probably "just stress."

During the next year, her symptoms did not change significantly but did occur more frequently. It was now common for her to have three to four days in a row of lower abdominal pain and discomfort associated with significant bloating and distention. Although she had always been slender, Meredith had to buy new clothes with elastic waistbands, because many of her clothes felt tight on the days when she was bloated. She began to plan her errands and social events more carefully, because sometimes the urge to go to the bathroom came on so suddenly that she was afraid she would have an accident. Meredith tried a variety of over-the-counter medications without any relief. One friend told her that she probably was not digesting her food properly and that enzyme supplements would help her. She tried these for a month, but they did not seem to help. Another friend told her that she wasn't getting enough fiber in her diet. Meredith became a strict vegetarian and eliminated all animal products from her diet. This only seemed to make the bloating worse. Another friend told her that her symptoms sounded just like her aunt, who had celiac disease (an allergy to wheat products; see Chapter 10).

After researching the topic online, Meredith thought that her symptoms could be the result of a wheat allergy, so she eliminated all wheat products from her diet, which was very hard to do. After two months without any improvement in her symptoms, she abandoned this strict wheat-free diet. Meredith next tried acetaminophen and a variety of over-the-counter anti-inflammatory medications in an attempt to help with the lower abdominal pain, but none of them alleviated her symptoms, and most of them upset her stomach. Out of frustration, she finally made an appointment to see her family practitioner.

Dr. Berkes listened to Meredith's story, carefully examined her, and reassured her that everything was normal. She ordered some simple laboratory tests, all of which yielded normal results. She told her that this was really "nothing to worry about" and said that maybe she was just overly stressed and a little anxious. She suggested that an exercise program and stress management might be helpful.

Meredith joined a health club, started yoga, and even learned to meditate, but her symptoms continued. The next time she discussed her chronic problem with several of her friends, they told her that all of her complaints were common symptoms of ulcerative colitis, an inflammatory bowel disease. This greatly concerned her, especially after one friend described how her brother needed multiple surgeries to help with his inflammatory bowel disease. The next day, Meredith called her family practitioner and told her that she was concerned that she had inflammatory bowel disease and wanted to see a specialist in stomach and bowel disorders. Dr. Berkes reassured her that her symptoms did not sound worrisome, but she agreed that seeing a gastroenterologist would be a good idea.

In my office, Meredith described her symptoms: lower abdominal cramps and discomfort; sudden urges to go to the bathroom; loose, watery bowel movements; and feelings of being very bloated and distended. She said she was concerned that she had inflammatory bowel disease and was also worried that she might have ovarian cancer (she had visited several websites that described abdominal discomfort and bloating as common signs of ovarian cancer).

I reviewed her history carefully. Her weight had been stable for the first five years of her symptoms, and during the last three years, she had actually gained eight pounds. The character of her pain and discomfort had not changed, although the episodes were now more frequent. A recent test of her complete blood count (CBC) was normal, and Meredith had never been anemic. She stated that no one in her family had a history of ovarian cancer, inflammatory bowel disease, celiac disease, or any type of cancer in the gastrointestinal tract. Meredith had not been camping or traveling, had not been taking antibiotics, and had been drinking water that came from the city water supply (all of these factors decreased the likelihood that she had developed diarrhea due to an infection in her colon). She did admit that she had problems with mild insomnia and that she felt stressed at work. I performed a complete physical examination and did not find anything abnormal.

I explained to Meredith that she had irritable bowel syndrome. Her long-standing symptoms of bloating, abdominal distention, and abdominal cramps and spasms preceding loose, watery bowel movements were fairly classic symptoms. Meredith had brought a long list of questions to her appointment that she wanted answered. The two questions at the top of her list were short but difficult ones: "Why me?" and "Why now?" Meredith also wanted to know if her IBS would turn into some other disease, like colon cancer. I answered her questions as best I could and reassured her that she was not alone with her symptoms. I told her that IBS is a common, chronic disorder that affects many women and men. I explained the natural history of the disorder (see Chapters 4 and 5) and gave her some written information as well.

When I asked Meredith what her worst symptom was, she said it was the urgency to go to the bathroom and the loose, watery bowel movements. She was less concerned about the abdominal pain and the bloating because, she said, she had "just learned to live with it." I advised Meredith to lower the amount of fiber in her diet, as her very high fiber diet was probably making her symptoms of bloating and diarrhea worse. I also advised her to avoid caffeine and fructose-containing liquids, because these can cause diarrhea and fecal urgency in some people who have IBS. We discussed a special diet called a low-FODMAP (Fructans, Oligodisaccharides, Disaccharides, Monosaccharides, and Polyols) diet, which excludes foods that may cause excessive fermentation in the gastrointestinal tract (see Chapter 15). Because Meredith didn't want to change too many things in her diet at once, she instead decided to schedule more regular meals and routine trips to the bathroom so that she wouldn't be afraid of having an accident when she felt the sudden urge to go to the bathroom. We agreed that she would take half an Imodium (loperamide) tablet each day after breakfast and again after dinner and would track her symptoms for the next four weeks, at which point she would return for an office visit.

When Meredith returned, she had a mixed report. She felt better overall. She had fewer episodes of diarrhea and some days even felt a little bit constipated after taking just the two half-tablets of Imodium each morning and evening. However, on two different days she had noted some blood in the toilet after having a bowel movement, and she feared that she might have colon cancer because her mother had told her that blood in the stool was a common sign of colon cancer. She also reported that the abdominal pain was becoming more of an issue. I reassured Meredith that colon cancer, although a significant medical problem in the United States, was unlikely in a young woman who was not anemic and did not have a family history of colon cancer. However, I also told her that it is not normal to have bleeding and that the best thing to do would be to schedule a colonoscopy to examine her colon and determine where the bleeding had come from. In addition, we agreed that she would start taking a low dose of a new medication, desipramine, each night before bedtime. This medication, one of a class of medications called tricyclic antidepressants (TCAs), is commonly used to treat abdominal pain in people who have IBS. In addition, this medication would likely improve her insomnia (see Chapter 17).

Meredith had her colonoscopy three weeks later. As expected, it was completely normal, except for a small internal hemorrhoid, which was likely the source of bleeding. She reported that her abdominal pain wasn't gone, although it was much better on the desipramine. In addition, she was sleeping better, and she felt more rested and better able to cope with some of the daily stressors in her life. Meredith was reassured by her normal colonoscopy and encouraged that by taking some simple medications, her symptoms had dramatically improved after many years of suffering from pain, bloating, and diarrhea. We discussed a few more ideas regarding diet and exercise, and I increased her dose of desipramine. She called back four weeks later to say that she felt dramatically better.

Like Meredith, people who have IBS have many questions about their condition. They are concerned that their symptoms indicate a very serious or life-threatening disease, such as colon or ovarian cancer. They worry that their symptoms may continue and evolve into a more serious disease, like inflammatory bowel disease. People who have IBS are often concerned that they will pass the condition on to their children. In addition, they are frustrated that they have not been able to get their symptoms under control by changing their diet or by using simple medications available over the counter. Finally, many people who have IBS feel confused, because they have been given contradictory, misleading, or even incorrect advice from family members, friends, nurses, and physicians.

This book seeks to answer questions, correct misperceptions, and alleviate concerns of people who have IBS and their family members and friends. In short, the goal of this book is to make sense of IBS.

Summary

- IBS is one of the most common medical conditions seen in primary care practice today.
- IBS is one of the most common reasons for a person to be referred to a specialist in digestive disorders (a gastroenterologist).
- IBS is found worldwide. It affects men and women of all ages, nationalities, races, and religions.
- IBS is not a new disorder but is now more widely recognized and more commonly diagnosed than it was in the past.
- People who have IBS characteristically suffer from lower abdominal pain or discomfort in association with either constipation or diarrhea (or both).

CHAPTER 2

What Is IBS?

When a patient is first diagnosed with a medical condition, one of the health practitioner's most important goals is to provide as much information as possible about the new diagnosis. This educational process includes carefully conveying the diagnosis to the patient, explaining terms, reviewing the natural history of the disease, and discussing treatment options. It is also an appropriate time to address the patient's individual concerns and fears.

Many people who have irritable bowel syndrome are inadequately informed about their disorder, are given incomplete information, or are given conflicting or confusing advice. When patients have insufficient or confusing information, they naturally can become frustrated, discouraged, and anxious. Having too little or wrong information can make symptoms seem unmanageable and even overwhelming at times. The fear stemming from believing that you have a seemingly murky medical problem is often much worse than dealing with a well-understood disease. The following case illustrates some of the pitfalls encountered in the new diagnosis for a person who has IBS. The case begins by presenting some of the typical symptoms of IBS.

Dr. Heckelman is a young doctor with a busy internal medicine practice in a large city. He is regarded by his colleagues as an intelligent, hardworking clinician who can accurately diagnose some of the most difficult diseases. He routinely sees 40 to 50 patients a day, and sometimes even more on a busy day. He recently saw Kimberly, a first-year college student at a local university, who came in at the urging of her mother. Kimberly told Dr. Heckelman that during the last several months she'd had lower abdominal discomfort, with a lot of bloating and gassiness, several times a week. In addition, Kimberly had developed diarrhea. She would often have urgent bowel movements that occurred after her abdominal pain began. Kimberly said that this was a change in her health, because as a high school student, she never had abdominal pain and never had a bowel movement more than once a day.

Dr. Heckelman listened to her story for a few minutes and then told her, "You have IBS. It is really nothing to worry about. I want you to get on a regular schedule at school, avoid all milk products, and take one Imodium (loperamide) tablet every morning. Call me in four to six weeks if you're not feeling better." Kimberly, a little confused by the rapid pace of the appointment, asked "Well, what is IBS? I've never heard of it." Dr. Heckelman replied, "You have a nervous gut. I'm sure a lot of your classmates have it too. We used to call it spastic colitis. That's all it is, a spasm. It's really nothing to worry about. Don't forget to call in a few weeks if you're still having problems." And with that, he rushed from the room on to the next patient, leaving behind a confused and disappointed Kimberly.

What Are Typical Symptoms of IBS?

The two symptoms of IBS that characterize and truly define this disorder are lower abdominal pain or discomfort and disordered bowel habits (constipation, diarrhea, or alternating symptoms of both). Abdominal pain is the hallmark of IBS—if a patient does not have abdominal pain, then he or she cannot be formally diagnosed as having IBS (see the formal definition later in this chapter). The pain or discomfort is usually located in the lower half of the person's abdomen, not the upper abdomen. Upper abdominal pain is more likely to indicate some abnormality in the structure or function of the stomach, liver, pancreas, or gallbladder.

People who have IBS differ on which of the predominant symptoms—abdominal pain or disordered bowel habits—are more bothersome to them. They may emphasize one or the other to their health care provider, depending on the intensity of the symptom, their reaction to it, and how much the symptom disrupts their life. For example, some people are not really bothered by abdominal pain but are perturbed by urgent diarrhea, which interferes with their job or social activities. Other people are more concerned with abdominal pain and are able to work around the problems of constipation or diarrhea.

The pattern of symptoms with IBS varies considerably from person to person but remains fairly consistent in a given individual, although there may be some variations in the intensity or the frequency of symptoms. Typically, symptoms are intermittent, with symptom-free periods lasting days, weeks, or (rarely) months. However, a small number of people will have daily symptoms without remission.

As noted previously, abdominal pain must be present for a health care provider to diagnose IBS accurately. The abdominal pain should coincide with having a bowel movement (defecation). Abdominal pain related to urination, menstruation, or exertion is *not* characteristic of IBS and suggests a different diagnosis. The character of the pain varies among people who have IBS, although for individuals it usually remains fairly stable over time. Some people who have IBS describe the pain as "crampy" in nature, whereas others describe it as sharp or burning. The location of the pain may vary from person to person but, again, remains fairly consistent over time in the same person. The abdominal pain of IBS is most likely to occur in the left lower side of the abdomen; it can occur on both sides but is less likely to occur only on the right side of the abdomen. Some people who have IBS have pain in the area above their pubic bone; others describe a deep-seated pain in their pelvis that moves toward the rectum and eventually remains there or pain that moves into their lower back, similar to labor pains. For some people who have IBS, the pain is difficult to locate, because it does not occur in a specific area.

The abdominal pain of IBS generally occurs in association with a bowel movement (either before, during, or after). Some people who have IBS have pain that occurs at other times as well. Unpredictable and unexpected episodes of abdominal pain can be frustrating for people who have IBS. The pain usually represents either a spasm of the smooth muscle that lines the GI tract or a GI tract that is overly sensitive to stretch, or distention. It is not uncommon for people with severe IBS to describe severe, debilitating, daily abdominal pain that develops from the time they wake up in the morning and then disappears at night.

In the United States, the generally accepted pattern of normal bowel activity ranges from three bowel movements a day to three bowel movements a week. People who have IBS have altered patterns of bowel activity. As with lower abdominal pain, the altered patterns of defecation may be variable from person to person but are fairly consistent for each individual. People who have IBS usually have one of three predominant patterns of altered defecation: predominantly constipation, predominantly diarrhea, or alternating constipation and diarrhea. Many people who have IBS and diarrhea find that the first stool in the morning is of normal consistency but subsequent bowel movements become increasingly loose and are associated with significant urgency, abdominal cramping, bloating, and gassiness. The extreme urgency and abdominal cramping may be temporarily relieved by the passage of stool; however, these symptoms often quickly return and precipitate yet another bowel movement. When the episode of diarrhea finally ends, the stool is usually all liquid or mostly mucus, and many people are left feeling exhausted. In contrast, people who have IBS and constipation often report the passage of rocky, hard, pellet-like stools called scybala. They may have symptoms of straining and incomplete evacuation (the feeling that you have not completely emptied your lower colon after having had a bowel movement). Mucus may cover the stools or be passed alone.

People who have IBS also often describe fecal urgency (the sudden urge to go to the bathroom, *now!*), increased stool frequency (more bowel movements than usual during a given time period), and severe lower abdominal cramps and spasms during the postprandial period (after a meal). These symptoms are just an exaggeration of a normal reflex. Almost everyone has the urge to have a bowel movement after at least one meal per day. This urge is a normal gastrocolic reflex (*gastro* refers to the stomach, and *colic* refers to the colon). The gastrocolic reflex develops when food in the stomach stimulates sensory receptors, which then send signals to the colon, telling it to contract. A normal reflex typically occurs 30 to 45 minutes after eating a medium-to-large meal. In people who have IBS, however, especially those who have IBS and diarrhea, this urge can be very exaggerated, and patients can develop an extreme sense of urgency that feels uncontrollable. This heightened gastrocolic reflex may occur within only a few minutes of beginning to eat and may force a person to hurry to the bathroom during the meal. Fecal incontinence occurs in up to 20 percent of people who have IBS and most likely results from extreme fecal urgency in association with repetitive spasms of the lower colon, rectum, and anal canal.

Bloating (a sense of fullness and gassiness in the abdomen) and abdominal distention (a visibly bulging abdomen filled with gas) are common symptoms in people who have IBS. Bloating and distention may reflect the presence of increased amounts of abdominal gas, delayed transit of gas through the GI tract, or, more commonly, increased sensitivity to normal amounts of intestinal gas.

What Is the Definition of IBS?

During the course of the past century, IBS has been given various labels, including nervous colitis, spastic colitis, mucus colitis, unstable colon, and irritable colon. These labels should all be discarded, as they are confusing, imprecise, and inaccurate. In addition, the labels may be distressing to patients, because they can be confused with other disorders, such as ulcerative colitis. In Kimberly's case, Dr. Heckelman told her that she had IBS without explaining what that term was and inappropriately referred to it as spastic colitis. Providing her with another term didn't help Kimberly at all, because she still did not know anything about what was causing her symptoms.

The name *irritable bowel syndrome* has led many patients—and physicians—to believe that this disorder is just a vague conglomeration of complaints. Some people suspect that IBS is an easy term for doctors to use if a patient's symptoms are vague, confusing, or not typical of any other specific disease or if the cause of the symptoms cannot be detected by laboratory tests or diagnostic studies. However, the name remains an appropriate description. First, this disorder truly is a constellation of symptoms (which is why it is called a syndrome) rather than a single isolated symptom. Second, IBS can affect multiple areas of the gastrointestinal (GI) tract and is not just limited to the colon. Third, the intestinal tract of a person who has IBS does at times seem "irritable." For these reasons, *irritable bowel syndrome* is an appropriate and descriptive title.

IBS is classified as a functional GI disorder (also called a functional bowel disorder). "Functional" means that even though people who have IBS have symptoms that seem to represent a problem in the GI tract, no testing (laboratory tests, x-ray studies, and endoscopic procedures like colonoscopies) can identify such a problem (such as an ulcer, a blockage, or even a malignancy). "Functional" is an accurate word for IBS because although the GI tract may look normal in patients who have IBS and all currently available relevant tests are normal (see Chapters 7 & 8), it clearly does not always function normally. When there are no abnormal findings on physical examination, and test results are normal, symptoms of abdominal bloating and distention with either constipation or diarrhea can be frustrating and sometimes confusing for patients and physicians. However, like many other medical conditions, a concise definition for IBS does exist, and physicians may use this definition to diagnose IBS in their patients.

The definition of IBS has evolved considerably over the past three decades. In the late 1970s a list of symptoms called the Manning criteria was used to diagnose IBS. The Manning criteria were used to guide clinical research and patient care; generally, the more symptoms (criteria) a patient had, the more likely it was that the patient had IBS. The Manning criteria included:

- Abdominal pain easing after a bowel movement
- Looser bowel movements after the onset of pain
- More frequent bowel movements at the onset of pain
- Distention of the abdomen
- Passage of mucus when having a bowel movement
- Feelings of not having completely emptied after having a bowel movement

In 1989, a group of experts met in Rome and published a revised set of criteria for the diagnosis of IBS. These modifications, identified as the Rome criteria (later called Rome I), were meant to simplify the Manning criteria and to clarify the relationship between the presence of abdominal pain and disordered bowel habits. The Rome I criteria have been revised twice since the original meeting, and clinicians and researchers now use the Rome III criteria to accurately diagnose IBS in men and women. According to the Rome III criteria, people diagnosed with IBS must have had their symptoms begin at least six months before diagnosis and, during the last three months before diagnosis, they must have had at least three days per month in which they experienced abdominal pain or discomfort associated with two or more of the following:

- Symptom relief with defecation
- Change in stool frequency
- Change in stool form (appearance)

In addition, for physicians to accurately diagnose IBS and to categorize it appropriately (IBS with constipation, diarrhea, or mixed symptoms of alternating constipation and diarrhea), their patients should have one or more of the following symptoms at least 25 percent of the time:

- Abnormal stool frequency (less than three times a week)
- Abnormal stool form (lumpy/hard)
- Abnormal stool passage (straining, incomplete evacuation)
- Bloating or feeling of abdominal distention
- Passage of mucus
- Frequent, loose stools

In everyday clinical practice, many physicians use criteria that are less strict and less cumbersome than described above. For example, if a patient has chronic symptoms of lower abdominal pain or discomfort associated with disordered bowel movements, and these symptoms are relieved with defecation, then he or she has IBS. This simpler definition helps minimize the difficulty that patients have trying to remember their bowel habits and GI symptoms during the previous six months. A new definition of the Rome criteria (Rome IV) will likely be published in 2016; this change will be mostly important for physicians and scientists performing research studies.

What Is Causing My Symptoms of IBS?

Our understanding of the underlying body processes that cause IBS (that is, the abnormal physiology, or the *pathophysiology*, of IBS) has changed considerably during the last half-century. In the 1940s and 1950s, the medical community thought that IBS was a nervous disorder of the GI tract, which is why many people who have IBS were said to have "nervous colitis." Dr. Thomas Almy, who was regarded as a leading figure in gastroenterology at the time, was one of the first physicians to propose a connection between the brain and the GI tract. This concept, now called the brain-gut axis, led to a tremendous leap in our understanding of the pathophysiology of IBS (see Figure 2.1).

In his early experiments, Dr. Almy performed rigid sigmoidoscopy (an examination of the lower portion of the colon; see Chapter 8) on healthy volunteers and recorded a variety of information, including their respiratory rate (number of breaths per minute), heart rate, and blood pressure. He also recorded how many times their colons contracted during a certain period of time. After observing a volunteer's colon for some time, Dr. Almy gave the person some stressful news. Almost immediately, there were significant changes in the person's heart rate, blood pressure, and respiratory rate. These changes were not surprising, because stress has long been known to affect these bodily functions. What was not expected, given the information available at the time, was that the colon would also rapidly respond to stress, by changing its pattern of contraction. Shortly afterward, Dr. Almy told the volunteers that the stressful information was incorrect, at which point the heart rate, respiratory rate, and blood pressure all returned to baseline, as did the pattern of colonic contractions. This early experiment was one of the first to demonstrate the strong connection between the brain and the gut. Most people are probably not surprised by the existence of the brain-gut connection. Who has not felt a "sinking feeling" in the gut on hearing bad news or experienced "butterflies" in their stomach in anticipation of a stressful event?

More recently, researchers have found that people who have IBS process sensations from the GI tract differently than patients who do not have IBS. As Dr. Almy's and these experiments have shown, IBS is a com-

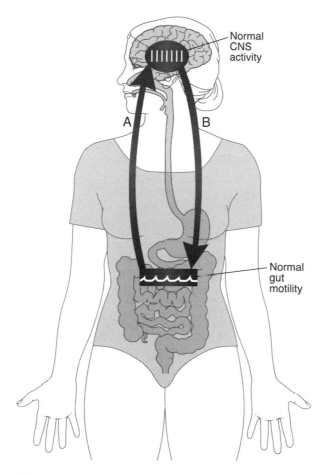

Figure 2.1. The Brain-Gut Axis

The brain and the gut are intimately connected via a pathway of nerves that lead from the gut to the brain (*A*) and from the brain to the gut (*B*). This bidirectional information highway is called the brain-gut axis. One of the largest nerves that connects the brain and the gut, the vagus nerve, is 90 percent sensory in nature. This proves what people who have IBS can attest—that the gut truly is a sensory organ. In a healthy gut, contractions in the GI tract are regular and not typically felt or sensed, and the areas of the brain involved in monitoring GI tract motility and sensation generally function at a low level of activation.

plex disorder in which multiple physiologic processes are involved. The three main processes involved in the generation of IBS symptoms include abnormalities in gut motility (the movement of food and liquids through the GI tract, also called peristalsis), alterations in sensory function of the GI tract (how nerves sense things within the gut), and changes in the way the brain processes sensory information from the GI tract (part of the brain-gut axis). The realization that the gut and the brain are intimately connected now plays a central role in the theory of IBS. This interplay between the central nervous system (CNS) and the GI tract, the brain-gut axis, is described in detail in Figure 2.1.

Gut Motility Abnormalities

For many years, the medical community thought that IBS was simply a case of abnormal motility of the GI tract. The term *motility* refers to how things move. Gastrointestinal motility is a complicated process. When GI motility is normal, foods and liquids are propelled easily through the GI tract, from the point of food ingestion at the mouth to the expulsion of waste at the rectum. Normal GI tract motility depends on normal functioning of the muscles and nerves within the GI tract.

The muscle in the GI tract is called smooth muscle (in contrast to the striated muscle seen in muscles that attach to the skeleton, and cardiac muscle seen in the heart). The smooth muscle of the GI tract forms a tube approximately 25 to 30 feet long that stretches from the mouth to the rectum. This tube is designed to propel contents through the GI tract (see Chapter 6).

More so than muscle function, normal motility relies on an intact and functioning nervous system. The human nervous system is generally described as having several distinct parts: the central nervous system, which includes the brain and the spinal cord, and the peripheral nervous system, which includes the somatic nervous system and the autonomic nervous system (see Figure 2.2). The somatic nervous system includes all of the nerves that supply skeletal muscles—these are the muscles that you can voluntarily control. The autonomic nervous system (ANS) functions autonomously, or without conscious thought; the nerves of this system regulate heart rate, blood pressure, sweating, and GI function. Nerves of the ANS originate within the spinal cord and ganglia (collections of nerve

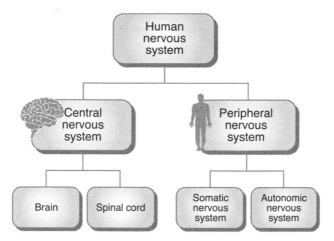

Figure 2.2. The Nervous System—An Overview
The human nervous system can be classified into two major subdivisions, the central nervous system (CNS) and the peripheral nervous
system (PNS). The CNS, consisting of the brain and spinal cord, is safely
encased within the skull and the spinal column. The brain is involved in
conscious thought, emotions, memory, movement, and sensation. The
spinal cord is a bundle of sensory and motor nerves that carry information back and forth from the brain to the rest of the body. The PNS also
can be divided into two parts, the somatic nervous system and the autonomic nervous system. The somatic nervous system receives sensations
from the skin, joints, and muscles and transmits this information to the
brain. It also carries signals from the brain to the skeletal muscle system
and joints to initiate and coordinate voluntary movement. The autonomic
nervous system is described in the caption for Figure 2.3.

---

cell bodies); these nerves are found extensively within the abdominal cavity. The ANS can be broken down further into the sympathetic nervous
system, the parasympathetic nervous system, and the enteric nervous system (ENS; see Figure 2.3).

The ENS is a network of nerve cells and connections that line the GI
tract (see Figure 2.4). The ENS is often called the "second brain" because
there are more nerve cells in the ENS than there are in the spinal cord.
The ENS is what makes your gut work effortlessly and without any conscious thought—food, liquids, and nutrients are propelled down your GI

tract without you ever having to think about it. You only become aware of the ENS not working properly when you develop symptoms such as bloating, constipation, diarrhea, or abdominal pain.

Technological advances in the 1970s enabled researchers to directly measure motility patterns of the stomach and small intestine. When people who have IBS participate in motility studies of the stomach and small intestine, they are sometimes found to have unusual patterns of activity called discrete clustered contractions. These discrete clustered contractions are isolated bursts of rhythmic contractions and are typically found in the small intestine. The contractions can be associated with episodes of abdominal pain in some people who have IBS. Other people who have IBS have prolonged muscle contractions within the colon or small intestine, or they have severe contractions within the colon, especially after a meal (see Figure 2.5). These contractions may also be associated with episodes of abdominal pain. Although people who have IBS may

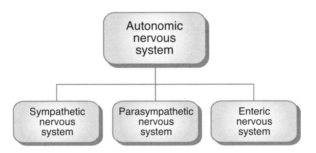

Figure 2.3. The Autonomic Nervous System
The autonomic nervous system (ANS) was formally recognized and described over 100 years ago. The ANS is responsible for automatic responses in the body (ones that happen without our thinking about them) such as breathing and our heart beating. The ANS can be broken down into three sections: the sympathetic nervous system, the parasympathetic nervous system, and the enteric nervous system. The sympathetic nervous system originates in the spinal cord, and the parasympathetic nervous system originates in the brainstem and the lower spinal cord. In the GI tract, the sympathetic nervous system is generally responsible for slowing down motility, while the parasympathetic nervous system is generally responsible for speeding it up.

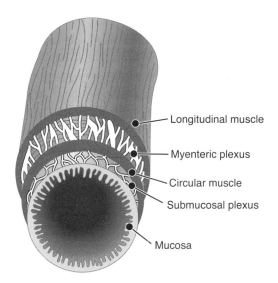

— Longitudinal muscle

— Myenteric plexus

— Circular muscle

Submucosal plexus

Mucosa

Figure 2.4. The Layers of the GI Tract
There are two layers of smooth muscle in the GI tract, the inner layer, which is circular muscle, and the outer layer, containing longitudinal muscle. These layers are involved in the muscular contractions (peristalsis) required to move materials through the GI tract. Two other layers contain the nerves of the enteric nervous system (ENS). The submucosal plexus is a highly complex pathway of interconnected nerve cells and their processes. It lies between the circular muscle layer and the innermost layer, the mucosa. The submucosal plexus processes sensations within the GI tract. The myenteric plexus, between the two muscle layers, is primarily involved in coordinating peristalsis. The mucosa contains cells that produce and secrete mucus and other cells that absorb fluid and nutrients.

experience different patterns of abnormal GI motility, no single pattern is routinely found in all people with this disorder. In general, the symptoms of IBS and the alterations in GI motility that are associated with them reflect an exaggeration of normal patterns of GI motility. This means that everybody—people who do and do not have IBS—has similar patterns of motility in the GI tract, although some of these patterns are exaggerated and amplified in people who have IBS.

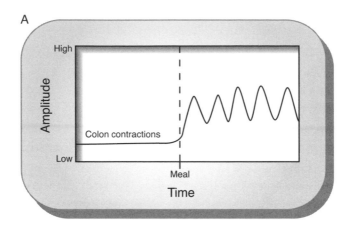

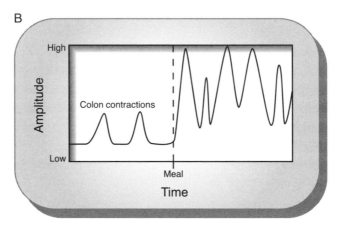

Figure 2.5. Colonic Motility before and after a Meal
A, Healthy volunteers. On the left side of the panel, the motility of the
colon is stable, without any contractions. After the person eats a meal,
smooth muscle contractions occur as part of the normal gastrocolic
(stomach-colon) reflex. The contractions are of modest strength and do
not cause pain or discomfort. *B,* Patients who have IBS. Occasional scat-
tered contractions are noted on the left side of the panel, even before a
meal. These contractions are felt as painful in some people. After eating
a meal, many people who have IBS have very strong, high-amplitude
contractions that can be uncomfortable or painful. Some experience urgent diarrhea and cramps immediately after eating a meal, and in these
persons, the contractions in the colon may be excessively strong and
prolonged.

Alterations in Sensory Function

As discussed previously, lower abdominal pain is a critical part of the definition of IBS. When evaluating people who have symptoms of IBS, physicians first try to understand why they are experiencing chronic abdominal pain. In the past, these people were often subjected to multiple tests, including blood work, x-rays, computed tomography (CT) scans, barium enemas, and colonoscopies. When all of these tests came back normal for people who have IBS, physicians often told them that the pain was "all in their head."

Physicians now know that people who have IBS have an increased sensitivity to pain within the GI tract. The concept of altered sensitivity to pain within the GI tract is called visceral hypersensitivity. The term "viscera" refers to internal organs within the body (stomach, colon, etc.). In essence, visceral hypersensitivity means that people who have IBS generally have a lower threshold for pain in the GI tract than do people who do not have IBS.

Researchers have completed many different studies that demonstrate the concept of visceral hypersensitivity. In several of these studies, they used a special technique involving balloon distention of the GI tract to measure the heightened sensitivity. During this procedure, a small balloon is placed in the GI tract and gradually inflated. People who have IBS sense the balloon being inflated (distended) much earlier in the process (that is, at very low levels of balloon inflation) than do people who do not have IBS (see Figure 2.6). In addition, people who have IBS also describe the distention as more painful.

These experiments show that people who have IBS sense painful stimuli within the gut at much lower levels, and with more pain, than people who do not have IBS. Some health care providers use the analogy that people who have IBS can hear a radio (their GI tract) at even the lowest volume, whereas people who do not have IBS need to turn the volume up to hear all of the signals from their GI tract. In essence, people who have IBS have particularly acute sensitivity: they sense things in their gut that other people do not.

Visceral hypersensitivity may lead people who have IBS to interpret normal sensations in their GI tract as abnormal and painful. The mis-

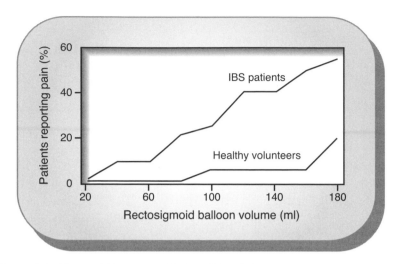

Figure 2.6. Visceral Hypersensitivity of the GI Tract
People who have IBS are frequently overly sensitive to stimulation from within the GI tract. Hypersensitivity in the GI tract can be easily assessed by inflating a small balloon in the GI tract and measuring a patient's response. The graph above records how healthy volunteers and patients who have IBS compared in their responses to balloon distention of the rectum.

A small percentage of healthy volunteers first began to sense the balloon inflation as painful after approximately 80 to 100 ml of air had been instilled into the balloon. It was not until approximately 160 to 180 ml of air had been instilled into the balloon that a larger percentage of normal volunteers began to feel the inflated balloon as a painful sensation.

In contrast, many patients who had IBS could sense the balloon inflation at very low levels. About a third of patients who had IBS reported that at even modest levels of balloon inflation (100 ml) the pressure is very uncomfortable. Similar results were obtained when the balloon was inflated in the esophagus, stomach, small intestine, or colon. These findings are all consistent with the notion that people who have IBS are hypersensitive in the GI tract.

interpretation of normal sensations as painful is a condition called allodynia. Health care providers do not know why some people who have IBS have allodynia and others do not. One theory is that a previous illness, infection, or surgery could have somehow injured the sensory nerves from the GI tract and made them more sensitive.

Influences of the Brain on the Gut

People who have IBS may also process sensory information abnormally in places outside of the GI tract. In particular, they may process sensory information differently in the brain than do people who do not have IBS. As part of a study published several years ago, people who had IBS underwent a special x-ray study of the brain called a positron emission tomography (PET) scan. PET scans measure the metabolism of individual organs and cells and thus can be used to measure the activity of a specific organ. During the study, researchers performed PET scans before and during balloon distention of a person's rectum. These images of the brain were then compared to those of people without IBS who underwent similar testing. The results showed that people who had IBS had increased activity in the prefrontal cortex, which is an area of the brain associated with anxiety and increased vigilance. In addition, people who had IBS had less activity in the anterior cingulate cortex, an area important for opioid (narcotic) binding.

The findings of this PET study confirmed that people who have IBS process and interpret gut sensations differently than do people who do not have IBS. One theory as to why this occurs is that people who have IBS cannot block out painful sensations as well as people who do not have IBS. Another theory is that people who have IBS have difficulty separating out, or discriminating, the normal sensations of gut motility that we all have from the abnormal sensations that may arise from an overly strong contraction or spasm in the GI tract. Thus, the nervous systems of people who have IBS misinterpret the normal sensations as painful or unpleasant. This theory of misinterpretation becomes relevant later in the book when we discuss treatments for IBS (see Chapter 13).

Finally, it is now well recognized that other stimulation, such as stress, anxiety, or depression, may regulate sensory processing in the brain and thus influence a person's perception of pain. These findings have significant implications, especially in regard to treatment of IBS. IBS treatment that focuses only on the GI tract may not be nearly as successful as a multisystem approach that treats both the GI tract and the central nervous system (see Chapters 13, 14, 16, and 17 for more information about the treatment of IBS).

What Is the Brain-Gut Axis?

As mentioned previously, research studies and physicians' observations during the last several decades have discovered a significant and critical connection between the brain (the central nervous system) and the gut (the GI tract) in people who have IBS (see Figure 2.7). Although some physicians suspected a connection between the brain and the gut as many as one hundred years ago, Dr. Almy's study was one of the first to scientifically demonstrate this connection in humans.

The brain-gut axis can best be described as an information highway that connects these two vital structures. This information highway is not unidirectional, meaning that it does not run only from the gut to the brain, or only from the brain to the gut. Rather, messages are transmitted bidirectionally. Information about GI function, motility, and visceral sensation is constantly sent from the gut to the brain. In the other direction, information about emotions, mood, conscious and subconscious thoughts, and sensations elsewhere in the body is constantly sent from the brain to the gut.

Sensory information within the GI tract is first recorded by sensory nerves that line the gut wall. These specialized cells that collect information about sensations in the GI tract are called sensory afferent neurons. They send the collected information through the spinal cord and up into the brain. Within the brain, there are many specialized structures responsible for collecting sensory information from the gut. These structures may relay the information to other areas of the brain, where the information can be grouped with, and interpreted alongside, information from other parts of the body. It is here, within the brain, that external influences such as stress can affect the interpretation of signals from the gut or the content of messages sent to the gut. Signals from the brain are sent to the gut by a series of nerves, including the vagus nerve and the sympa-

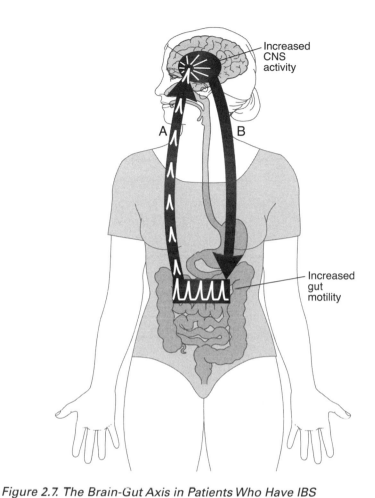

Figure 2.7. The Brain-Gut Axis in Patients Who Have IBS
In people who have IBS, the brain-gut axis may be more active than in
people who do not have the disease. Increased activity in the gut is common in patients who have IBS; contractions may be more frequent and
stronger. As messages are sent from the gut to the brain via any of the
millions of sensory nerves in the GI tract (via pathway *A*), increased sensations of discomfort or pain register in the brain. This increased brain
activity may in turn lead to an increase in the number, type, or intensity
of signals to the gut (pathway *B*). These signals may then further stimulate gut motility, worsening pain or causing diarrhea.

thetic and parasympathetic nerves. Through these pathways, information is constantly being sent back and forth between the brain and the gut.

When this intricate and delicate system functions normally, gut motility occurs effortlessly, digestion occurs painlessly, and neither constipation nor diarrhea dominates a person's GI function. When this interconnected pathway is disrupted or malfunctions, GI dysfunction is bound to occur and cause the typical symptoms of IBS: abdominal pain, bloating, and constipation or diarrhea.

Summary

- IBS remains widely misunderstood. Misconceptions and misperceptions about IBS are common.
- IBS is defined by the presence of abdominal pain or discomfort in association with disordered defecation (that is, either constipation or diarrhea or both). The sensation of abdominal pain or discomfort is a key part of the definition of IBS.
- Other typical symptoms of IBS include bloating, gassiness, abdominal distention, feelings of extreme urgency to use the bathroom, excessive straining while having a bowel movement, feelings of incomplete evacuation after having had a bowel movement, and the passage of mucus during evacuation.
- IBS symptoms develop from abnormalities in both gut motility and visceral sensitivity. In some cases the GI tract contracts too quickly and too forcefully; in other cases, it may not contract enough. Nearly all people who have IBS are hypersensitive in their GI tract, which means that they sense things too well in their gut.
- The brain-gut axis plays a critical role in IBS.

CHAPTER 3

Why Do I Have IBS?

Health care providers understand the underlying cause or causes of many common medical conditions. For example, we know that elevated levels of cholesterol in the bloodstream can lead to narrowing of the coronary (heart) arteries, which may then lead to reduced blood flow to the heart and a heart attack. We know that a long history of excessive alcohol intake will damage the liver and lead to cirrhosis (scarring of the liver). Multiple research studies have found that obesity is a key factor in the development of adult onset diabetes. The medical community, however, still does not understand the precise cause, or causes, of irritable bowel syndrome. At some point, all people who have IBS ask their doctors why they developed this common condition. Many people wonder whether they were born with IBS, and others ask their doctors if they developed IBS because of something they did to themselves, such as eating the wrong foods or taking the wrong medication. Unfortunately, the precise etiology (cause) of IBS remains unknown. Given the complexity of this disorder and its multiple symptoms, it is reasonable to assume that IBS does not develop from a single cause. Rather, there are likely several factors involved in the development of IBS, and these may be different in different individuals. Data are emerging that suggest that some people are exposed to certain conditions that predispose them to develop IBS later in life.

In this chapter, I review some of the current theories about how and why IBS develops, try to address commonly asked questions about the development of IBS, and present a hypothesis for why IBS occurs in some people but not others. The following case study illustrates some of the typical issues that people face after a new diagnosis of IBS.

Susan is a 25-year-old law student. She was referred to Dr. Kaufman because of her recurrent episodes of bloating, abdominal pain, and diarrhea. Susan explained that these problems started more than six months ago with only occasional episodes of abdominal cramps; she currently has lower abdominal pain, cramping, diarrhea, and bowel urgency nearly every morning. She stated that she feels very bloated and has resorted to wearing sweat pants most of the time because other pants feel too tight. One of her friends recently joked that she looked pregnant. Her weight has been stable during this time period. Susan saw a doctor at the law school student health clinic who told her that stress was causing these symptoms and that if she eliminated caffeine from her diet and got more rest, she would feel better. Susan was frustrated by this advice because she had researched her symptoms carefully on the Internet and didn't believe that more rest would solve her problems. During her appointment, she had asked the doctor what she thought were some simple questions, such as: "Why do I have this? Did I do something to cause this? Will it get better? And will it go away?" Unfortunately, the doctor wasn't able to answer her questions.

Unsatisfied, Susan made an appointment with Dr. Kaufman, a specialist at a university hospital near her parents' home in Washington, D.C. Susan told Dr. Kaufman that she has always been successful: she was at the top of her class in high school and again in college. She has a reputation for working hard and for being very competitive, whether in school or on the sports field, where she is also quite accomplished. She stated that ever since junior high school, her stomach has always been "a little twitchy." Before exams, trips, and major athletic events, she would frequently have a lot of stomach growling and grumbling, followed by bouts of diarrhea. She attributed this to "a nervous stomach" and said that at other times, she did not have any problems with diarrhea. Susan said that her recent problems of bloating, lower abdominal pain, and urgent trips to the bathroom with loose, watery bowel movements had started nearly six months earlier. At first, she could not recall anything out of the ordinary about this time period. However, Dr.

Kaufman felt that there were several important pieces of information in Susan's history that might help answer some of her questions. He learned that Susan's symptoms appeared to start shortly after a spring trip to Mexico. She went on the trip on the spur of the moment because she had just ended a long-term relationship with her boyfriend. The break-up was very stressful to her and she decided to join a group of her former sorority sisters on a cruise to Mexico. Unfortunately, Susan and all of her friends got sick on the trip. They each had several days of low-grade fevers, abdominal cramps, and diarrhea. Their illnesses began with nausea and vomiting, although Susan considered herself fortunate because, although she was nauseated, she did not vomit. Susan and all of her friends believed that they had food poisoning or developed some type of an infection onboard the ship. By the time they returned home, everybody felt better except for Susan. She continued to experience abdominal cramps, urgency, and diarrhea. The doctor at the student health clinic ordered some blood tests and had Susan collect samples of her diarrhea to see if there was any evidence of bacteria or parasites. All of the tests came back normal.

Dr. Kaufman carefully reviewed Susan's medical history and could not find any information that made him especially concerned (such information is sometimes referred to as warning signs, or "red flags"; see Chapter 7). He did note that both her mother and a sister also had problems with abdominal pain, spasms, cramps, and diarrhea, although they had not been formally diagnosed with a specific disorder. His careful physical examination did not reveal anything abnormal. Dr. Kaufman told Susan that all of her symptoms were compatible with irritable bowel syndrome. He carefully explained the meaning of IBS, described the typical symptoms, and reviewed the natural history of the disease. He reassured her that her symptoms would likely improve with a combination of diet, exercise, and medications.

Dr. Kaufman then told her some surprising news. He said that she likely developed IBS because of the infection she had while in Mexico. He told her it was likely that she and all of her sorority sisters had developed some type of viral or bacterial infection of the gut (that is, a gastroenteritis). In most cases, such an infection resolves without causing any long-lasting injury, but in her case, it may have caused some persistent inflammation to the GI tract or might have injured the nerves contained within the lining of the GI tract (the enteric nervous system; see Chapter 2). Dr. Kaufman found it interesting that whereas her friends all got better, Susan did not—possibly because all of them vomited at the onset of the illness. He said that it was unfortunate that she didn't vomit at the beginning of the illness, as this may have significantly decreased the amount of virus or bacteria to which her GI tract was exposed.

Finally, Dr. Kaufman suggested that there were three other reasons why Susan might have developed such long-lasting symptoms: (1) she had two family members with similar symptoms, which raised the issue of a genetic tendency to develop IBS; (2) she had a history of a "nervous" or "twitchy" gut and the addition of a stressful event to her system could have overwhelmed her body; and (3) some people are more susceptible to developing IBS if they are stressed at the time of an infection. Two stressors (an emotional break-up with her boyfriend and an infection in her GI tract) going on at the same time might have overwhelmed the normal defense systems in her body.

Susan asked a few more questions and then discussed treatment options with Dr. Kaufman. She felt that she now had a good grasp of the problem at hand and that some sense had been made of her symptoms and problems. She was now ready to deal with the problem of IBS.

What Causes IBS?

The etiology of an illness refers to the underlying event (or events) that cause an illness to develop. In the case of IBS, the initial event may be something simple, such as a viral or bacterial illness, which is often not even noticed or remembered by the patient. However, this precipitating incident may then lead to a cascade of events, eventually resulting in the gut dysfunction that produces the typical symptoms of IBS. In contrast to just a decade ago, the medical community now has a much better understanding of the abnormal physiologic processes that produce the symptoms associated with IBS (pain, bloating, and either constipation or diarrhea). IBS is a particularly complex disorder in which many physiological processes are involved, including abnormalities in intestinal motility (the movement of materials through the gastrointestinal tract), alterations in visceral sensory function (awareness of sensations within the GI tract), and changes in central nervous system (CNS) processing of sensory information. This relationship between the CNS and the intestinal tract has been labeled the brain-gut axis (see Chapter 2).

Although physicians may understand the physiologic processes that produce symptoms of IBS, why those processes begin in some people and not others is still unknown. Many different theories have been explored, and these are discussed below.

Genetics

A thorough medical history always includes a review of a patient's family history. During this part of the interview, the physician focuses on medical conditions present in the patient's first-degree relatives (mother, father, brothers, sisters), although more distant family members may be included as well. The purpose of the family medical history is to look for inherited disorders, disorders that are transmitted from one generation to the next.

Some information about the growth and development of a person is found on structures called chromosomes. Chromosomes consist of tightly coiled and compacted DNA (deoxyribonucleic acid). Specific segments of DNA make up genes, which are responsible for producing certain proteins and directing the growth and development of a person.

Every human being has 23 pairs of chromosomes. Children receive 23 chromosomes from the mother and 23 from the father: one from each parent's 23 pairs. These include one set of chromosomes that determines a person's sex (the X and Y chromosomes) and 22 other pairs of chromosomes, referred to as autosomal chromosomes. Autosomal chromosomes determine body characteristics such as eye color, hair type, body shape, and height. These characteristics and diseases are transmitted from parent to child in a number of distinct patterns. One of the easiest patterns to recognize is the autosomal dominant pattern (when only one of two chromosomes in a pair must have the gene present for the specific condition to develop). Some examples of autosomal dominant disorders include familial hypercholesterolemia (1 in 500 people in the United States have this disorder), polycystic kidney disease (1 in 1,250), Marfan syndrome (1 in 20,000), and Huntington's disease (1 in 2,500).

Another common pattern of inheritance is the autosomal recessive pattern (when both chromosomes, one from each parent, have the abnormal gene, and one copy of the gene is not enough to cause the condition). Examples of autosomal recessive disorders include sickle cell anemia (1 in 625 African American people have this disease), cystic fibrosis (1 in 2,500 people), Tay-Sachs disease (1 in 3,000 people), and phenylketonuria (PKU; 1 in 10,000 people).

Many people who have IBS believe that they've inherited the disorder from their parents or grandparents because these family members have symptoms similar to their own. When interviewing patients and reviewing their family history, I am often told by patients that their problem must be inherited because their mother "always had bowel problems" or because their father had stomach problems "all of his life." Although interesting, the stories of different family members and their gastrointestinal (GI) symptoms do not prove that their problems are genetically linked to a patient's IBS. To determine whether a patient has a genetically linked disorder, the first question a physician must ask is whether that patient's symptoms are truly similar to that of his or her family member or members. Many people lump "abdominal problems" together, such as acid reflux disease (gastroesophageal reflux disease, or GERD), ulcer disease, chronic constipation, and IBS. These individual problems likely develop as the result of separate processes, however, and should be viewed as separate medical conditions. In addition, there are many other symptoms and disorders that commonly occur in association with IBS, although they do not appear to be genetically linked.

If a patient does have first-degree relatives with symptoms of IBS, then her or his physician should make a careful note of these symptoms. However, it takes much more than just having another family member with similar symptoms to prove that a disease is genetically linked. This is especially true with a common disorder such as IBS. If two family members have Marfan syndrome, which occurs in only 1 in 20,000 people, it is probably not just a coincidence. IBS, on the other hand, is found in nearly 15 percent of the U.S. population. Thus, in a large family of seven or eight people, two family members who have IBS does not necessarily indicate a genetic link.

What do research studies show about the genetic basis of IBS? Some of the best research data about genetics come from twin studies. Twins occur in approximately 1 in 90 live births worldwide and can be one of two types: monozygotic (identical) or dizygotic (fraternal). A *zygote* is a fertilized egg. A monozygotic (*mono* means "one") twin develops when one egg is fertilized and then splits into two identical eggs that continue to grow and develop into two genetically identical individuals. Dizygotic (*di* means "two") twins develop when two different eggs are fertilized by two different sperms and hence are not identical.

If there is a strong genetic link in IBS, then researchers would expect that if IBS develops in one monozygotic, or identical, twin, it will develop in the other identical twin as well. Studies have shown that there is a statistically significant higher incidence of IBS in identical twins than in the general population. In addition, identical twins are twice as likely as fraternal twins to develop IBS. However, if one identical twin develops IBS, the incidence of the other twin developing it is not 100 percent, which it should be if the disorder is completely genetically transmitted. Many scientists who focus their research efforts on understanding IBS believe that the findings from the twin studies mean that there is a genetic predisposition for the development of IBS. This predisposition means that if a person has a specific gene (or genes), then there is an increased likelihood that he or she will develop IBS. It is unlikely that there is a single gene that predisposes people to develop IBS later in life; there may be several abnormal genes that act together to cause people to develop IBS. One theory, discussed at the end of this chapter, is that some people have a genetic factor or factors that places them at increased risk of developing IBS during their lifetime. Unless some other event or events occur, however, IBS will not develop. A genetic tendency or predisposition for IBS is not an absolute guarantee that IBS will develop.

Environment

Several research studies have shown that having a mother or father who has IBS increases the likelihood that you will develop IBS. This does not necessarily indicate a genetic link, because the risk of developing IBS is greater if your mother or father has symptoms of IBS than if you are a fraternal twin and your twin has IBS. Although there are some data that support a genetic predisposition (but not a guarantee) for the development of IBS, the comparison between the twin and parental findings raises the issue of whether the environment could also contribute to the development of IBS.

Environmental influences may include where a person lives, climate, socioeconomic status, race, religion, and the number of family members present in the household. Because behavior and personality are primarily formed during the early childhood years, is it possible that different social environments influence the likelihood of a person developing IBS later in life? This is a difficult subject to tackle because there are so many variables involved; for example, different parenting methods, educational level of the parents and the child, stability of the parents and their marriage, and the effects of schooling on the child all may have an effect on the etiology of IBS.

Despite the great prevalence of IBS, very little research has been done about environmental influences on this disease. Where one lives in the United States does not appear to affect the likelihood of developing IBS: it is just as common in the North as in the South and in urban areas as opposed to rural areas. Race does not appear to be a major factor either: IBS is as prevalent in African Americans as it is in European Americans and nearly as common in Hispanics and Asian Americans as it is in white people. In addition, studies from around the world have shown that IBS is found in a large number of people in Africa, Asia, and the Middle East. This reinforces the ideas that race, climate, and geography do not play a role in the development of IBS. To my knowledge, there are no studies that have focused solely on religion and IBS. The assumption is that because IBS is found throughout the world, in many different cultures with many different religions, then it is unlikely that religious practices play a role in the development of IBS.

Researchers currently agree that global environmental factors likely do not influence the development of IBS. On a more basic level, could individual differences at home increase the risk of developing IBS? The answer, although exceedingly difficult to measure, is quite possibly yes. How can researchers objectively measure different parenting skills and styles and compare these different styles in a standardized manner? Parenting skills may develop in response to the child's behavior, further complicating the issue. One way to look at this would be to study differences in the prevalence of IBS during specific, contrasting time periods in our nation's history. For example, if we knew that people were more likely to develop IBS during the Victorian era as compared to the1960s, then some people might argue that a more rigid upbringing (popular during the Victorian era) increases the likelihood of IBS developing. Unfortunately, few such studies are available during either of these time periods, and because the research methods employed are so different, they cannot be directly compared.

We do know that parenting skills can significantly influence the development of IBS in children. IBS may develop in children because of direct influence from their parents or through more indirect influences, such as children observing that whenever their mother or father has an unpleasant task or assignment, then he or she develops abdominal pain, diarrhea, and has to stay home from work. Children model their parents quite faithfully, and before long, those children learn to have abdominal pain and diarrhea before an unpleasant assignment is due at school or work. Direct influences may be the result of parents "rewarding" their children for being ill. Staying at home because of abdominal pain may result in a reward by the parent, such as a special treat, meal, or toy (whether the illness is real or not). This reward reinforces the child's view that being ill is desirable. Most physicians who treat people who have IBS strongly believe that parents can teach their children to develop poor coping skills and poor responses to being ill, which increase the likelihood of developing a functional bowel disorder such as IBS later on in life.

Stress

For many years, physicians told people who had IBS that the disease was caused by stress, depression, and anxiety. It was not uncommon for physicians to tell people that the symptoms of IBS were "all in their head." The theory that stress, anxiety, and depression could cause IBS probably developed for many different reasons. First, testing at the time could not identify any organic or structural problem that could account for the multiple symptoms of IBS. Thus, if a problem could not be found, it was common practice to diagnose the patient with either a psychosomatic or a psychiatric disorder. Second, very little information was available about the brain-gut axis before the 1970s, and until 15 years ago, this concept was not widely discussed. Neither physicians nor patients were cognizant of the strong connection between the brain and the gut. Because this phenomenon was not well understood, it was difficult for physicians to account for this vital connection in their diagnostic studies or treatment plans. Finally, functional bowel disorders are a difficult concept to understand. In the past, the medical community did not really embrace this complex concept and was still operating under the rubric that the physical symptoms of IBS had to be based on some structural or biochemical abnormality that could be identified by laboratory tests or x-ray studies.

Most physicians now recognize that stress, anxiety, and depression do not cause IBS but that these emotional factors can dramatically influence the brain-gut axis. During times of emotional stress, IBS symptoms may flare up or worsen. This concept probably does not come as a surprise—we are all aware of how easily emotions affect our general well-being and state of health. For example, if your friend has a mild cold on a beautiful spring day and he has been looking forward to a planned outing for weeks, then it is very likely that he will find the mental and physical energy to go. On the other hand, if you have another friend with those same symptoms on a gray, rainy day, and she is obligated to go to some dreadfully boring meeting, you wouldn't be surprised if she decides not to go and to stay home to nurse her cold symptoms instead. Both positive and negative emotions can greatly influence the physical state of a person. In fact, during the last decade researchers have found that positive emotions can influence the immune system in a beneficial manner.

In short, the connections between the brain and the gut are strong. The brain-gut axis is susceptible to external influences, such as stress (see Figure 3.1). In addition, internal influences such as mood and emotions (anxiety, fear, depression) can also dramatically affect the brain-gut axis. These emotions can directly influence GI activity. An example of this influence would be a lawyer who develops urgent diarrhea only before stressful court appearances.

Emotions can also modulate how the brain senses gut activity, which may be a major reason why people who have IBS have more severe symptoms when depressed or anxious. In reality, they may be having the same symptoms they normally have, but the coexisting stress (or anxiety or depression) makes it difficult for them to properly interpret the signals from their gut. Their threshold for sensing gut sensations may be lower during these stressful periods, and thus they may perceive not only more signals from the gut but also more intense signals.

Although physicians now realize that stress and anxiety do not cause IBS, when we evaluate a person who has IBS, we do let them know that they may experience a flare-up of their symptoms during times of stress. For people experiencing a flare of their typical IBS symptoms, a symptom diary may help pinpoint the stressful event (or events) that triggered the aggravation (see Chapter 13). By using a symptom diary, it is not uncommon for a person to pinpoint an event that coincided with the onset of more severe symptoms. This may be a stressful situation at home (fight with spouse, financial problems, problems with children at school) or at work (major projects, deadlines, job security). Although discussed at length in Chapter 7, pinpointing a triggering event is critical in the overall IBS treatment plan, which involves treating the coexisting life stressors along with the IBS symptoms. Until these coexisting stressors are treated and under control, they will continue to negatively affect the brain-gut axis and make symptoms worse—and they may actually increase the likelihood of developing IBS in the first place (see below and Figure 3.1).

Diet

The topic of diet is usually raised by people who have IBS because eating so often produces symptoms of bloating, gas, abdominal pain, or even diarrhea. Many people think that different foods seem to cause IBS symptoms. Certainly, many people who have IBS develop a worsening of their symptoms after eating; however, this is probably just an exaggerated physiologic response to eating (see Chapter 6). Some people who have IBS may be intolerant of certain foods, especially lactose and fructose, and these can produce symptoms that mimic IBS. Celiac disease (an allergy to wheat) can cause symptoms of gas, bloating, and diarrhea and therefore resembles IBS (see Chapter 10). Other food allergies rarely produce symptoms that mimic IBS, but they may worsen IBS symptoms (see Chapter 15). True food allergies are uncommon, but IBS is quite common. At present, there are no good data to support the view that any

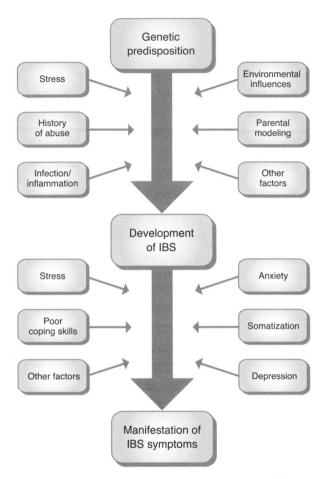

Figure 3.1. Contributing Factors in the Development of IBS
Although the precise mechanism that leads to the development of IBS
remains unknown, this diagram illustrates likely influences in a sequence. Research studies have shown that some people have a genetic
predisposition to develop IBS. This predisposition is not a guarantee that
IBS will develop, but it does increase the likelihood that IBS will occur.
One theory is that, for IBS to develop, a second or third inciting factor
needs to be present as well. For example, a common infection of the GI
tract early in life (such as a "stomach flu") followed by a period of stress
might produce the right setting for IBS to develop.

particular diet causes IBS. However, as noted in the treatment section of this book (see Part III and particularly Chapter 15), there is some good evidence that specific diets may improve IBS symptoms in some people.

Medications

Medications may be over the counter, prescription, herbal, homeopathic, allopathic, or naturopathic. Their goal is to treat a specific problem as effectively as possible while producing as few side effects as possible. Unfortunately, practically all medications have side effects. Some side effects are more severe than others, but no medication is without risk. The power of medication is so strong that in some research studies even a placebo (a "sugar" pill) produces side effects in some people. A common opinion in the medical community is that if aspirin were a new medication and was brought before the Food and Drug Administration (FDA) for approval now, it would never be approved because of the large number of known side effects. But hasn't aspirin been shown to have many benefits, and isn't it sold all over the world? As you can see, the topic of medications and side effects is extremely complicated.

Some types of medications used for other medical problems may produce side effects that mimic symptoms of IBS, and other medications may worsen the symptoms of IBS. Medications used to treat constipation (lactulose and sorbitol) may produce significant bloating. People with chronic pain are often prescribed narcotics, which slow down the normal movement of gut contents (called peristalsis) and frequently lead to constipation. People with migraine headaches or chronic functional GI pain may be prescribed a tricyclic antidepressant (TCA), commonly used to treat chronic nerve pain and sometimes very effective in the treatment of IBS (see Chapter 17). However, in some people who take a TCA, increased dosage can cause constipation. At present, there are no good data available to suggest that any specific medication causes IBS.

Infectious Illnesses

Several research studies have shown that an infectious gastroenteritis (an inflammation of the lining of the stomach and intestine) can increase the likelihood of a person developing IBS later in life. Everyone has friends, relatives, or neighbors who developed an infectious gastroenteritis (often labeled "traveler's diarrhea" or "tourista") while on a trip abroad. Although most recover completely, some people with infectious gastroenteritis continue to have persistent symptoms of bloating, abdominal pain, and altered bowel habits for months or even years after the acute illness. These people typically undergo blood work, specialized stool studies, and even procedures such as colonoscopy or a computed tomography (CT) scan in an attempt to diagnose the problem. By the time they see a physician, the active infection has usually gone away, but their symptoms continue—a medical condition known as post-infectious IBS. Although the precise mechanism is unknown, researchers have several theories as to why IBS may persist after an acute episode of infectious gastroenteritis. For example, the infection may temporarily or permanently injure the nerve supply within the GI tract that is responsible for coordinating the movement of contents in the gastrointestinal tract (peristalsis). Injury to the nerves could lead to either diarrhea or constipation and may also lead to increased abdominal pain and an increased awareness of pain in the GI tract (called visceral hypersensitivity). Another possible reason why IBS persists after infectious gastroenteritis is immune hypersensitivity, whereby recurrent exposure to a previously benign substance causes an inflammatory state in the GI tract. This persistent state of inflammation could then alter intestinal motility and lead to diarrhea.

In one of the most telling examples of post-infectious IBS, a large number of people in a small town in Canada developed severe gastroenteritis after the town water supply was contaminated with runoff from local farms. Many people were hospitalized and treated with antibiotics for their infectious gastroenteritis. Several people died, including one of the town's doctors. Two years later, nearly one-third of the townspeople had developed symptoms of IBS, and nearly 10 years after the outbreak, more than one-third of the population continued to have symptoms of IBS, although they did not have these symptoms before the outbreak of gastroenteritis.

Abuse

During the last decade, many published scientific studies have explored the role that a history of previous physical, emotional, or sexual abuse plays in the development of IBS. Studies revealed a higher incidence of physical or sexual abuse in people (primarily women) who have IBS than in control groups of people who do not have IBS. This difference may be a result of self-selection (people with histories of abuse are more likely to seek health care), increased severity of symptoms, high levels of psychological distress, or poor coping skills. Physicians at academic medical centers and large university hospitals tend to see a significantly larger population of people who have IBS and report a history of sexual or physical abuse than physicians in community practice settings. Clearly, a history of abuse is an important factor to consider in people with functional bowel disorders. A person's decision of when to discuss abuse with a doctor is a highly personal one, but he or she should definitely mention the abuse, because it is a vital piece of information that may lead to a major change in the overall treatment plan.

One cautionary note: if you have been abused and decide to discuss this issue with your doctor, make sure there is adequate time for an appropriate discussion. This emotionally charged issue should not be brought up as you are leaving the office with coat on and hat in hand.

How Does IBS Develop?

Although there are many different theories about why some people develop IBS and others do not, the information presented throughout this chapter allows us to diagram a proposed pathway for the development of IBS. A common starting point is the genetic predisposition to develop IBS, which probably involves the interaction of multiple genes (not just the actions of a single gene). Genetic predisposition is not a guarantee that a person will develop IBS, but it does increase the likelihood for her or him.

If a person is genetically predisposed to develop IBS, he or she should be aware of the following factors that may increase the likelihood of developing the disease: significant stress, an infection in the GI tract, a history of abuse (emotional, physical, or sexual), and environmental and parental influences. The precise role that each of these factors plays in the development of IBS is unknown. In addition, there are other factors that explain why some people who have IBS develop more severe symptoms than others. I discuss these other factors throughout the book.

Summary

- We do not know why IBS develops in some individuals but not others.
- IBS probably develops as a result of many different factors (see Figure 3.1).
- Certain individuals may be genetically predisposed to develop IBS. It is not guaranteed that these individuals will develop IBS, but their genetic predisposition increases the likelihood.
- There is no good evidence that a specific diet or type of medication can cause IBS.

CHAPTER 4

How Common Is IBS?

Irritable bowel syndrome is one of the most common medical conditions encountered by health care providers of all types—nurse practitioners, physician assistants, internists, and physician specialists like gastroenterologists, obstetricians, gynecologists, surgeons, and psychiatrists. It affects more than forty million adult Americans. Each week, 12 percent of all patient visits to a family practitioner or internal medicine physician are for symptoms related to IBS. During the course of one week, more people see physicians for IBS than for other common medical conditions such as asthma, diabetes, or heart disease. In addition, at least 40 percent of the people referred to gastroenterology specialists have IBS. Thus, contrary to popular perception, IBS is a common disorder that occurs not only in Western societies, such as North America and Europe, but throughout the world (see Figure 4.1).

Hank's story illustrates some of the misconceptions about IBS and the people who have it.

Hank is a 47-year-old truck driver from Oklahoma. He spends most of his time on the road hauling cattle and farm supplies. During the last several years he's had frequent problems with constipation and abdominal pain. On many days, he notices a persistent ache or discomfort in his lower abdomen. His abdominal pain is relieved temporarily after he has a bowel movement, but his trips to the bathroom are few and far between. If he's lucky, he has a bowel movement twice a week. When he does go to the bathroom, he has to strain a lot, and he passes rocky, hard stools. Hank's friends told him that he is "too uptight" and that he should drink some prune juice and eat more fruits and vegetables. Unfortunately, Hank has difficulty eating fruits and vegetables because his meals are mostly at fast food restaurants and truck stops while he is on the road.

Hank went to his local pharmacy and the pharmacist told him to take some fiber pills, which didn't seem to help (although he only tried them for a week). His wife told him that he probably had irritable bowel syndrome (she had read about it in a magazine), but he laughed and said that irritable bowel was very uncommon and never happened in men. His symptoms persisted for several more months, and despite trying a variety of over-the-counter products (milk of magnesia, magnesium citrate) and herbal remedies (senna and cascara), he didn't feel any better.

Hank went to see his doctor for his yearly check-up. After a physical examination (which was completely normal) and some simple laboratory tests (blood count), Dr. Liu asked if there was anything else he wanted to discuss. Although he was somewhat embarrassed to discuss his symptoms, Hank told Dr. Liu about his abdominal pain and constipation. Dr. Liu listened carefully, double-checked a few important points in Hank's medical and family history (see Chapters 3 and 7), and then told him that because of his symptoms and his normal examination, it was quite likely that he did have IBS. Hank was skeptical and told Dr. Liu that he didn't think that he could have IBS if he was constipated. Dr. Liu reviewed some of the facts and figures about IBS (discussed below) and reassured Hank that IBS is a common problem that occurs in both men and women. Hank seemed reassured and they spent the remaining time discussing different treatment options (see Chapter 15).

Of all the people in the United States who have IBS, only about 30 percent visit a health care provider for treatment of this disease. There are several reasons why people who have IBS may avoid the doctor's office. One, they have mild, intermittent symptoms that they either ignore or treat at home with over-the-counter medications. Two, they are too embarrassed to discuss their symptoms with a doctor or other health care provider. These people may feel uncomfortable describing their symptoms because they think the symptoms are uncommon or because they

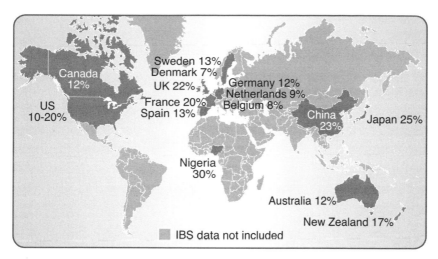

Figure 4.1. The Worldwide Prevalence of IBS
Although many people think of IBS as a problem only in the United States, people the world over have this condition. Research studies have demonstrated that IBS is quite common worldwide, including in Europe, Japan, China, Australia, and New Zealand. This map provides an estimate of the percentage of the population that has IBS in each country for which data are available. The variation in percentages may be caused by the use of different questionnaires and different definitions of IBS in the studies, but true differences in the prevalence of IBS may also exist, based on ethnicity, social customs, and geography.

---

do not know the proper terms to describe them. Three, many people who have IBS avoid going to a doctor because they worry that their symptoms indicate a serious illness, and they don't wish to hear bad news. Ordinarily, you would think that if you had a medical problem that might be serious, you would want to see a doctor and have a thorough evaluation. However, some patients are so fearful of hearing bad news that they put things off as long as they can. A recent study found that nearly 17 percent of people who have IBS incorrectly believe that they will develop cancer. Finally, some people who have IBS don't see a doctor because of financial reasons. This may be due to a lack of insurance, the inability to pay the copayment for an office visit, or concerns that they won't be able to pay for medications, laboratory studies, or diagnostic tests.

How Do We Know How Many People Have IBS?

People who have IBS usually have a lot of specific questions: How common is it for someone to develop IBS? What are my risks for developing IBS? How many other people in the community have IBS? What is the natural history of IBS? In answering these questions, it is best to start by defining the two most common ways to measure the extent of disease: incidence and prevalence. Although these terms are frequently used in the media and in the medical literature, they can still be confusing.

Incidence refers to the number of new cases of a specific disease that develop within a certain time period (such as a given year). For example, if members of a small community (10,000 adults) answered a health questionnaire and 100 said that they had been newly diagnosed with IBS during the past year, the incidence would be 1 percent per year (100/10,000). A study performed in the United States over 10 years ago found that the incidence of IBS was 9 percent (that is, 9 new cases of IBS diagnosed for every 100 people surveyed; see Figure 4.2). A European study performed using a different method found the incidence of IBS to be lower, approximately 2 percent (2 of 100 people had been newly diagnosed with IBS during the previous year). Most likely, the incidence of IBS differed in these two studies because the types of questions physicians used to diagnose IBS were different, and the study populations themselves were also somewhat different (Europeans vs. Americans).

Incidence only describes the number of *new* cases of a disease during a certain time period. Researchers use incidence to determine the frequency of IBS in a given population, not to study why the disease develops, its natural history, or the nature of its symptoms. Because people with typical symptoms of IBS are not always formally diagnosed and therefore cannot be accurately counted in a study, incidence may underestimate the frequency of the disease. As noted above, only 30 percent of people who have symptoms of IBS ever see a doctor for their problems; thus up to 70 percent of people who have IBS may not be included in research studies or surveys.

Another common way of measuring the extent of disease, which may be more familiar to people and is often more useful, is prevalence. The

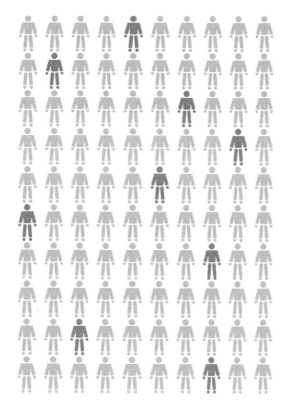

Figure 4.2. Incidence
This diagram illustrates the statistical term *incidence*. Incidence is defined as the number of people who develop a disease during a specific time period. Typically, incidence is defined as the number of new cases that develop over the course of a year. In this example, at the start of the year, 100 people were surveyed and none had symptoms. At the end of the year, the same 100 people were surveyed and 9 had developed symptoms. This means that the incidence of the disease in this particular population is 9 percent (9/100).

prevalence of a disease is a measure of how many people have the disease at any given time. The prevalence of IBS is commonly derived from survey studies involving large groups of people. In these surveys, various populations (young, old, European, American, Asian, etc.) are asked a series of questions to determine whether they have symptoms of IBS at the present time. The prevalence of IBS is the percentage of people who, at the time of the survey, have all of the symptoms consistent with IBS. So, if the same community mentioned earlier (population of 10,000) fills out a questionnaire asking if they currently have IBS (or have symptoms that fit the definition of IBS), and 1,500 people say yes, the prevalence would be 15 percent (1,500/10,000; see Figure 4.3). Health care providers often use the concept of prevalence because it lets them know how many people with the disease are in the community.

People often wonder about the relationship between incidence and prevalence. It seems logical to think that if the *incidence* of a disorder was 5 percent, then at the end of 10 years, the *prevalence* should be 50 percent because 5 percent of the population develops the disease each year (incidence of 5 percent per year x 10 years = prevalence rate of 50 percent). However, this equation assumes that the population never changes. As we all know, our local population is changing all the time. People move into our communities and people leave. People who have IBS may have their symptoms disappear over time, and other people may develop new symptoms consistent with IBS. So, this seemingly logical line of thinking is flawed, because it is based on the assumption that once a person is diagnosed with the disorder, that person will always have it. Fortunately, that is not the case for people who have IBS.

If we look at the example of incidence and prevalence in Figure 4.4, we can see that there are 17 people who currently have symptoms of IBS and have been formally diagnosed with this problem (prevalence). At the same time, three people have been newly diagnosed with IBS. This should raise the prevalence to 20 percent (20 of 100 people), but we also need to take into account 3 people who were previously diagnosed with IBS but whose symptoms have since changed. These three people no longer fit the definition of IBS: one person had all of her symptoms resolve, one person died of a medical condition not related to IBS, and one person had the diagnosis of IBS changed to celiac disease. (Please note that IBS is never a lethal disease and it does not shorten someone's lifespan. In addition, physicians rarely diagnose IBS as another disorder [see Chapter 7]).

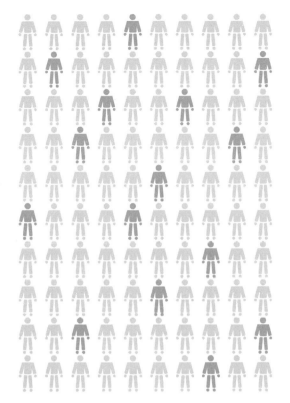

Figure 4.3. Prevalence
This diagram illustrates the statistical term *prevalence.* Prevalence is defined as the number of people who have a disease at a specific point in time. In this diagram, 100 people were asked if they had the symptoms consistent with a specific disease. Fifteen people said yes, and thus the prevalence is 15 percent (15/100). Note that this is different from incidence, since prevalence does not signify how many people developed the disease or disorder during a given time but rather how many people have symptoms of the disorder at a specific point in time.

Who Gets IBS?

If you review the map of the world in Figure 4.1, you may notice that the prevalence rates of IBS seem to differ in various parts of the world. The prevalence rates of IBS from different research studies vary for many reasons, including what type of questionnaire was used, how the ques-

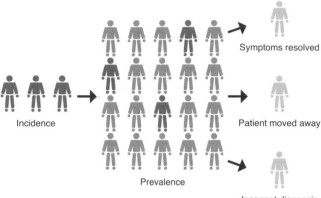

Figure 4.4. How Prevalence Changes over Time
This diagram illustrates how the prevalence of a disorder can change
with time and why the incidence of a disorder does not mean that eventually everyone will develop that disease. On the left side of the diagram,
3 people develop IBS during the course of one year, so the incidence is
3 percent. If more and more people develop the disease, then the prevalence will increase. In the middle portion of the drawing, a survey of the
population (20 people) shows that 3 people are afflicted, and thus the
prevalence is 15 percent (3/20). However, as time progresses, the prevalence may change as the population changes. Some people's symptoms
may resolve, some patients may have been incorrectly diagnosed, and
some people may move away. In addition, some people will be newly
diagnosed while other people have their diagnosis changed, move away,
or get better. Thus, the prevalence of a specific disease in a given population may change over time or it may remain the same.

---

tionnaire was administered (in person, by phone, by mail), and what
definition of IBS was used. Overall, the worldwide prevalence of IBS is
approximately 10 to 35 percent. Multiple studies from the United States
have consistently found a prevalence rate of 10 to 20 percent, with an
average of 15 percent (see Figure 4.1). This prevalence rate means that between one in six to one in seven adult Americans suffers from IBS. Most
people who have IBS begin to develop symptoms in their late teenage
years or early twenties, although the problem may not be diagnosed for
many years (see Chapter 7). The prevalence of IBS peaks in the third and

fourth decades of life and decreases in the sixth and seventh decades of life. The prevalence of IBS in people over age 60 is approximately 11 percent (11 of 100 people over 60 years old have IBS, based on symptoms). Physicians may diagnose IBS in some people who are well into their seventies and even in their eighties, although this is not common (see Figure 4.5), and they are quite cautious about doing so because other diseases (colon cancer, diverticulitis) may have similar symptoms.

In regard to other factors that may influence who gets IBS, race/ethnicity does not appear to play a major role in the development of IBS. Several studies have reported a similar prevalence among European Americans and African Americans, and two studies have reported that the prevalence of IBS is somewhat lower in Asians and in Hispanics when compared to European Americans or African Americans.

Socioeconomic status may play a role in the development of IBS, although data from research studies are not very clear on this issue. One study showed that people in a lower socioeconomic group were more likely to develop IBS symptoms than people of higher socioeconomic status, but this study was not designed to determine why finances appear to be related to the development of IBS. It is quite possible that finances, as a single, specific issue, do not play any role in the development of IBS. Someone who is better off financially can afford to see a physician or take medications that relieve symptoms of IBS; thus, people in a higher socioeconomic group might be more likely to have their symptoms improve or resolve. Conversely, a person who is financially more stressed might not be able to see a physician or afford medications that improve their symptoms of IBS; thus, their symptoms might persist for a longer period of time. In addition, we already know that stress and emotions can affect the GI tract through the brain-gut axis (see Chapter 2), so it seems logical that financial stress could worsen IBS symptoms.

In large population studies, women are at least twice as likely as men to be diagnosed with IBS. In studies conducted at referral medical centers (usually large, university-associated or university-owned medical centers), the ratio of women to men who have IBS and are enrolled in research studies is usually three to one and may be as high as four to one. Researchers have found that throughout the world, women consistently outnumber men when it comes to having IBS—except in India and Sri Lanka.

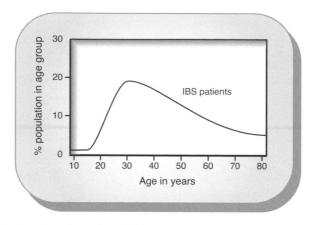

Figure 4.5. The Relationship of IBS to Age
This diagram illustrates the prevalence of IBS in relation to age. IBS is uncommon in children. The peak prevalence of IBS is in people in their late twenties to late thirties. After that, the prevalence slowly decreases. Older individuals can have IBS, although it is much less common than among younger adults.

Studies performed in these two countries have shown that IBS is actually more common in men than in women, most likely because men generally have much greater access to health care than do women in this area of the world and are thus more frequently diagnosed.

The disparity in the diagnosis of IBS in men and women may occur for a number of different reasons. One, in most countries women are more likely than men to make routine health care visits, usually to see a gynecologist or an obstetrician. Many young women use their gynecologist as their primary health care provider. During these visits, women may be asked about the presence of other symptoms, including a change in bowel habits, bloating, or abdominal pain. Two, women who see a physician more regularly (such as a gynecologist) may be more willing to discuss IBS-related problems, as opposed to men, who are less likely to see a physician on a regular basis and who may wish to focus on other health issues during these less-frequent visits. Three, some studies have showed increased health care–seeking behavior in women who have IBS. However, the results of these studies probably represent only a small fraction of all women who have symptoms of IBS and describe only people with the most severe symptoms, rather than all women (or men) who have IBS.

Differences in hormone levels might also explain the gender disparity in diagnosis of IBS. Elevated hormone levels (estrogen and progesterone) during pregnancy can cause smooth muscles in the GI tract to relax, which partially explains the increase of acid reflux disease and constipation in pregnant women. Emerging data show many women experiencing changes in their IBS symptoms that fluctuate with their menstrual cycle. One recent study found that 50 percent of women note a worsening of IBS symptoms at the onset of menses. In addition, there is now a small amount of data showing that some women who have IBS note an improvement in their symptoms after menopause, a time when levels of hormones drop significantly. In summary, hormones are likely to play a key role in the presentation and severity of IBS symptoms, and they should be factored into current and future treatment programs.

Summary

- IBS is very common. Approximately 15 percent of adult Americans (1 in 7) suffer from this disorder.
- Although IBS can develop and be diagnosed at virtually any age, the most common time of diagnosis is in the third or fourth decade of life.
- Women are more likely to be diagnosed with IBS than men. The reasons for this are not clear, and this issue is an active area of research.
- Because many people who have IBS never see a physician or other health care provider for their problems, IBS is underreported.
- IBS *does not* increase a person's risk of developing cancer and does not shorten a person's lifespan.

CHAPTER 5

What Is My Prognosis?

When your doctor uses the term *natural history*, he or she is talking about how a disease will progress if it goes untreated. Most people are familiar with the natural history of common diseases. For example, they know that the average cold lasts 5 to 10 days, a typical viral flu that affects the intestinal tract may last 2 to 4 days, and high blood pressure left untreated will increase a person's risk of a stroke or a heart attack. But what you may not know is that the natural history of disease is not the same in everyone. You may catch a cold with symptoms that last for weeks, whereas your husband feels better after only a few days. If you get migraine headaches, perhaps your symptoms go away after 2 to 3 hours. Other people with migraines are known to have symptoms for 12 to 36 hours.

Another term that doctors frequently use is *prognosis*, meaning the long-term outcome of a medical problem. The prognosis of a medical disorder depends on natural history and whether or not the disease evolves into other medical problems. For example, the prognosis of the common cold is excellent. Although a cold can be frustrating and annoying and produce symptoms that may make you feel crummy for a few days, the common cold never turns into another disease (although it may make you more susceptible to other diseases, such as pneumonia). Migraine headaches can certainly be debilitating, but no matter how frequently you get them, they will not increase your risk for a stroke or other life-threatening medical condition.

In contrast, long-standing type I diabetes (diabetes that must be treated with insulin) does not have as good a prognosis as the common cold. If you have this type of diabetes, you are more likely to develop eye problems (such as retinopathy), kidney damage (nephropathy), and nerve injury to your hands and feet (peripheral neuropathy). Similarly, if you have chronically high cholesterol, you are at an increased risk of developing heart disease. If you have an untreated infection in your stomach (*Helicobacter pylori*), you have an increased risk of developing an ulcer in either your stomach or small intestine or even developing stomach cancer.

People who have irritable bowel syndrome frequently ask about the natural history and prognosis of the disease. How long does IBS last? Will IBS evolve into another disease? Does IBS increase my risk of developing other medical problems, especially cancer? In this chapter, I address the most common concerns about the natural history and prognosis of IBS. Keep in mind that the natural history and prognosis of a disease varies from person to person, as illustrated by the examples given above.

What Is the Natural History of IBS?

Although researchers working on different studies may address the same question—such as "What is the natural history of IBS?"—they may come up with different answers. Research results may vary because of differences among study populations, for example. Researchers may carefully screen participants to include only people who have IBS in a study, but types of IBS vary from person to person, as well as among study populations at different research centers. For instance one center may recruit people from the general community who have IBS. Many of these people would have mild IBS symptoms or have had IBS symptoms for only a short time. In contrast, some research studies recruit people who are hospitalized and have IBS. These people likely have severe IBS symptoms, because they have already tried some simple remedies at home, did not see their symptoms improve, and thus sought a physician's advice. Finally, some IBS-related research studies only enroll people who have seen a gastroenterologist or been treated at a specialized clinic for IBS. These people typically have had severe symptoms for a longer period than people from the general community who have IBS, and they have usually tried different types of treatments without success.

When we do research to learn about the natural history of IBS, we need to keep in mind the potential differences among study populations. In addition, we should consider the answers to two separate questions. One, what is the natural history of a single episode or flare of IBS? Two, what is the long-term natural history of this disorder over the course of several years or over the course of a person's lifetime?

Flares of IBS

For the most part, the natural history of a single episode (called a "flare") of IBS depends on the person and whether she or he suffers from IBS with constipation or IBS with diarrhea. Some people find that a flare of IBS may last 3 to 5 days and then resolve by itself or with the use of medications. For other people, flares may last weeks or, rarely, even months. Many people who have IBS track their symptoms during the course of months or years to see if there is a pattern to their flares. As discussed in Part III, tracking these episodes using a diary or calendar can be helpful, because it allows you to identify the precipitating event or events that may have caused the flare. Just like people who have migraine headaches or episodes of arthritis, people who have IBS have flares that last for a specific period, with fairly reproducible and consistent symptoms. The predictability of the flares is reassuring for many people who have IBS, because it helps them learn coping strategies.

Long-Term IBS

IBS is a chronic disorder for most people. In one study, researchers found that during the course of two years, nearly 70 percent of people who had IBS continued to have some symptoms. The results of this study do not mean that 70 percent of people had daily, persistent symptoms during the 2-year period, but rather that they still had some symptoms at the end of the study period that classified them as having IBS. This research study was performed at an academic medical center, however, and people who have IBS and are referred to academic medical or research centers for evaluation and treatment are likely to have more intense or persistent symptoms than people in the general community who have IBS.

Other researchers have measured the persistence of IBS symptoms in people during a two-year follow-up period and even a five-year follow-up period. Although their study populations were not large, researchers from both studies found that approximately 66 percent of people continued to have IBS symptoms during the follow-up periods. These data only apply to people who have IBS, see a doctor, and then enroll in a research study. As discussed in Chapter 4, nearly one in seven adult Americans have some symptoms of IBS, but most of them (approximately 70 percent) never see a doctor for their problems. Unfortunately, we have little information about the natural history of IBS in this large group of people from the community who never seek medical advice. People who have IBS but avoid the doctor's office may have mild symptoms that resolve on their own after several months or years. Thus, although a seemingly discouraging percentage of people have persistent symptoms of IBS, the data from the studies described above may not accurately reflect the entire population of people who have IBS.

What Is the Prognosis for IBS?

People who have persistent symptoms of IBS often worry about whether IBS will transform into other medical problems. Whereas some people's symptoms resolve completely over time, other people who have IBS may have their symptoms go away just as other, new symptoms appear. For example, people who have IBS may experience relief from their lower abdominal pain only to develop new symptoms of recurrent upper abdominal pain or discomfort. Chronic symptoms of upper abdominal pain or discomfort (often associated with eating a meal) are characteristics of dyspepsia, which frequently goes hand-in-hand with IBS (see Chapter 9 for more information). The appearance of new symptoms, however, does not indicate that IBS has changed into another medical disorder.

Fortunately, there is only good news for people who have IBS and are worried about their prognosis. There are absolutely no data in the medical or scientific literature to show that having IBS increases the risk of developing another medical disorder. IBS *does not* increase the risk of developing cancer of the colon or rectum. In fact, there is no evidence to suggest that having IBS increases the risk of developing cancer anywhere in the body. There are also no data to suggest that having IBS shortens a person's lifespan or that IBS can transform into another disorder, such as inflammatory bowel disease (Crohn's disease or ulcerative colitis; see Chapter 12).

Although many people who have IBS have symptoms that can last for months or even years, everyone experiences symptoms differently: some people's symptoms resolve completely; others have symptoms that resolve while other, new problems develop; and some have symptoms that do not resolve completely but become less intense or less frequent over time. Regardless of the length or severity of their symptoms, people who have IBS can be reassured in the knowledge that IBS does not increase their risk of developing another medical condition.

Having IBS does not keep anyone from developing other disorders, of course, and you and your doctor still need to work together to schedule the routine tests recommended for people your age. This includes routine screening for breast cancer (this may include regular breast examinations, mammograms, or even thermal imaging) and pap smears (for women), vaccinations, and colonoscopies (colon cancer screening needs to start at age 50 in the average-risk Caucasian individual and 45 in African Americans).

Summary

- For most people who have IBS and go to see a doctor, IBS is a chronic condition with persistent symptoms that may last for months or even years.
- Flares of IBS are different for each person, and most people who have IBS are familiar with their typical symptoms. For each person who has IBS, the nature and duration of symptoms are usually fairly consistent.
- The prognosis for IBS is excellent. IBS has never been shown to increase the risk of developing inflammatory bowel disease or colorectal cancer or to decrease a person's lifespan.

CHAPTER 6

The Anatomy of Digestion

The human body is amazing in its structural and functional design. Like any complicated structure, it is made up of many different systems, each of which is responsible for specific activities and functions. These specialized areas are referred to as organ systems. There are ten major organ systems in the body:

respiratory (lungs, trachea)
cardiovascular (heart, arteries, veins, lymphatics)
musculoskeletal (skeletal muscles, bone)
nervous (brain, spinal cord, nerves)
integumentary (skin, hair)
immune (spleen, tonsils, bone marrow, appendix, lymph nodes)
urologic (kidneys, bladder)
endocrine (thyroid gland, pancreas, adrenal gland)
hematological (red blood cells, bone marrow)
gastrointestinal (GI)

As a gastroenterologist, I have no doubt that the GI system is the most fascinating organ system in the body. The GI system encompasses not only the GI tract (described in this chapter), but also the salivary glands, the liver, the pancreas, and the gallbladder. In the following section, I provide a brief overview of the normal anatomy and physiology of the GI tract. An understanding of the normal physiology of the GI tract creates the context for understanding problems within this complicated system that lead to symptoms of irritable bowel syndrome. In addition, having a working knowledge of the anatomy and physiology of the GI tract will help you better understand many of the medical terms used by health care providers, improving your ability to communicate with your doctor, and he or she with you. In this chapter, I also provide a brief description of normal digestion and a discussion of what causes intestinal gas.

Anatomy of the GI Tract

You may be surprised to learn that your lips and mouth are technically the beginning of your GI tract. Without these two key structures, you could not chew solid food or swallow liquids. After solid food is ingested, it must be chewed, mixed with saliva, pushed to the back of the throat (oropharynx) by the tongue, and then swallowed. Although you probably don't think about the act of swallowing, it is a complicated process. Swallowing begins when the muscle in your upper esophagus (upper esophageal sphincter) relaxes so that chewed food can enter your esophagus when pushed backwards by your tongue. At the same time, your vocal cords snap shut, your soft palate elevates (to prevent food from going up into your nose), and your voice box (larynx) changes position. All of these actions ensure that food passes into your esophagus and not into your trachea and lungs.

The esophagus is a muscular tube approximately 10 inches in length that connects the mouth to the stomach. It is located in the chest (thoracic) cavity with the heart and lungs. Strong muscular contractions, called peristalsis, push food and liquids from your upper to lower esophagus and then into your stomach. After you begin to swallow and food enters the upper part of your esophagus, the rest of the process is performed under the direction of different divisions of the nervous system (the autonomic nervous system and the enteric nervous system) that supply the GI tract, without any conscious thought or effort on your part. Solid foods pass through your esophagus and enter your stomach in approximately 3 to 8 seconds. At the end of the esophagus is a muscular ring called the lower esophageal sphincter (LES). This muscular ring is normally contracted to prevent acid, bile, food, and other chemicals from entering the esophagus from the stomach. However, when you start swallowing, the LES relaxes to allow the rhythmic muscle contractions of the esophagus to push food into your stomach.

The stomach is a J-shaped organ located in your abdominal cavity (below the diaphragm, or breathing muscle). The stomach has many different functions: it produces acid to help break down food, stores food temporarily, mixes and grinds food up into smaller pieces, and moves food and liquids into the small intestine.

The small intestine is separated from the stomach by a thick muscular ring called the pylorus. The pylorus opens and closes in coordination with the stomach to allow food to enter the small intestine at the appropriate time. The small intestine is approximately 20 to 25 feet long and is divided into three areas: the duodenum, the jejunum, and the ileum. The last part of the small intestine, the ileum, is directly connected to the colon via the ileocecal valve. This narrow, angled connection between the small intestine and the colon prevents the backward flow of contents from one part of the GI tract to another.

The colon, also called the large intestine, is a muscular tube approximately four feet long. The colon begins in the right, lower part of the abdomen, where it is connected to the small intestine through an area called the cecum (the cecum also includes the opening of the appendix; see Figure 6.1). As the colon moves into the upper abdomen (here it is called the ascending colon), it takes a sharp turn (the hepatic flexure) near the liver and then travels across the abdomen from the right side to the left side (this part of the colon is called the transverse colon). Near the spleen, the colon makes another sharp turn (the splenic flexure) and heads down into the lower abdomen (here it is first called the descending colon and then the sigmoid colon). The sigmoid colon eventually becomes the rectum, which merges into the anal canal.

Normal Digestion

A common misconception about the digestive process is that it only involves the stomach. In reality, many different parts of the GI tract help change the food that you eat into a form that your body can use.

The digestive process begins as soon as you start to chew your food. Chewing breaks food down into smaller pieces and lubricates it with saliva, making it easier to swallow. Saliva contains amylase, a digestive enzyme that breaks down starch and glycogen (the storage form of sugar). After you chew and swallow your food, peristalsis pushes the food through the esophagus and into the stomach, where it may remain for some time. During this period, strong muscular contractions of the stomach help grind up the food and mix it with stomach acid—a process that can take several hours, depending on the size of the meal, the proportion of liquids to solids, and the nutritional content of the meal. Larger meals leave the stomach more slowly than smaller meals, and liquid meals (such as soups) leave the stomach faster than solid meals (such as sandwiches). In addition, meals higher in fat content are pushed from the stomach more slowly than meals containing little fat.

The stomach only sends food into the small intestine when the food particles are small enough to be further broken down by digestive enzymes and absorbed. Food particles are typically 2 to 3 mm in size before

---

Figure 6.1. Anatomy of the Gastrointestinal Tract
The gastrointestinal tract begins at the mouth and ends at the anal canal. The esophagus is a 10-inch-long muscular tube that runs from the mouth to the stomach. The esophagus lies in the thoracic (chest) cavity. Shortly before reaching the stomach, the esophagus passes through an opening in the diaphragm. The diaphragm is the muscle that is vital for breathing and separates the thoracic cavity from the abdominal cavity. The remainder of the GI tract resides within the abdominal and pelvic cavities. The stomach empties into the small intestine. The small intestine is approximately 20 to 25 feet long and is responsible for absorbing nutrients (vitamins, minerals, proteins, carbohydrates, and fats). The small intestine ends at the ileocecal valve, which connects the end of the small intestine (the ileum) to the beginning portion of the colon (the cecum). The appendix is attached to the cecum. The colon is approximately 4 to 5 feet long. The ascending colon extends from the lower right, in the pelvic cavity, up into the abdominal cavity, where it turns near the liver (the hepatic flexure). As the transverse colon, it then crosses from right to left in the abdominal cavity, turns at the spleen (the splenic flexure), and continues, as the descending colon, down into the pelvic cavity, where it turns again and becomes the sigmoid colon. The GI tract terminates in the rectum and anal canal.

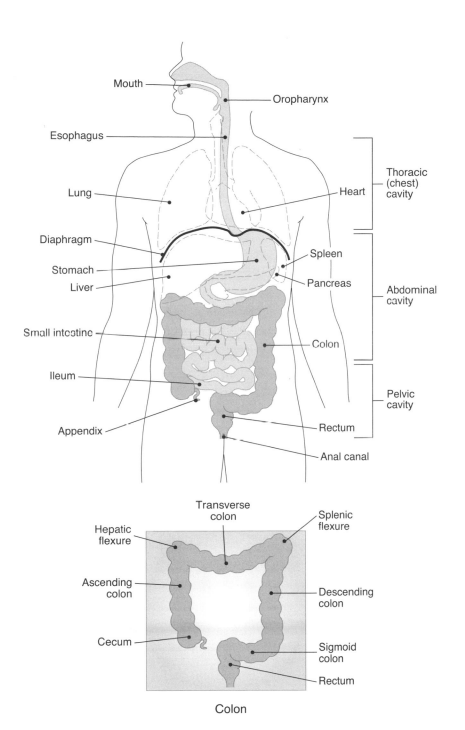

Mouth

Oropharynx

Esophagus

Lung

Heart

Thoracic (chest) cavity

Diaphragm

Spleen

Stomach

Pancreas

Liver

Abdominal cavity

Small intestine

Colon

Ileum

Pelvic cavity

Appendix

Rectum

Anal canal

Transverse colon

Hepatic flexure

Splenic flexure

Ascending colon

Descending colon

Cecum

Sigmoid colon

Rectum

Colon

they leave the stomach. When particles of food are small enough, they enter the small intestine in small amounts—approximately 1/2 to 1 teaspoon (2.5 to 5 ml) at a time. This liquefied food then mixes with fluid and secretions from the small intestine and pancreas.

The pancreas is an organ that is especially important to the digestive process because it produces many different enzymes (amylase, lipase, trypsin, chymotrypsin, and elastase) that further break down small particles of food. The liver secretes a substance called bile that also helps digest food, specifically helping in the digestion and absorption of lipids (fats).

The liquid material comprised of secretions from the digestive organs is called chyme (pronounced "kyme"; it rhymes with "lime"). Chyme is propelled through the small intestine by peristalsis, which is crucial to digestion in the small intestine. As the muscles of the small intestine contract, liquid chyme is exposed to the very large surface area of the small intestine, allowing fluids and nutrients to be slowly absorbed. The small intestine functions, to some degree, like a sponge, and it has many tiny villi that greatly increase its surface area. If the 20 to 25 feet of small intestine were removed and completely spread out, they would just about cover the surface of a tennis court. The primary function of the small intestine is to absorb nutrients, including vitamins, minerals, fats, carbohydrates, and proteins. At the end of the small intestine, the remaining liquid chyme passes into the large intestine, where the material will be further concentrated and eventually eliminated as stool. The time it takes for the first bite of food to travel from the stomach to the colon varies dramatically because of volume, fat content, and proportion of liquids to solids. On average, this process occurs within 3 hours of eating a meal.

Evacuation

Evacuation of stool from the rectum (a process called defecation) is normally an easy process that functions smoothly. Many people have a complete, spontaneous bowel movement each day without straining, pain, or feelings of incomplete evacuation. However, defecation is a complicated, learned process that requires an intact nervous system (central, autonomic, enteric, and peripheral) and normal muscle function (within the GI tract and the pelvic floor). The process of defecation is also greatly influenced by societal norms, familial customs, and personal behavior.

Defecation involves certain steps that must occur in a precisely coordinated sequence. One, stool must be propelled from the sigmoid colon into the rectum (requiring normal motility in the colon). Two, distention (stretching) of the rectum by stool must be detected by the body and the brain (requiring an intact nervous system). Third, the person's body and brain must recognize that it is a socially appropriate time to defecate. (People can normally block the urge to defecate if it occurs at an inappropriate time, such as during a meeting or a car ride.) Four, the person will usually assume a squatting or sitting position, thereby straightening the anorectal angle and making evacuation easier. Five, the internal anal sphincter normally automatically relaxes when the rectum is stretched, and then the person must consciously relax the external anal sphincter. Finally, the person performs a valsalva maneuver, increasing intra-abdominal and intra-rectal pressure and permitting the evacuation of stool. A valsalva maneuver is when you take a deep breath and contract your abdominal muscles without letting your breath out.

Although having a bowel movement should be an easy process, it now seems quite complicated, doesn't it? It's little wonder that toilet training is so difficult for some children. In addition, because all of these complicated steps must occur in a precise sequence, injury to any one part of the system can affect the entire process, leading to constipation, diarrhea, or incontinence.

Normal Colon Function

Many people think the colon is simply a pipeline for material to pass through on the way from the small intestine to the rectum. But the colon has a variety of functions. One, it helps concentrate stool by absorbing large amounts of water. The colon can easily absorb 4 to 5 liters of fluid per day, if necessary. It also has the ability to absorb electrolytes (for example, sodium, potassium, and chloride) and some nutrients. Two, the colon is responsible for the continued breakdown, fermentation, and absorption of certain carbohydrates. Three, the colon acts as a reservoir to store stool (one of the major functions of the sigmoid colon).

The colon is normally quite active; it contracts and relaxes in a coordinated pattern throughout the day. Specific patterns of neuromuscular activity within the colon depend on the time of day, whether you are awake or sleeping, the volume and timing of your most recent meal, your level of physical activity, the presence of coexisting medical problems, medication use, and the time of your most recent bowel movement. Normal colonic motility, or movement, involves mixing the liquid material from the ileum within the ascending colon and then propelling the material from the right side of the colon to the sigmoid colon and rectum, where it can be concentrated further, stored, and then evacuated. The normal transit of material through the colon takes approximately 36 hours (although it can differ dramatically from one person to the next), which is equally divided between the right colon (ascending colon), transverse colon, and left colon (descending colon, sigmoid colon, and rectum).

Normal Pelvic Floor Function

Aside from the GI tract, there are other areas of the body that must function normally to avoid problems such as diarrhea, constipation, pain, and bloating. The pelvic floor is a group of muscles that support the internal organs of the lower abdomen and pelvis (the urethra, bladder, vagina, cervix, uterus, prostate gland, anal canal, and rectum; see Figures 6.2 and 6.3). The muscles of the pelvic floor include the pubococcygeus, iliococcygeus, and puborectalis. When viewed in cross-section, these muscles form a gently sloped funnel that stretches from the coccyx (tail bone) to the pubic bone. When viewed from the front (anterior) to the back (posterior), the pelvic floor muscles run from both sides of the inner hip bones and blend together in the midline.

Healthy pelvic floor muscles support the internal organs, keeping them in proper position and assisting them in normal functions. These muscles play an especially important role in the health and normal function of the bladder and rectum: they assist in the complete emptying of both of these organs. In addition, pelvic floor muscles prevent leakage from the bladder (urinary incontinence) and rectum (fecal incontinence). If a person's pelvic floor muscles are injured, or if the muscles do not work in a coordinated manner, then she or he may experience constipation, fecal incontinence, or urinary incontinence.

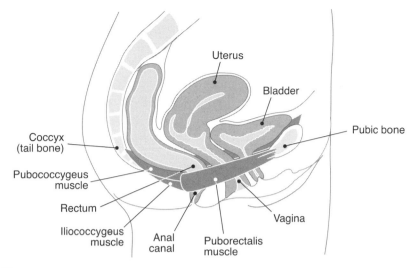

Figure 6.2. Anatomy of the Pelvic Floor
This cross-sectional view shows the muscles of the pelvic floor and the organs supported by it in a woman. The pelvic floor consists of a group of muscles that form a funnel-shaped structure stretching from the pubic bone at the front to the coccyx (the tail bone) at the back and to the pelvic bones on the sides. The muscles of the pelvic floor are the pubococcygeus, iliococcygeus, and puborectalis. The organs supported by the pelvic floor in women are (from front to back) the bladder, vagina, uterus, anal canal, and rectum; in men, the bladder, prostate gland, and anorectal area are supported by the pelvic floor.

Abnormal Colon Function

Constipation and diarrhea are not diseases; they are symptoms of abnormal colon function. Although several different conditions may cause these symptoms (see Tables 6.1 and 6.2), IBS is one of the most common causes of either constipation or diarrhea. How does IBS cause these two contradictory processes?

People who have IBS can develop constipation for many different reasons. One, the movement of material through the colon may be very slow (this can occur when either the muscles or the nerves that supply the colon have been injured). Two, there may be poor coordination between the muscles and nerves in the colon. (The muscle and nerve sys-

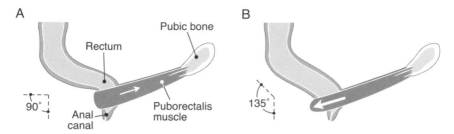

Figure 6.3. Pelvic Floor Changes during Evacuation
Many steps need to occur in an intricate and properly timed sequence
in order to evacuate stool easily and effectively. In *A*, the puborectalis
muscle is contracted, producing a tight "turn" at the junction of the anal
canal and rectum. This turn, called the anorectal angle, is usually approximately 90 degrees when evacuation is not occurring. The relative tightness of the angle helps maintain continence. At the time of defecation,
the puborectalis muscle relaxes, opening up the anorectal angle to approximately 135 degrees (as in *B*). This wider angle, in combination with
relaxation of the external anal sphincter and the internal anal sphincter,
makes evacuation of stool much easier.

tems may be normal, but if their actions are not coordinated, they won't
function normally as a group.) Three, people who have IBS may become
constipated because their pelvic floor muscles do not function or coordinate normally. In some people who have IBS, especially younger women,
the complex signals required to have a normal bowel movement become
mixed up or confused (see pelvic floor dyssynergia, described later in the
chapter). Finally, some people who have IBS and chronic constipation
have GI tracts that function normally, even when evaluated by many different tests (see Chapter 8). These people are said to have normal transit
constipation, which is constipation (infrequent stools, bloating, fullness,
abdominal pressure) without evidence of a mechanical obstruction or any
abnormalities in colonic motility or pelvic floor function. Understand-
ably so, normal transit constipation is a difficult concept for patients and
physicians to comprehend. Normal transit constipation may represent
an undefined neurochemical or hormonal problem; alternatively, it may
represent a sensory disorder. This type of constipation is an active area
of research within the field of gastroenterology, and physicians may have

Table 6.1. Common Causes of Constipation

Anal fissure	Neurologic disorders
Anatomical obstruction	Pelvic floor dysfunction
Colorectal cancer	Psychiatric disorders
Compression of the colon caused	Rectal prolapse
by an abdominal or pelvic mass	Rectocele
Irritable bowel syndrome	Slow intestinal motility
Medications	Stricture caused by Crohn's disease
Metabolic disorders	Stricture caused by diverticulitis
Muscular disorders	Stricture caused by ischemic colitis

Table 6.2. Common Causes of Diarrhea

Abnormal GI tract motility
Dietary changes (for example, excess fiber; lactose, fructose, or gluten
   intolerance)
Functional bowel disorders (for example, IBS)
Increased secretion of fluid in the small intestine
Infections (viral, bacterial, parasite)
Inflammatory bowel disease (Crohn's disease or ulcerative colitis)
Injury to the lining of the GI tract that prevents normal absorption
Medications
Metabolic disorders (for example, hyperthyroidism, long-standing diabetes)
Osmotic agents (sugars that can't be absorbed, such as sorbitol)
Prior gallbladder surgery
Short gut syndrome

a better understanding of why this condition develops sometime in the next decade.

People who have IBS and diarrhea may also have malfunctioning colons. The colon may contract too vigorously, especially in the sigmoid colon, which can lead to cramps and spasms in the rectosigmoid area and a sense of urgency to defecate. In some people who have IBS and diarrhea, materials move too quickly through the colon, which minimizes how much time the colon has to absorb water and concentrate stool. When materials move too quickly through the colon, people will have softer, more liquid stools.

Abnormal Pelvic Floor Function

People who have pelvic floor dysfunction often complain of excessive straining, prolonged or excessive time spent in the bathroom attempting to have a bowel movement, and feelings of incomplete evacuation ("I went a little but still feel like I need to go more"). Some people need to assist evacuation with digital stimulation (inserting a finger into the rectum), pushing on the perineal body (the small muscular area just in front of the rectum), or vaginal splinting (placing a finger or fingers in the vagina to assist with defecation).

Pelvic floor dyssynergia is one of the most common pelvic floor disorders to cause constipation. In people who have pelvic floor dyssynergia (primarily women), the internal anal sphincter does not relax properly and/or the external anal sphincter contracts inappropriately during attempted defecation. People may develop the sensation that they need to have a bowel movement, but when they push or strain, they tighten the external anal sphincter muscle and block the normal evacuation of stool. This condition does not respond well to medications; it is treated most effectively with physical therapy and a bowel retraining program.

There are many other problems that can develop in the pelvic floor or anorectal area and lead to constipation: rectal prolapse (a portion of the lining of the rectum is pushed out, usually with severe straining), intussusception (the lining of the rectum folds on itself and impedes or prevents normal defecation), or the formation of a rectocele (a bulging of the rectal wall; this usually occurs in the anterior direction, toward the vagina). Less commonly, people who are constipated may have descending perineum syndrome (abnormal descent of the pelvic floor) or weakened muscle contractions in the rectum.

Intestinal Gas

What's Normal?

Gas in the intestinal tract is normal, although it can be uncomfortable or embarrassing for some people. Intestinal gas is usually one of five types of gas: nitrogen, oxygen, carbon dioxide, hydrogen, or methane. Most intestinal gas is nitrogen, with oxygen being the second most common.

Whereas nitrogen and oxygen are present in the intestinal tract because they have been swallowed, carbon dioxide, hydrogen, and methane are present because they are formed within the GI tract. Gas may develop after a person ingests different foods or liquids. People who drink large amounts of carbonated beverages may find that they have more problems with upper intestinal gas than people who drink only water or noncarbonated beverages. Most intestinal gas develops during the normal digestive process, when sugars and simple carbohydrates are broken down and completely absorbed while other sugars and carbohydrates are only partially broken down. The remaining sugars and carbohydrates are then fermented by bacteria in the intestinal tract, which produces hydrogen and, to a lesser degree, methane. As proteins and fats are broken down during the digestive process, they may produce carbon dioxide and small amounts of methane. Less commonly, gas can develop within the GI tract as a result of a chemical reaction. For example, gastric acid can react with bicarbonate, creating an end product of carbon dioxide. The carbon dioxide may be expelled during a burp, or it may diffuse through the stomach wall and into the bloodstream, from which it is breathed out during normal respiration.

Researchers have developed special devices to measure the amount of gas within the GI tract. Their studies have shown that the normal individual has 200 to 300 ml of gas within their intestinal tract at any one time (although not a perfect comparison, a typical 12-oz can of soda contains approximately 350 ml of liquid). Over the course of 24 hours, people release approximately 750 ml of gas from their rectum (technically referred to as flatus). Flatus typically occurs 10 to 15 times per day in a normal person.

Gas and the Upper GI Tract

Some people have problems with upper intestinal gas and recurrent or persistent belching and burping (the technical name for belching and burping is eructation). Nearly all gas present in the upper GI tract (that is, the stomach and upper small intestine) is there because people swallowed it, typically because they ate or drank too fast. Eating or drinking in the car, eating while talking on the phone, or eating while walking to a meeting are some of the most common ways of unintentionally swallowing a large amount of air. Some people easily swallow 2 to 3 liters of air during a single meal. Swallowing air (called aerophagia) can develop in some people as a nervous habit. In others, it may occur because oral stimulation (smoking, chewing gum, sucking on candies or mints) causes large amounts of saliva to be produced, which then leads to repetitive swallowing of both saliva and air.

Belching occurs when gas within the stomach produces a sensation of upper abdominal fullness, pressure, or discomfort. To release this gas, the lower esophageal sphincter must relax, temporarily forming a common cavity or connection between the stomach and the esophagus. This connection allows gas to rise up and move from the stomach into the esophagus. The upper esophageal sphincter then reflexively relaxes, and a noisy release of gas occurs. Belching or burping after a meal is considered a compliment in some countries but rude in others. Belching is not usually dangerous, but it can become part of a vicious cycle. Venting gas from your stomach may initially provide relief from the sensation of fullness or pressure, but some people end up swallowing more air at the end of the burp or belch. This air then creates more pressure or discomfort in the upper abdomen, forcing the person to belch again and subsequently swallow more air. This cycle can be broken in most people who have aerophagia by first recognizing the behavior and then modifying the maladaptive behavior that leads to air swallowing.

Gas and the Lower GI Tract

Some people seem to have a lot of intestinal gas, usually as a result of the breakdown and fermentation of dietary substances in their GI tract. Carbohydrates not completely broken down and absorbed in the small intestine will eventually pass into the colon. At this point, the bacteria that normally reside in the colon will ferment these undigested substances, leading to the production of lower intestinal gas. Typical undigested substances include the nonabsorbable carbohydrates stachyose and raffinose (found in beans and legumes), lactose (milk sugar), and poorly absorbed carbohydrates such as fructose and sorbitol (found in fruit juices, sports drinks, "energy" drinks, and fruit).

You may be surprised to learn that people who have IBS generally have the same amount of intestinal gas as people who do not have IBS. This fact has been confirmed by x-rays and by measuring the amount of gas in the intestinal tracts of both groups of people (those who have and those who do not have IBS) who complain of feeling bloated or gassy. Many people who have IBS, however, seem to be very sensitive to even small amounts of gas within their intestinal tract. This gas may make them feel bloated or distended, and it can occasionally cause crampy pain and discomfort.

That some people who have IBS are hypersensitive to gas in the intestinal tract should not be surprising, since we know that people who have IBS are generally more sensitive to pain throughout their intestinal tract, compared to people who do not have IBS. This hypersensitivity to distention caused by gas in the GI tract was confirmed by several research studies. During these studies, a small tube was inserted into the colon of both healthy volunteers and people who had IBS. Increasing amounts of gas were then infused through the tube, and the study subjects were asked to indicate when they could begin to sense the gas distending their colon and when they considered the pressure uncomfortable or painful. These studies all showed that people who had IBS sensed the distention sooner and felt discomfort at lower amounts of pressure during the procedure than did the healthy volunteers. People who had IBS reported that even small amounts of gas in the colon were uncomfortable or painful, whereas the healthy volunteers did not have any complaints of pain or discomfort. These studies support the view that people who have IBS sense things differently in their GI tract, whether it be gas, peristalsis, or pain.

Finally, data collected during the last several years have shown that many people who have IBS, especially those with chronic diarrhea, do not digest fructose well. This is an important finding, because fructose is a common additive to a large number of food products in the United States. Treatment options for gas and bloating are reviewed in Chapters 15 and 19.

Summary

- The GI tract extends from the mouth to the anus and is 25 to 30 feet long.

- The process of digestion begins in the mouth, accelerates in the stomach via mixing and grinding and the addition of various enzymes, and continues in the small intestine with additional enzymes secreted by the pancreas.
- Constipation and diarrhea are symptoms rather than diseases. There are many different medical conditions that can produce symptoms of constipation, diarrhea, or both.
- The role of pelvic floor dysfunction is often overlooked during the evaluation of a person who has IBS and constipation. This disorder can be identified by history, a careful physical examination, and anorectal manometry. Pelvic floor retraining is the best therapy for this disorder; medications are rarely effective.
- Intestinal gas is a problem for many people, and people who have IBS are frequently more sensitive to the effects of intestinal gas than others. Dietary factors (lactose, fructose, artificial sugars, fiber) are often the culprits.

PART II

Diagnosing Irritable Bowel Syndrome

CHAPTER 7

How Is IBS Diagnosed?

Making an accurate and timely diagnosis of irritable bowel syndrome is critical for the proper treatment of this condition. First, an accurate diagnosis identifies and provides a name for the multiple symptoms that have been troubling the patient, sometimes for years. Second, the patient learns that there are many other people who have similar symptoms; people who have IBS often suffer in silence, not realizing that others share similar problems. Third, a definitive diagnosis provides the opportunity for the patient to become informed about this medical condition. He or she can then research the topic and talk to family members, friends, and coworkers, probably discovering that some of them also have IBS symptoms. Knowledge truly is power for anyone with a chronic medical condition, and being informed significantly improves communication between patients and their health care providers and enhances the effectiveness of treatments. Fourth, making a definitive diagnosis of IBS often ends the need for further testing (see Chapter 8) and the parade of normal results, which can be confusing ("Why are all of these tests normal if I feel so crummy?"), time consuming, expensive, and at times, even risky. Finally, and most important, once a clear diagnosis of IBS is made, appropriate treatment can be initiated.

The accurate diagnosis of any medical condition is based on three key components: a thorough review of the patient's history, a careful physical examination, and, when necessary, appropriate diagnostic tests or studies. This principle of performing all three components is followed whenever a health care provider begins evaluating a patient for any type of medical problem. However, the amount of time spent on each component will vary greatly, depending on the type and complexity of the problem. For example, with a patient who has a simple urinary tract infection (UTI), the doctor will want to know what the symptoms are, when they started, and if the symptoms are similar to UTIs the patient had in the past. An abbreviated physical examination is usually performed, and a urine sample is sent to a laboratory for analysis (typically a urinalysis and urine culture). For a more complicated problem, such as infertility due to endometriosis, an extensive list of questions will need to be answered, a comprehensive medical examination will need to be performed, and extensive testing, possibly including exploratory surgery, will be required.

In some cases, the diagnosis of a particular problem can be made in a single office visit using only a brief focused history and physical examination, without performing any tests. Examples include a classic migraine headache, low back pain from overuse, or a sinus infection that develops after a cold. In other cases, the diagnosis of a problem may require multiple visits, with repeated and more focused examinations, and extensive and specialized testing. The latter is often the case with diseases that have vague, intermittent, or fluctuating symptoms (such as multiple sclerosis) or diseases that progress very slowly over time (like Alzheimer's disease).

For many patients, unfortunately, the diagnosis of IBS can be an unnecessarily lengthy, difficult, and expensive experience. In part, this is because people who have IBS are often given an inaccurate diagnosis at first. It is not uncommon for patients who have IBS to be told that their symptoms represent acid reflux disease, inflammatory bowel disease (such as Crohn's disease or ulcerative colitis), or a food allergy. This misdiagnosis occurs because many of the symptoms of IBS (abdominal discomfort, bloating, and diarrhea) are quite "nonspecific," that is, they are found in many different disorders rather than being specific to IBS. This is the case with many medical problems, which is why combining a careful history with a thorough physical examination and the use of appropriate tests is so important. Also, in the past, many patients who had IBS were told that their symptoms were "all in your head." Fortunately, this statement is rarely made by doctors now. The mistaken belief that many or all IBS symptoms were imagined by a patient developed because the tests available at the time were unable to identify an organic process that could account for the patient's symptoms, the way pneumonia can be diagnosed by a chest x-ray. This misimpression was reinforced by the fact that it is common for people who have chronic illnesses to become depressed or anxious. The unfortunate combination of diagnostic test results that were normal and symptoms of psychological distress led many frustrated doctors to believe that IBS symptoms were the result of a "nervous" disorder, like the anxiety or depression that the patient was experiencing.

In addition to the problem of misdiagnosis, many people who have IBS receive a delayed diagnosis. Although many people who have IBS first note symptoms in their late teenage years or early twenties, for patients with moderate symptoms the average time between the onset of symptoms and the diagnosis of IBS is at least three years. This delay in diagnosis and treatment occurs for a number of reasons. Many patients are uncomfortable discussing bloating, diarrhea, and abdominal pain, even with their doctors. They feel awkward describing these somewhat personal and intimate bodily functions to strangers, and they are not familiar with the vocabulary commonly used to effectively discuss their symptoms. Some people hesitate to voice their fears and concerns to their doctors, not wanting to be thought of as "complainers" by their doctor, so they minimize their illness. People who do not discuss their symptoms, even with family or friends, may believe they are the only one with these worrisome symptoms and assume that there is nothing a doctor could do for them. These feelings can lead to a sense of isolation and further reluctance to discuss symptoms. Many people avoid consulting a professional about symptoms of illness because they are concerned that their symptoms represent a severe problem, such as cancer, and they don't want to receive bad news. Finally, in the case of chronic illnesses, many patients become accustomed to their symptoms, no matter how disabling, managing them in their own way or surrendering to them, and only seek care when their typical symptoms change for the worse or become overwhelming.

The diagnosis of IBS should not be a lengthy and difficult process. With a detailed history, a careful physical examination, and appropriate tests, IBS can be accurately diagnosed at the first office visit in the vast majority of patients.

A Detailed History

At your initial office visit with any health practitioner—internist, family practitioner, physician's assistant, nurse practitioner, gynecologist, or gastroenterologist—the first part of the appointment will be spent reviewing your medical, surgical, medication, and family history. The doctor will also ask about your habits (exercise, diet, tobacco use, alcohol use, drug use), your social situation (single, married, widowed, separated, partnered, children), your work history (employed, working at home or volunteering, retired, disabled), and whether you have any allergies to medications or foods. However, the focus will be on your current problem. Many physicians greet their patients with an open-ended question such as "What brings you in today?" or "How can I help you today?" This is your chance to let the doctor know, in your own words, what symptoms you are currently experiencing and why you called for an appointment. It is also a good time to let the doctor know of any previous physician visits for the same problem, to express your thoughts and concerns, and to bring up any specific questions you want answered.

The first few minutes of a doctor's visit are important, because they set the tone for the rest of the visit and for future visits as well. Here are two examples of first office visits to the same specialist; they differ dramatically in their tone, content, and outcome.

David, a 23-year-old law student, was referred to Dr. Hannah Rose, a gastroenterologist, for the evaluation of abdominal pain, bloating, and diarrhea. David had already been shown to a chair in the examination room by the nurse when Dr. Rose entered. She introduced herself: "Good morning. I'm Dr. Rose. What brings you in today?" and David replied that he had a one-year history of lower abdominal pain that appeared to be associated with diarrhea. He said that he also felt very bloated at times, despite watching his diet and working out at the gym, where he did a lot of sit-ups. He admitted that he was a little embarrassed to see a doctor about these problems because he thought he was quite healthy, but his father had died of colon cancer in his early sixties, and David wanted to make sure that he was okay.

For the next five minutes, David carefully related his symptoms, reviewed how he had tried to treat these symptoms with diet and exercise, and mentioned how the symptoms affected his everyday life. Dr. Rose listened carefully without interrupting and then asked David if there was anything else he wanted to discuss before she started asking him some specific questions about his problem. David confessed that he had brought a list of questions that he wanted answered but said he would be happy to hold them until the end of the visit, as he was sure most would be addressed during the rest of the interview.

Colin was a 27-year-old computer engineer. He was referred to Dr. Rose by his internist for evaluation of chronic abdominal pain, bloating, and diarrhea. He was seated in the examination room when Dr. Rose entered and said: "Good afternoon, I'm Dr. Rose. What brings you in today?" Colin replied, "Didn't my doctor tell you?" "Well, yes," said Dr. Rose, "I do have some notes from your doctor, but I always like to hear the story firsthand from the patient. Can you tell me about this pain you've been having?" Colin answered, "Well, it hurts a lot." A period of awkward silence ensued while Dr. Rose waited for Colin to elaborate on this initial comment. When no further details were forthcoming, Dr. Rose asked Colin if he could tell her when the pain began. Colin replied, "A long time ago." Again, a period of silence followed. Realizing that using open-ended questions was not likely to elicit the information she needed, Dr. Rose continued the interview with a long list of questions that could be answered with a simple "yes" or "no."

These two cases, both involving young men with similar symptoms seeing the same doctor, reveal how important, and how much in control, the patient can be during the first part of the interview. David was open, told his story in his own words, voiced his concerns, and let the doctor know that he had some questions he wished to have answered. This turned out to be a productive visit, and David left feeling confident that Dr. Rose would be able to assist him with his problem. Colin, on the other hand, was not able to tell his story in his own words. He did have some questions and concerns, but he was never able to voice them, because Dr. Rose had to spend nearly the entire visit drawing out of him information that

Colin likely could have provided in just a few minutes if he had given it some thought beforehand. Colin left the office later that afternoon feeling unsatisfied and somewhat frustrated. Dr. Rose finished the interview feeling unsatisfied and drained.

The point of describing these two interviews is to highlight three important facts about doctor-patient interviews. First, patients are in control of the interview to a large degree, within constraints like the scheduled length of the visit. Second, by being open, being prepared, voicing your concerns, and bringing a list of questions, you can ensure that the interview will be informative and productive for both you and the physician. To help you prepare, some tips are listed in Table 7.1 (see also Chapter 23). Third, some doctors do not have a good bedside manner, and you can find this out during the initial interview. If your doctor is not able to answer your questions or treats you in a rude or brusque manner, find another doctor. Ask friends and family members for names of doctors they have had good experiences with. Remember that your doctor does not need to be your best friend; however, you need to have confidence that your doctor will do her or his best on your behalf.

During history taking at an office visit to evaluate symptoms of IBS, the two key symptoms to bring to the doctor's attention are abdominal pain and altered bowel habits. Which of these two components is emphasized by the patient usually depends on which the patient finds most disturbing. Let's look in detail at the IBS symptoms that a patient and doctor should discuss.

Abdominal Pain

The presence of abdominal pain is required for the diagnosis of IBS. Clinicians often use specific guidelines (called the Rome II criteria) to help make the diagnosis of IBS (see Table 7.2). These guidelines state that people diagnosed with IBS should experience symptoms of IBS at least six months before diagnosis and that these symptoms should be active (present) during the preceding three months. Patients frequently ask me how many days they should be experiencing abdominal pain or discomfort to be correctly diagnosed as having IBS. Somewhat surprisingly, abdominal pain does not have to be present every day to meet criteria for having IBS. Abdominal pain or discomfort should be present at least three days

Table 7.1. Tips to Maximize Your First Visit to Your Doctor

- Bring a list of the prescription and over-the-counter medications you take and any vitamins and herbal supplements you may use. Note the dosages and the time of day when you take them.
- If you have taken other medications in the past for the same symptoms, bring a list of those as well. Note the dosages and how long you took the medications, if you remember.
- If you have seen other doctors for the same problem, bring a list of their names and specialties.
- If you have had any tests for this problem in the past, have your other doctor(s) send them to this doctor in advance of your arrival. These might include the results of blood work, x-ray studies, endoscopy reports, or more specialized testing. If the tests were done recently, you may be able to avoid having to repeat them.
- Think about your symptoms before you come in for your appointment. Make a list of your symptoms. Try to answer the following questions: When did the symptom start? How would you describe the symptom? What makes your symptoms better? What makes them worse?
- Bring a list of your concerns or fears. You may think they would never leave your mind, but for many reasons they might not get discussed without such a reminder.
- Bring a list of questions that you want answered. Put these questions in the order of importance to you. Because of time limitations, the doctor may be able to get to only some of the questions on the first visit, although other questions on the list can be addressed at follow-up appointments.

Table 7.2. The Rome III Criteria Defining Irritable Bowel Syndrome

- Recurrent abdominal pain or discomfort
- Onset of symptoms at least six months earlier
  - Symptoms must be present at least three days per month within the last three months
  - Symptoms of abdominal pain or discomfort must be associated with at least two of the following:
    - Improvement with defecation, and/or
    - Onset associated with a change in stool frequency, and/or
    - Onset associated with a change in stool form

of the month, for the last three months. People who have IBS may have lower abdominal pain one or two days of the week, and then have one week with minimal or no discomfort, followed by a week with three to four days of severe pain or discomfort. It is common for people who have IBS to have periods of "good" days or weeks followed by periods of "bad" days or weeks. Of course, every person is different, and some people who have IBS do experience daily abdominal pain or discomfort in addition to their symptoms of constipation or diarrhea.

To be accurately diagnosed with IBS, patients should note an association with abdominal pain or discomfort and altered bowel habits. People who have IBS experience abdominal pain or discomfort with at least two of the three following symptoms: changes in stool frequency, changes in stool consistency, and improvement in pain or discomfort after having had a bowel movement. In less scientific terms, abdominal pain should be related in some way to having a bowel movement. For many patients who have IBS, the abdominal pain happens just before having a bowel movement. The pain may occur as a crampy sensation or discomfort in the left lower quadrant of the abdomen, along with the urge to empty the bowels. Often this pain goes away after evacuation. Sometimes the pain develops during, or is made worse by, having a bowel movement. The exact reason why this pain develops is unknown, and it may represent any of a variety of processes, including spasm in the colon, persistent contractions in the colon, stretching of the colon, or increased awareness of normal peristalsis (the concept of increased vigilance or hypersensitivity in the gut).

For other patients who have IBS, however, the pain occurs unpredictably, without any rhyme or reason, at any time of the day. This unpredictability is frustrating to patients and can be quite worrisome and socially inhibiting. Finally, although some patients who have IBS have disordered sleep, many patients who have IBS note that pain occurs immediately on awakening in the morning but is absent at night. Physiologically, this makes sense, since the GI tract is quietest at night, because most food is eaten during the day and first half of the evening.

Although the chronic abdominal pain of IBS can be discouraging, frustrating, exhausting, and even depressing to some patients, *it is not dangerous*. However, the presence of abdominal pain can, in some situations, mean that something dangerous is developing in the abdominal cavity (or elsewhere, in unusual circumstances). For example, in a teenager, the development of new abdominal pain in the lower right portion of the abdomen along with fever and an elevated white blood cell count often indicates the presence of appendicitis. Abdominal pain in the right upper quadrant of the abdomen with nausea, vomiting, and abnormal liver tests may indicate hepatitis (inflammation in the liver) or gall bladder disease. The careful history and physical examination performed by the health care provider helps differentiate the abdominal pain of IBS from that caused by a variety of other medical conditions.

Altered Bowel Habits

The second most common complaint voiced by patients who have IBS is that of abnormal bowel habits. Large-population studies conducted over the years have shown that the majority of healthy people report having anywhere from three bowel movements per week to three bowel movements per day. For most people who do not have IBS, their individual pattern of bowel habits is fairly consistent for a given individual over time. In people who have IBS, one of the first symptoms they notice is a change in their usual bowel pattern. This is worrisome to many patients, because they've heard that a change in their bowel habits could indicate colon cancer. In addition, nearly a quarter of patients who have IBS have fluctuating bowel habits during the course of the year. Keeping track of bowel habits is important, because if the patient alternates between symptoms of constipation and diarrhea, it is difficult to decide which type of treatment will be best. (Part 3 of this book discusses treatments.)

People who have IBS usually have one of three patterns of defecation: constipation predominant, diarrhea predominant, or alternating constipation and diarrhea, sometimes called a mixed pattern. Patients who have IBS and constipation often report the passage of rock-hard, pellet-like stool called scybala. In addition, they may describe excessive straining in an attempt to move their bowels, prolonged time spent in the bathroom (hours in some cases), feelings of incomplete evacuation, and pain or discomfort with defecation.

IBS patients prone to diarrhea often find that the first bowel movement in the morning is of normal consistency but subsequent bowel movements become increasingly loose and are accompanied by significant urgency and gassiness. Urgency is best defined as the feeling of having to race to the bathroom out of fear of having an accident. The urgency and cramps may be temporarily relieved by the passage of stool; however, these feelings may quickly return and precipitate yet another bowel movement. Mucus may cover the stools or be passed alone. As described previously, patients who have IBS often have fecal urgency and lower abdominal discomfort during the period following a meal (the postprandial period). This reflects an exaggerated or heightened gastrocolic reflex (see Chapter 6).

Bloating

Bloating and abdominal distention are also common symptoms experienced by people who have IBS. Bloating is a sense of gassiness or fullness throughout the abdomen. Distention is enlargement or stretching of the abdomen. Patients often say that their abdomen feels "tight" and that on days when they are very bloated they can't wear certain form-fitting clothes because their belly is so distended. These symptoms may reflect the presence of increased amounts of abdominal gas or an increased sensitivity to normal amounts of intestinal gas. Increased gas production can occur in patients who have lactose or fructose intolerance, in people who ingest large amounts of fiber (whether dietary fiber or a fiber supplement), and in those who ingest legumes (beans, for example) that contain stachyose and raffinose (see Chapters 10 and 19). Some patients who have IBS also suffer from aerophagia, an uncommon condition in which air is inadvertently swallowed rather than inhaled.

Although bloating and distention are frequent and troubling symptoms, they rarely reflect a dangerous problem. Contrary to popular belief, most people who have IBS do not produce more intestinal gas than people who do not have IBS. People with IBS do, however, have a decreased tolerance of distention from normal amounts of intestinal gas. Some studies have shown that patients who have IBS have difficulty evacuating intestinal gas, so the gas remains in the GI tract longer, leading to feelings of fullness, bloatedness, and tightness across the abdomen.

Other Topics

During the history-taking part of your office visit, your doctor may ask you a series of questions that do not immediately seem relevant to your problem. These questions are designed to see if you have a dangerous organic problem, such as a bleeding ulcer, liver disease, or cancer, rather than the troublesome but nondangerous condition of IBS. The doctor may ask you about your weight. When people lose weight without trying to, it may reflect a serious medical problem, especially in older patients. Weight loss is not associated with IBS, and thus unintentional weight loss cannot be blamed on IBS and always warrants further investigation by your doctor. Your doctor will also ask about symptoms that would indicate anemia (a low red blood cell count), about evidence of blood in your stool, and about prior episodes of bleeding from your gastrointestinal tract. Anemia and bleeding are also not directly associated with IBS, and thus any evidence of bleeding or anemia will trigger an investigation to determine the underlying cause. If you have diarrhea, your doctor will take a careful travel history to look for evidence of a recent viral, bacterial, or parasitic infection, including giardia and entamoeba histolytica (amebiasis). In addition, your doctor will ask about your diet, recent antibiotic use, and medications, because all of these can cause diarrhea.

As the interview progresses, your doctor may ask you about the presence of what are called "constitutional symptoms." These symptoms include: fatigue, myalgias (muscle aches), arthralgias (joint aches), fevers, chills, and night sweats. Although occasionally present in patients who have IBS, these symptoms can occur for a variety of reasons. There is no evidence that IBS directly causes these symptoms; typically they result from other medical problems, such as a viral infection, fibromyalgia, arthritis, hypothyroidism, or, rarely, cancer.

The doctor will ask you about your family history and pay particular attention to whether any first (mother, father, sister, brother) or second degree (grandparent, aunt, uncle, cousin) relatives in your family had inflammatory bowel disease, celiac disease, or any type of gastrointestinal cancer (colon cancer, stomach cancer, esophageal cancer). Patients with symptoms of IBS who have a first degree relative with any of these diseases may need to have specialized laboratory or diagnostic tests.

As the interview progresses your doctor will likely ask a series of questions related to other parts of the gastrointestinal tract, such as, Do you have burning in your chest that moves up into the mouth or throat? (acid reflux); Have you ever had pancreatitis? Have you ever been jaundiced? (liver problems). In addition, he or she will do what is commonly referred to as a "review of systems." These questions are a way to quickly review a patient's general medical condition and locate any other medical problems that may need to be addressed. This list includes questions related to the heart, lungs, kidneys, musculoskeletal system, vascular system (arteries and veins), central nervous system, endocrine system (glands like the thyroid and pituitary), and genitourinary system.

Your doctor may also ask whether you have ever suffered any type of abuse. The term *abuse* is not limited to just physical abuse but also includes any form of mental, emotional, or sexual abuse. Although this question surprises many patients, many research studies have shown that patients who have functional bowel disorders like IBS are more likely to have a history of abuse than patients who have other medical conditions. Some doctors will raise this issue at the time of the first office visit, while others may wait until a doctor-patient relationship has been established, after several visits. If you have experienced abuse, you can improve your doctor's ability to care for you by bringing this to his or her attention. The timing of this discussion depends on both the patient and the physician. When you decide to bring this issue to your doctor's attention, it should be done when there is enough time for the issue to be dealt with carefully, not at the end of the visit as you are walking out the door.

A Careful Physical Examination

The next part of the office visit is the physical examination. The physical generally starts with some simple measurements, such as height, weight, blood pressure, heart rate, and respiratory rate. The extent of the physical examination will depend on whether you are seeing your primary care doctor (internist, nurse practitioner, physician assistant, obstetrician, gynecologist, or family practitioner) or a specialist (for suspected IBS, a gastroenterologist). In addition, the extent and complexity of the examination will depend on the nature of your symptoms and whether this is your first visit or a follow-up visit.

The physical exam is important for many reasons. It is a critical part of the search for the cause of your symptoms; it can determine that another condition, not IBS, is causing your problems. For example, patients who have celiac disease may also have diarrhea and bloating, but a careful physical examination may reveal evidence of anemia and characteristic skin lesions, often seen in people who have a wheat allergy but not in people who have IBS. Patients who have inflammatory bowel disease (IBD) will exhibit symptoms of abdominal pain and diarrhea, just like those who have IBS, but will often reveal characteristic changes in the mouth, skin, eyes, or skeletal system that people who have IBS do not have. Also, people can have more than one disease at the same time. Although a single unifying diagnosis would be easier for both doctor and patient, it is not uncommon for patients to have several ongoing processes at once. Thus, a physical examination for symptoms of IBS may uncover a malignant skin lesion or an enlarged lymph node that otherwise would have gone unrecognized. Even if a patient has been diagnosed with IBS in the past, a repeat examination is important to verify the response to treatment and to see whether or not new problems have developed.

The physical examination of patients being evaluated for IBS is safe, and many people find a careful exam by an experienced doctor reassuring. Your doctor will probably examine your head and neck first, inspect your mouth, and then focus on your heart, lungs, skin, extremities (arms and legs), and nervous system. The nervous system is assessed by checking your reflexes and determining whether you can feel different sensations, such as pressure, in your extremities. Most doctors, especially gastroenterologists, will center their examination on the abdomen. This is appropriate, because all of the symptoms of IBS are related to the abdomen. The initial part of the examination begins with the doctor simply looking at your abdomen. This is done to check for scars, to check for asymmetry (generally the abdomen is fairly symmetrical, meaning that the left and the right side look alike; if it is asymmetrical it could indicate some underlying problem), and to look for evidence of obvious structural problems such as a mass or tumor. Then, putting a stethoscope to your abdomen, the doctor will listen for the normal sounds associated with peristalsis in the intestinal tract. These sounds will reveal if there is an obstruction of the intestinal tract. The doctor will also be able to hear the blood pulsating through some of the arteries in your abdominal cavity; if partially blocked, these arteries sound very different from arteries that are wide open.

The doctor will then "palpate" the abdomen, gently pressing with her or his hands. Palpation may reveal some tenderness or firmness, especially in the left lower quadrant over the sigmoid colon. (The anatomy of the GI tract is discussed in Chapter 6.) Stool is often present in the sigmoid colon, in patients who have and do not have IBS, and this can usually be felt. Patients who have IBS often have spasms in the sigmoid colon, which may account for tenderness. If the examination is very painful, or if the doctor finds evidence of an enlarged liver or spleen or evidence of fluid in the abdominal cavity (ascites), then further investigation will be called for, since these findings are not compatible with the diagnosis of IBS and will need to be explained. The doctor may tap on ("percuss") your abdomen, listening for different sounds. This gives information about the size of organs and whether the area under the skin is hollow, solid, or fluid filled.

Although not the most popular part of the examination for patients, a rectal exam should be performed at the initial office visit (unless recently performed by another doctor and completely normal). This part of the exam is important because it can detect a variety of medical problems that have symptoms that mimic those of IBS. Most doctors perform this part of the examination with the patient lying on his or her left side (on the left hip and shoulder) with both knees partially drawn up toward the chest. This allows the doctor to get a clear look at the area around the anus (the muscular area at the end of the rectum [see Chapter 6]). Some doctors prefer to perform this examination with the patient on the right side or standing up. During the rectal examination, hemorrhoids (dilated blood vessels) may be seen; these are especially likely in patients who strain significantly during bowel movements. Fissures, or small tears, may be seen, which might indicate the passage of hard stool or an alternative diagnosis, such as Crohn's disease, a form of inflammatory bowel disease. The presence of an anal fissure may explain a history of rectal bleeding, especially in patients who have constipation and straining. The doctor may test sensation in the anal area and check to see if reflexes are normal in this area. With a lubricated, gloved finger, the doctor will check the anal canal and the rectum for signs of bleeding, internal hemorrhoids, a blockage from impacted stool, a stricture (narrowing), or a mass. Patients who have IBS often have some tenderness in the rectum, due to visceral hypersensitivity and muscular spasms. Significant tenderness, evidence of a mass, or the presence of blood in the rectum warrants further investigation.

Appropriate Diagnostic Tests

The third component of the initial office visit involves diagnostic tests. Most people who have IBS do *not* need extensive laboratory, radiological, or invasive testing. In the past, patients were often subjected to multiple diagnostic studies in an attempt to find out why they were suffering from abdominal pain, bloating, and constipation. It was not unusual for a patient who has IBS to have undergone a whole series of tests, only to be told that everything was normal and that nothing was wrong. These studies often included blood tests, x-rays of the abdomen and chest, an ultrasound of the gall bladder, an x-ray of the small intestine, a CT scan of the abdomen and pelvis, a barium enema or colonoscopy, and an upper GI series or upper endoscopy. That these tests usually all had normal results confirms what we now know, that IBS is a functional disorder of the gut and is not caused by an organic lesion or structural problem in the GI tract.

Our greater understanding of IBS has led to a dramatic change in the way doctors evaluate patients for this condition. We now realize that extensive testing rarely turns up a cause of patients' chronic symptoms of abdominal pain, bloating, constipation, or diarrhea. Several studies have shown that extensive testing of all patients who have IBS rarely provides a new diagnosis or uncovers a different medical problem.

We generally recommend a few simple tests as part of the initial evaluation of a patient with symptoms of IBS (as long as the studies have not recently been performed elsewhere). These tests include simple laboratory tests, many of which can be done with a single blood sample, such as red and white blood cell counts and tests to measure blood sugar, kidney function, and electrolytes in the blood. For patients who have severe symptoms of constipation, blood testing for thyroid disorders is reasonable, and for patients who have persistent diarrhea, checking the erythrocyte sedimentation rate (ESR) is a simple way to look for evidence of inflammation in the body (an abnormal ESR will be seen in patients who have IBD but not in those who have IBS). In addition, patients who have persistent diarrhea will be asked to collect stool samples with a simple specially designed kit. These samples will be checked for white blood cells (fecal leukocytes). If that test is positive, the stool samples should be sent for further tests, to check for the presence of bacteria or parasites that might explain the diarrhea. (People who have persistent diarrhea who do not respond to standard IBS therapy should have their blood tested for celiac disease, because celiac disease can occasionally mimic IBS.)

When patients have symptoms that are severe enough or confusing enough, or if symptoms fail to respond to what is thought to be appropriate treatment, the doctor will want to have a look inside the intestinal tract. Direct visual examination can be performed using either a flexible sigmoidoscope or a colonoscope (see Chapter 8). Both of these devices are lighted tubes with a miniature camera attached.

Putting It All Together

During the initial office visit, your doctor will be generating what is called a "differential diagnosis," a list of medical conditions that could account for your symptoms. One reason for preparing for the initial visit and giving your doctor as much information as possible is that the list of disorders that can cause symptoms of abdominal pain and altered bowel habits is long. Table 7.3 provides just some of these possibilities. As the interview progresses and the physical examination is performed, the doctor is able to narrow the list because of the presence or absence of certain information and findings. In the case of a patient who has IBS, when the interview establishes the chronic nature of the symptoms and the physical examination appears to rule out organic disease, the differential diagnosis narrows considerably. In most cases, given enough information, the diagnosis of IBS can be made at the time of the first office visit.

Table 7.3. A Brief Differential Diagnosis of IBS Symptoms

Inflammatory bowel disease	
Crohn's disease	Ulcerative colitis
Microscopic colitis	
Collagenous colitis	Lymphocytic colitis
Malabsorption	
Celiac disease	Small intestine bacterial overgrowth
Tropical sprue	Lymphoma
Pancreatic insufficiency	Amyloidosis
Lactose, fructose, or gluten intolerance	
Food sensitivities	
Food allergies	
Urologic sources of pain	
Kidney stones (nephrolithiasis)	Prostatitis
Interstitial cystitis	
Gynecologic sources of pain	
Ovarian cysts	Uterine fibroids
Endometriosis	Pelvic inflammatory disease
Interstitial cystitis	
Other disorders	
Colonic inertia	Mastocytosis
Viral gastroenteritis	HIV enteropathy
Diabetic diarrhea	Whipple's disease
Intestinal ischemia	Eosinophilic enteritis
Cancer	Pelvic floor dysfunction

Early diagnosis of IBS is an important goal, because it allows appropriate treatment to begin right away and minimizes expensive, time-consuming, and sometimes risky testing. In several good research studies, patients diagnosed with IBS based on a normal physical examination and a predefined definition of IBS were followed for several years. In these studies, the accuracy of the diagnosis was more than 97 percent. In one study, patients were followed for nearly 30 years, and the initial diagnosis of IBS remained accurate during that long follow-up period. The high accuracy of making a diagnosis resulting from a simple definition and a careful history and physical examination should be reassuring to people who think they may have IBS. Although this combination of definition, history, and examination for diagnosis is not perfect, in the few cases where a patient had not been correctly diagnosed with IBS, nothing serious was missed, such as colon cancer or inflammatory bowel disease. These results support our contention that IBS can be safely, efficiently, and accurately diagnosed in the office.

Summary

- The average patient who has IBS sees three different doctors during three years before the diagnosis of IBS is made.
- IBS can be accurately diagnosed by using a formal definition of IBS (the Rome criteria), taking a careful medical history, performing a thorough physical examination, and using selected diagnostic tests, as appropriate.
- IBS cannot be diagnosed by a CT scan, an ultrasound, or a colonoscopy. Because IBS is a *functional* bowel disorder, the GI tract may look normal but not function normally.
- For patients who have IBS with chronic symptoms, repeated testing is seldom helpful and rarely leads to a change in diagnosis or treatment.

CHAPTER 8

Diagnostic Tests and What They Mean

A diagnosis of irritable bowel syndrome can be made by any of several types of medical practitioners and with fewer or more tests, depending on what symptoms the person is experiencing. Some patients are diagnosed with IBS by their primary care provider after a careful history is taken, the symptoms are reviewed, and a physical examination is performed and doesn't reveal another cause for the symptoms, as described in Chapter 7. Other patients are diagnosed with IBS only after they have been referred to a specialist for evaluation. Typically, that specialist is a gastroenterologist: a physician who, after finishing four years of medical or osteopathy school, undertakes a three-year training program in internal medicine and then completes an additional three or four years of specialized training in gastroenterology, the study of the digestive tract and the internal organs associated with digestion. Gastroenterologists are well versed in treating people who have IBS.

During the evaluation of a patient who has IBS, doctors and other practitioners sometimes perform diagnostic studies or tests. These tests may be done because information gleaned from either the patient's history or the physical examination makes the physician suspect that there may be another condition causing the symptoms. For example, a middle-aged woman who has symptoms of IBS and constipation and states that she feels cold all the time and that she has noticed a change in her voice may have a thyroid disorder. A patient who has abdominal discomfort and diarrhea may indeed have IBS, but these symptoms could also be signs of an infection in the colon. In this situation, the provider would request that samples of stool be collected and analyzed to check for an infection.

In the evaluation of a patient who has symptoms of IBS, some tests are fairly simple, such as having a sample of blood drawn for blood tests. Others are a little more complicated, such as getting a CT scan of your abdomen. Some tests are more invasive, such as flexible sigmoidoscopy or colonoscopy. Occasionally, patients will have persistent symptoms that fail to respond to dietary interventions or medical therapy. Such patients are referred to large hospitals or academic medical centers for sophisticated tests that might include anorectal manometry and defecography (video or magnetic resonance).

It is surprising to many people that experts in the field still disagree quite a bit about what tests should be used in the evaluation of a patient who has IBS symptoms. Some doctors believe that no tests are required for a young person who has classic symptoms of IBS, as long as the history and physical examination are completely normal and the warning signs ("red flags") of more serious diseases with similar symptoms have been carefully looked for. Other doctors believe that all patients should have certain simple tests to exclude other conditions, that is, to make sure that another problem is not masquerading as IBS. These tests would probably include some simple blood tests and either flexible sigmoidoscopy or colonoscopy. Another approach is to go ahead and begin treatment if a patient has classic symptoms of IBS and no warning signs of other conditions and to have tests done only if the patient does not improve with treatment. Finally, some doctors believe that IBS is a "diagnosis of exclusion," that it can only be diagnosed after other possible causes have been eliminated with a battery of tests, all producing normal results.

Several studies have looked at the value of performing certain laboratory or diagnostic studies in the evaluation of patients who have IBS symptoms. In one study, when more than 1,400 people with symptoms of IBS underwent laboratory tests and diagnostic studies, the rate of significant medical problems was the same in the people who had IBS symptoms and in the control (or comparison) group of healthy volunteers who did not have IBS symptoms. More specifically, when the group with IBS symptoms had blood work done to look for anemia ("low blood count"), infection, thyroid disease, or evidence of inflammation in the body, all of their tests were as normal as the group of healthy volunteers. Furthermore, when the patients who had IBS symptoms were given specialized tests for lactose intolerance and a problem in the colon, once again the results were no different from the healthy volunteers. Thus, if people who have IBS symptoms keep coming up with the same test results as people who do not have those symptoms, one wonders how useful it is to put the patient through the trouble and expense of the tests. A recently published study from several major medical centers in the U.S. confirmed these results and also found that celiac disease was not more prevalent in people who had IBS than in people who were undergoing routine screening colonoscopy. There are currently no firm guidelines about which tests need to be routinely performed in the course of evaluating patients who have symptoms of IBS. For this reason, I'll review some of the most commonly recommended tests that your health care provider may discuss with you (Table 8.1). My own recommendations are given at the end of the chapter. Below we look in some detail at each of the tests mentioned above.

Laboratory Tests

The tests described below are all performed by having a blood sample drawn, which may be done in an outpatient laboratory or clinic or by your doctor or another practitioner in the doctor's office.

Complete Blood Count (CBC)

A complete blood count, usually called a CBC, measures many items of interest. The two items of most significance in the diagnosis of IBS are your red blood cell count, to see if you are anemic, and your white blood

Table 8.1. Tests Frequently Used in the Evaluation of Patients Who Have IBS Symptoms

---

Noninvasive tests
    Blood tests: CBC, electrolytes, ESR, TSH, LFTs
    Stool tests: fecal occult blood, stool cultures, O&P
    X-ray tests: UGI series, barium enema, sitz marker study, CT scan
Invasive tests
    Endoscopy: sigmoidoscopy, colonoscopy

---

cell count, looking for evidence of an infection. White blood cells help you fight an infection when it has gotten into your body. A normal white cell count ranges from 3,500 to 10,000 (commonly abbreviated as "3.5–10") white blood cells per microliter (one millionth of a liter) of blood. If you have an infection, your white blood cell count (WBC) is typically elevated. With IBS the WBC should be normal, since the GI tract is not infected, unless you have an elevated WBC as the result of another problem occurring at the same time. Thus, in a person with abdominal pain and diarrhea, an elevated WBC may indicate that the symptoms are being caused not by IBS but rather by another ailment, such as inflammatory bowel disease (IBD) or a bacterial infection in the colon.

The other important piece of information to look for in a CBC is whether or not you are anemic. Anemia refers to a low red blood cell count. This is determined by checking the hemoglobin (abbreviated Hgb) and hematocrit (Hct). Hemoglobin is a protein found in red blood cells; it chemically binds to oxygen and carries the oxygen through your bloodstream. Women typically have hemoglobin levels of 12 to 16 mg/dl (*dl* means "deciliter," about 3.4 oz), while normal hemoglobin levels in men are 14 to 18 mg/dl. Your hematocrit is the percentage of red blood cells in a sample of your blood. Hematocrit levels in women typically range from 37 to 47 percent, and in men these levels are usually slightly higher, at 42 to 54 percent. If you are anemic, your red blood cell count is typically lower than the norms described above. There are many causes for anemia, including not making enough red blood cells, losing red blood cells (by bleeding) somewhere in the body, or premature destruction of red blood cells (red blood cells typically last 120 days in the bloodstream, and new ones are constantly being made in the bone marrow). By definition, IBS does not cause anemia. Patients can certainly have IBS and be anemic for other reasons (for instance, low iron intake, poor absorption of vitamin B12, very heavy menstrual cycles, recurrent bleeding from elsewhere in the body). If anemia turned up during evaluation for IBS, it would need to be investigated.

Thyroid Stimulating Hormone (TSH)

The thyroid is a small gland in the front of the neck, shaped almost like a butterfly. It is responsible for producing thyroxine, a hormone that acts throughout the body and helps to regulate metabolism. Approximately 6 percent of people in the United States have problems with their thyroid. This percentage is not higher among people who have IBS. In some people the thyroid is overactive; these persons may feel anxious or jittery, lose weight unintentionally, notice changes in their vision, and have diarrhea. People who have an underactive thyroid may gain weight unintentionally, notice a deepening of their voice, feel sluggish or tired, and have problems with constipation. Many physicians routinely check TSH levels in patients who have chronic constipation or diarrhea, to determine whether the thyroid gland is a factor in their bowel patterns. If your level of thyroid stimulating hormone is abnormal, your doctor may refer you to a specialist called an endocrinologist.

Erythrocyte Sedimentation Rate and C-Reactive Protein

Many patients and their doctors are concerned that the symptoms of IBS, especially diarrhea, may indicate an inflammatory process in their intestinal tract. Many health care providers will therefore check the patient's erythrocyte sedimentation rate (ESR). This simple blood test is a reasonable (although not perfect) measure of inflammation and infection in the body. For the same purpose, other doctors check for C-reactive protein (CRP). It is important to note that neither of these tests reveals where the inflammation or infection is. Rather, both the ESR and the CRP simply give evidence that some portion of the body is inflamed or infected. A common cold will increase a person's ESR and CRP, as will an infected toe or an inflamed joint. Because with irritable bowel syndrome the intestinal tract is not chronically inflamed or infected, patients who have IBS should have normal ESR and CRP levels, unless there is inflammation or infection present from another cause. If either of these levels is high, your doctor may need to order other laboratory tests or schedule special studies to help find out why.

Electrolytes and Kidney Function Tests

Electrolytes are salts (sodium, potassium, and chloride) in your blood. Kidney function tests (blood urea nitrogen [BUN] and creatinine) measure how well your kidneys work—how well they filter your blood of toxins and whether they can produce urine normally. These two types of tests should be normal in patients who have IBS. Some doctors routinely order these tests, while other doctors use them only for people who have recurrent or prolonged diarrhea, to make sure that the patient is not becoming dehydrated. Again, patients can have IBS and also abnormal kidney function and abnormal electrolytes, but IBS by itself should not affect these levels.

Liver Function Tests (LFTs)

The term *liver function tests* refers to several separate blood tests, usually performed as a group, that measure the level of specific enzymes within the liver. Enzymes are chemicals that speed up chemical reactions within the body. Their presence in the blood increases if there is an infectious or inflammatory process in the liver, such as hepatitis, or there is obstruction of the ducts draining the liver, as with gallstones. The liver is not associated with IBS in any way. However, some patients who have IBS have abdominal pain or discomfort in the upper abdomen near the liver. For that reason, many providers check LFTs to make sure that the abdominal pain or discomfort does not reflect some underlying problem in the liver. If these tests show elevated enzyme levels, your doctor may schedule a special x-ray study of your liver (either an ultrasound or a CT scan) and may refer you to a specialist in liver disorders, a hepatologist.

Stool Studies

Three stool studies are commonly ordered by doctors during the evaluation of a patient who has altered bowel habits and abdominal pain. The first is a stool heme-occult test. The second is a group of studies that look for an infection in the colon. The third test is a specialized test for evidence of inflammation in the colon.

The heme-occult test is a simple test used to look for nonvisible (occult) blood (heme) in the stool. This test can be performed in your doctor's office, or your doctor may give you specially treated cards so you can perform this test at home. Testing for occult blood in the stool is often routinely done for patients over age 50 as a "screening" test for colorectal cancer. (A screening test is one that detects a medical problem early on in its course, so that it can be quickly treated to prevent a more serious condition from developing.) People who have persistent diarrhea are often tested for occult blood, because the diarrhea may indicate an inflammatory condition, such as Crohn's disease, that could cause the person to slowly lose blood. Heme-occults are also frequently performed for patients who have abdominal pain and constipation, because of the concern that the constipation is a sign of cancer of the colon or rectum. People who have cancer of the colon often become anemic because the growing cancer may slowly bleed. The blood shows up in the stool, giving a positive ("positive" in medical terms means that the substance being looked for is present, not that the result is good) heme-occult result.

The advantages of the heme-occult test are its simplicity, ease, safety, and low cost. The major disadvantage is that it is not very accurate. The test may give misleading results. It may show that blood is present even though no disease is there. On the other hand, the test may be negative—not showing the presence of blood—when there actually is a problem. In a variety of disorders of the colon (a polyp, an early cancer, inflammation) bleeding can be intermittent (come and go). Thus, on the day the stool sample is checked, the test may be negative (that is, no blood is present) if there has been no recent bleeding, but on another day it would be positive. Because heme-occult tests can miss serious disorders such as colon cancer, nearly all gastroenterologists recommend that everyone over the age of 50 undergo a screening colonoscopy to look for cancer of the colon or rectum. Due to an increased risk of colon cancer in African Americans, gastroenterologists now recommend that routine colon cancer screening start at age 45 for African Americans.

If there is evidence of blood in your stool, your doctor will probably suggest that you get a complete blood count, if one hasn't recently been performed. In addition, he or she will probably advise that you have either a flexible sigmoidoscopy or, in most cases, a colonoscopy (both described below).

The second most commonly ordered stool study is a panel of tests designed to look for evidence of an infection in the colon. If you have persistent diarrhea, your doctor may recommend that samples of stool be collected and sent to a laboratory to be tested for evidence of an infection. One test determines if there are fecal leukocytes in the stool. Leukocytes are white blood cells. People who have an infection or inflammatory process in the colon generally have a large number of white blood cells (fecal leukocytes) in their stool. If this test is normal (that is, no white blood cells are seen), then your doctor may not need to order any more stool studies, as it is very unlikely that you have an inflammatory or infectious condition in your colon. Patients who have IBS and diarrhea normally do not have fecal leukocytes in their stool, while with patients who have Crohn's disease, ulcerative colitis, or some kind of infection in their colon, large numbers are generally found in the stool. If your stool studies return showing that you have a high number of fecal leukocytes, your doctor may order additional stool studies, looking for common infections of the colon (*Salmonella*, *Shigella*, *Campylobacter*, *Yersinia*, and *Clostridium difficile*) or the presence of parasites (the O&P test, meaning "ova and parasites"). Giardiasis is a common parasitic infection (caused by *Giardia*) that can produce symptoms of abdominal discomfort and diarrhea that mimic the symptoms of IBS.

A new and, as yet, seldom performed study tests for lactoferrin in the stool of patients who have chronic diarrhea. This chemical is found much more commonly in the stool of people with an inflamed colon than in healthy people or patients who have IBS, so its presence could signal either inflammatory bowel disease or an infection.

Endoscopy

Endoscopy refers to any type of procedure that uses a thin, flexible, lighted tube to view the inside of the gastrointestinal tract. These tubes, called endoscopes (more specifically, sigmoidoscopes and colonoscopes), have both a light and a miniature video camera inside. In addition, endoscopes have thin channels that permit the passage of tiny forceps, with which the operator can take samples of tissue (biopsies) to be tested in a laboratory, if necessary.

In an upper endoscopy, the upper GI tract (esophagus, stomach, and duodenum) is examined using an endoscope. Endoscopies of the lower GI tract examine the colon and anorectal area. Patients who have IBS and either diarrhea or constipation are often referred to a gastroenterologist or a surgeon for endoscopy of the lower GI tract, either a sigmoidoscopy, which looks at the anorectal area, sigmoid colon, and descending colon, or a colonoscopy, which extends the examination to the full length of the colon. Both tests are usually performed in an outpatient setting; they can be done in a hospital, but they do not require an overnight stay. Both examinations are designed to allow your doctor to look directly at the lining of your lower intestine and rectum. They can be used to search for sources of bleeding, for evidence of an obstruction or blockage, or for the presence of diverticuli (abnormal pockets or pouches in the intestine), polyps, and cancerous tissue. These examinations are very helpful in revealing the presence of either an infection or inflammatory bowel disease. During endoscopy, the lining of the intestinal tract is clearly seen and can be carefully inspected. Photographs can be taken, either to document a problem or to provide a baseline so that a subsequent test can be compared to the conditions during the first test. If necessary, biopsies can be taken and polyps can be removed.

For both sigmoidoscopy and colonoscopy you need to prepare by taking medications or solutions to "clean out" the colon. This preparation is usually done the day before the test. With some methods of preparation, you may also be asked to consume only clear liquids for one or two days before the test or to work your way down in steps from solid food to clear liquids during a period of two to three days.

On the day of the exam, you will need to arrive an hour or two before the test. A nurse will check you in, and the physician performing the test, if it is not your own gastroenterologist, may take a brief history and do a limited physical examination. The endoscopy is usually performed in a special room. You will lie on your left side (on your left shoulder and left hip) with your right knee partially bent and brought toward your chest. The physician will perform a digital rectal examination before beginning to insert the endoscope.

Flexible Sigmoidoscopy

Sigmoidoscopy uses a shorter endoscope than colonoscopy. Because of that, the examination is limited to the lower colon and rectum, which includes the anal canal, the rectum, the sigmoid colon, and the descending colon (see Figure 8.1). On some occasions, depending on the patient's anatomy and level of comfort, the endoscope can be advanced past the splenic flexure and into the transverse colon, although this does not rou-

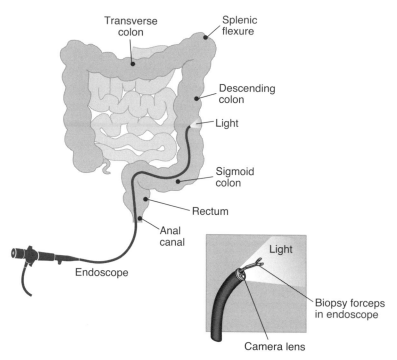

Figure 8.1. Flexible Sigmoidoscopy
Flexible sigmoidoscopy is performed to allow the doctor to see the lining of the lower gastrointestinal tract. The sigmoidoscope is a soft, flexible, lighted tube that is inserted through the anal canal and rectum and carefully advanced through the sigmoid colon and descending colon. Under ideal conditions, the sigmoidoscope can be advanced to the splenic flexure. This test is usually performed in an outpatient setting. If necessary, biopsies can be taken and polyps can be removed with tiny forceps inserted through the end of the sigmoidoscope. Reasons for having this test include rectal bleeding, rectal pain, chronic diarrhea, and lower abdominal pain thought to arise in the GI tract.

tinely occur. The test generally takes anywhere from 5 to 20 minutes, depending on the patient's anatomy, the patient's comfort, and whether or not biopsies need to be taken or polyps need to be removed. In contrast to colonoscopy (described below), flexible sigmoidoscopy is usually performed without sedation. This means that there is very little recovery time after the procedure; most patients can resume their regular activities, including driving a car, immediately afterward. Not using sedation also decreases the risks associated with the procedure.

Flexible sigmoidoscopy begins with the patient lying on her or his left side, with the right knee drawn up toward the chest. As described above, a rectal examination is performed first. During this initial part of the examination, you may have the feeling that you need to have a bowel movement. This is a normal sensation that occurs due to stimulation of nerves in the rectum. The sigmoidoscope is then gently inserted and carefully advanced to its fullest extent—usually the upper portion of the descending colon, near the splenic flexure. The sigmoidoscope is then slowly withdrawn, and the physician carefully watches the images of the colon displayed on a large video screen. In most endoscopy procedure rooms, the patient is also able to watch these images if he or she desires.

During this part of the procedure, the endoscopist may need to add a little air to your colon, a process called insufflation, because the colon, being empty, is typically collapsed. Inserting air into the colon enables the physician to better visualize its lining. You may feel some pressure in your abdomen when the air is introduced and may have some mild abdominal discomfort or cramps as the scope goes around a curve or bend in your colon, but most patients tolerate flexible sigmoidoscopy quite well. Although the air is removed at the end of the procedure as completely as possible, some patients feel a little bloated or gassy after the test. Some patients feel mild abdominal discomfort, which is usually caused by a spasm of the smooth muscle that makes up the lining of the colon. This spasm can occur in response to stretching of the colon, either by the air that is placed into the colon or by the endoscope. These sensations are unpleasant for some patients, but they rarely mean that anything significant is happening.

At the end of the procedure, which on average takes about 10 minutes, you can get dressed, and a nurse will check you before you leave. The doctor will be able to share the results of the visual examination with you right away, but if biopsies were taken or polyps removed, the pathology test results will take 5 to 10 days. No special diet is required after flexible sigmoidoscopy; you can return to your regular diet following completion of the test.

Colonoscopy

Because colonoscopy uses a much longer endoscope compared to flexible sigmoidoscopy, the entire colon can be carefully examined (see Figure 8.2). Often, we can even see the end of the small intestine (terminal ileum) and the area where the small intestine and colon connect (ileocecal valve), areas that are important if your doctor is concerned that you might have inflammatory bowel disease.

Another advantage of colonoscopy is that it is generally performed using mild sedation. This means that most patients either sleep through the exam or are partially awake but relaxed and quite comfortable. During "conscious sedation," you breathe on your own, and your vital signs (blood pressure, heart rate, oxygen content of your blood, respiratory rate) are constantly measured. Conscious sedation is considered very safe; it is quite different from general anesthesia, in which the patient is connected to a ventilator (breathing machine), sleeps deeply, and takes a long time to recover from the sedation.

Colonoscopy is considered the most effective screening test for colorectal cancer and is recommended for *everyone* over the age of 50 (although, as noted above, screening colonoscopies should start at age 45 in African Americans). Compared to sigmoidoscopy, the preparation is usually a little longer and somewhat more involved. In addition, due to the use of sedation, recovery time is longer, and you will not be allowed to drive until the following day. You will not be able to go to school or work after the test, because your thinking might be foggy from the sedation and your legs might be a little wobbly. Finally, because the test examines your entire colon, the risk of having a complication is slightly greater than in sigmoidoscopy.

Colonoscopy begins just like flexible sigmoidoscopy, with one major exception. Prior to the test, an intravenous (i.v.) catheter will be inserted into a vein in one of your arms. This is a thin needle connected to plastic tubing so that medications can be administered during your examination.

As with flexible sigmoidoscopy, the colonoscope is gently inserted and advanced, this time through the entire colon. If your doctor is concerned about the possibility of IBD (Crohn's disease or ulcerative colitis), then

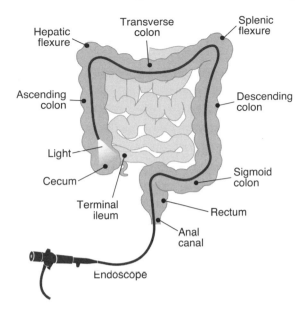

Figure 8.2. Colonoscopy
The colonoscope is just like the sigmoidoscope (see Figure 8.1), only longer. It enables viewing of the entire colon. Colonoscopy is usually performed using "conscious sedation," since the test takes longer and is more uncomfortable for some patients than sigmoidoscopy. As with sigmoidoscopy, if necessary, biopsies can be taken and polyps removed during the exam.

he or she will also inspect the lower small intestine (the terminal ileum). As the colonoscope is slowly withdrawn, the physician will likely need to add some air to the colon, as described above, to make sure that she or he can get a good look at the lining of the colon. If necessary, biopsies can be taken or polyps removed.

The doctor is able to learn a great deal by visual examination of the entire colon, and he or she will probably mention the findings to you after you are awake; but because you may be groggy from the sedation, a follow-up visit or phone conversation may be scheduled. If biopsies were taken, the pathology report on them will not be available for 5 to 10 days, and your doctor will review those results with you then.

Risks

Both of these examinations are considered very safe, and in the overwhelming majority of cases, the benefits far outweigh the possible risks. However, some minor reactions or side effects can occur with either test, such as irritation of the colon, nausea or vomiting shortly after the exam, or a persistent feeling of being bloated or gassy due to the introduction of air into the colon. As with any medical procedure, there is the possibility that some more serious unintended consequence could occur. The colon could bleed significantly, although this is usually a possibility only if a large polyp is removed during the procedure.

Perforation, where a hole is inadvertently made through the wall of the colon, although a real possibility, is very uncommon. It occurs in less than 1 in 3,000 procedures. If a perforation occurs, it can often be safely managed by admitting the patient to the hospital, giving intravenous fluids and antibiotics, and letting the bowel rest and repair itself.

Colonoscopy carries risks that are due to the use of sedation. The medications used to aid relaxation during the procedure can result in deeper sedation than expected, necessitating a longer recovery time, possibly admission to the hospital, the use of medications to "reverse" the sedating medications, or, very rarely, use of a ventilator to assist breathing.

Radiologic Studies

CT Scan of the Abdomen

Computed tomography (CT) scans use a small amount of radiation from a special scanner, combined with sophisticated computer software, to provide precise cross-sectional images of the body. This imaging technique is often performed for patients who have chronic abdominal pain, to look for problems that can't be detected using blood tests and to look in places inside the body that can't be viewed by endoscopy (upper endoscopy or colonoscopy). Usually, patients drink a special liquid before the test (called oral contrast) that coats the intestinal tract. A second type of contrast agent is usually injected through an intravenous (i.v.) catheter into a vein in your arm (intravenous contrast). These two different contrast agents enable the physician reading the study (a radiologist) to clearly identify the GI tract and the surrounding blood vessels (arteries and veins). Although this is a noninvasive test, use of the second contrast agent requires that an i.v. line be placed, which some patients find uncomfortable. The test typically takes three hours, which includes the time needed to drink the contrast and to have the i.v. catheter put in. No sedation is used during a CT scan. The results are usually available within 24 hours.

Upper GI Series

This examination allows evaluation of the structure, and provides some information regarding the function, of the upper gastrointestinal tract (esophagus, stomach, pylorus, and duodenum). It is usually performed in the morning after an overnight fast (no food or fluid after midnight). Patients swallow approximately 2 cups (16 oz.) of an oral contrast, usually a barium solution. (Barium is an inert [nonreactive], chalky white substance that shows up vividly on x-ray images.) The barium solution coats the lining of the GI tract, and then x-ray pictures are taken over the next 30 to 45 minutes. On some occasions, the x-ray pictures are taken during a longer period of time, 2 to 3 hours. This longer time period allows the contrast solution to pass all the way through your small intestine, so that images can be made of this area as well (this test is called an upper GI series with small bowel follow-through).

This test is noninvasive, does not require an intravenously injected contrast agent or any sedation, and is safe. It can provide significant amounts of information about the anatomy and structure of the upper GI tract. Your doctor may order this test if she or he is concerned that you have an ulcer or blockage of the GI tract. Results of this test are generally available within 24 hours.

Sitz Marker Study

This test measures how long it takes for material to move through the colon. As such, it is an indirect measure of colonic transit time and colonic motility. It may be requested for patients who have constipation, especially those who are not responding to treatment. Patients swallow a gelatin capsule that contains 24 small, spherical, radio-opaque markers.

Because these markers are radio-opaque, they show up on x-ray images (this test may also be called a "radio-opaque marker study"). These tiny markers do not dissolve in your gastrointestinal tract but are transported from the stomach to the small intestine and into the colon by peristalsis. They are normally evacuated along with stool anywhere from 1 to 5 days after being swallowed. We recommend that the capsule be taken on a Sunday morning. You then go to the radiology department 1, 3, and 5 days later for a simple abdominal x-ray, until the markers have been evacuated. These x-rays should be taken at approximately the same time of day that the capsule was swallowed. The location and the number of the markers are noted on each of the days, and this provides a good estimate of how fast, or how slowly, contents move through your colon and sometimes can show where they slow down or get hung up. Normally, at least 20 of the 24 markers are eliminated from the colon by the fifth day.

Overall, this is a very safe and easy test. Disadvantages include that you have several x-rays taken of your abdomen, which means that you receive a small amount of radiation each time. However, this amount of radiation is generally considered safe. If you live a long distance from a radiology clinic, the repeated visits can be inconvenient, but patients usually find the effort worthwhile. No sedation is needed for this test. Results of this study are typically available to the ordering physician within 24 hours after the last x-ray is taken.

Other Tests

Ultrasound of the Abdomen and Pelvis

Ultrasound imaging uses sound waves, organized by a computer, to create pictures of internal organs. A small device, approximately the size of a hand-held microphone, is placed on your skin over the area to be scanned. Sound waves are then transmitted through the skin and a recording is made as these sound waves are reflected by the organs. Ultrasound can produce a three-dimensional picture of the liver, gallbladder, pancreas, kidneys, uterus, and ovaries. These pictures can reveal the size and shape of each organ and can show the presence of an obstruction, cysts (fluid-filled pockets), or a solid mass, such as a tumor.

The advantages of ultrasound include that it is noninvasive, very safe, does not expose the patient to any radiation, and does not require sedation. It may require drinking large amounts of water and not going to the bathroom for a couple of hours, which can be uncomfortable for some people. Unfortunately, it cannot measure the function of an organ and it is not that helpful in evaluating the structure of the gastrointestinal tract. Results of ultrasound imaging are usually available within 24 hours.

Hydrogen Breath Test

People with bloating and gassiness occasionally have a medical condition that prevents them from properly digesting certain types of food, most commonly the sugars lactose and fructose. In an unusual condition that can also cause chronic gassiness, too many bacteria exist in the upper gastrointestinal tract. Although the colon is loaded with bacteria, there should be only a very small amount of bacteria in the small intestine. If you are having trouble digesting certain types of sugars, or if your doctor is concerned that you may have bacterial overgrowth, then a hydrogen breath test may be recommended (see Chapter 11).

This safe and easy test is usually performed in the morning after an overnight fast. Patients drink a small amount of a sugary liquid (lactulose, fructose, or lactose) and then blow into a special measuring device every 15 minutes during a period of about 3 to 4 hours. The amount of hydrogen in the expelled air is measured, and this can help determine whether one of the conditions noted above is the cause of the gas and bloating. The captured samples of exhaled air are sent to a laboratory for analysis. The results of the analysis are usually available within 2 to 3 days. If the results are positive, indicating that you have too many bacteria in your small intestine, your physician may decide to treat you with antibiotics.

Anorectal Manometry (ARM)

This test may be recommended for patients who have persistent severe constipation or who have experienced fecal incontinence. Fecal incontinence, the accidental leakage of stool from the rectum, may develop as a result of injury to the muscles or nerves in the pelvic floor or because of disease. Anorectal manometry is designed to evaluate muscle and nerve function in the anal canal, rectum, and pelvic floor (see Figures 6.1–6.3). It is generally available only at major medical centers and in large hospitals or clinics interested in research. Patients lie on their left side on an examining table and a small balloon attached to a tube is inserted into the anal canal and rectum. The patient is asked to contract specific muscles in the anorectal area and then relax those same muscles. This test provides an objective measure of muscle tone and strength. In addition, it can determine whether the nerves in the anorectal area are functioning normally. Anorectal manometry does not require any special preparation beforehand. The test typically takes 30 to 45 minutes, and the results are available within 3 to 4 workdays.

Defecography (Video or Magnetic Resonance)

Defecography is available at only a few specialized medical centers and university hospitals. It can help diagnose problems in the pelvic floor or in the anorectal area. It would be appropriate for a patient who has persistent and severe constipation or who has significant straining during evacuation or feelings of incomplete evacuation. In this study, thick barium paste is inserted into the rectum using a special tube. The patient then sits on a specially designed commode, and the patient is asked to evacuate the barium while x-ray pictures are taken. If an x-ray machine is used, the test is called video defecography. Physicians at some academic medical centers now perform this test in the magnetic resonance (MR) suite. The MR scanner, in contrast to a CT scan, does not use any radiation. MR defecography can provide more information about other organs in the pelvic cavity, such as the bladder, uterus, and vagina, than video defecography.

Although many patients find anorectal manometry or defecography a little embarrassing, neither test is uncomfortable. Defecography (video or MR) is excellent for diagnosing problems that may cause significant constipation and straining, such as a large rectocele (bulge in the rectal wall). Anorectal manometry is very safe; no special preparation is required beforehand, and the test typically takes 45 minutes to perform. The results are available within 1 to 2 days.

Recommendations

At the time of initial evaluation of a patient who has symptoms of IBS, the best diagnostic tool is a thorough and thoughtful history and careful physical examination. If the physical exam is normal and there are no warning signs of serious illness in the patient's history, then most clinicians can accurately and confidently diagnose IBS without routinely performing multiple diagnostic studies and tests. After the initial office visit, I generally ask that the patient have blood drawn for a CBC, a TSH (if constipated or having severe diarrhea), and an ESR (if diarrhea is present), *if* these tests have not been done recently. If these laboratory tests were recently performed by another health care provider, there is little value in repeating them unless, of course, symptoms have changed or there are warning signs from the history or physical examination. If a patient's predominant symptom is diarrhea, I also recommend stool studies for fecal leukocytes, routine bacterial cultures, and ova and parasites (O&P). Stool studies are of no value in evaluating people who have constipation.

Flexible sigmoidoscopy may need to be performed for younger patients (those younger than 40 years of age). This can be scheduled shortly after the initial evaluation for those people who have significant pain in the left lower abdomen, those who have rectal pain, and those who have significant diarrhea where there is concern that the patient may have IBD rather than IBS. Alternatively, sigmoidoscopy can be reserved until after the follow-up visit four to six weeks later and ordered only for those who have not improved with treatment.

For patients 50 years of age and older, the same laboratory tests (CBC, ESR, TSH) noted above should be planned, if not recently performed. However, given the high prevalence of colorectal cancer in the United States, a full colonoscopy should be performed on all patients in this age group. Several research studies have shown that *routinely* performing abdominal ultrasounds, upper endoscopies, breath hydrogen tests, or CT scans in all people who have IBS does not improve the diagnosis of patients who have IBS, nor does it improve their treatment. Other research studies have shown that when a clinician performs a thorough history and physical examination, and no warning signs are present, the diagnosis of IBS can accurately be made 95 percent to 97 percent of the time. In a long-range study, the diagnosis remained correct even 30 years later. Of course, if new symptoms develop, if warning signs appear, or if reasonable treatment does not improve the symptoms, then specialized testing may be required. For this reason, regular and routine office visits with a primary care physician are helpful and important.

Summary

- Most patients who have IBS can be safely and confidently diagnosed using standardized criteria (the Rome criteria) along with a careful and thorough patient history and physical examination. Many tests are not usually necessary.
- Because many of the symptoms of IBS are not specific to a single disease, many physicians routinely seek only basic laboratory tests (CBC, TSH, ESR) to ensure that an infectious or inflammatory process is not present.
- Stool studies are commonly ordered for patients who have IBS symptoms and diarrhea; they are of little or no value for people who have constipation.
- Specialized testing may prove useful in some patients who have IBS who have persistent symptoms despite dietary interventions and medical therapy. Which tests are appropriate will depend on the symptoms being manifested and their severity. These tests might include anorectal manometry and defecography (for patients with constipation).
- Colonoscopy should be performed in *everyone* over the age of 50 (and starting at age 45 for African Americans).

CHAPTER 9

IBS and Other Medical Disorders

Dozens of research studies have shown that people who have irritable bowel syndrome see doctors more frequently than do people who have other chronic medical problems. In fact, a person who has IBS is twice as likely to seek the advice of a doctor than a person who has other chronic medical problems. Given the recurrent symptoms of abdominal pain, bloating, and either constipation or diarrhea that plague people who have IBS, it does not seem unreasonable for people who have IBS to seek the care of a physician more frequently than others do.

However, what seems surprising is that people who have IBS are much more likely to have other medical problems, not related to the gastrointestinal (GI) tract. Both patients and doctors have noticed that many people who have IBS also have a variety of other conditions that do not appear to be related to disturbances in the GI tract. The large number of medical reports and scientific studies that document an increased occurrence of other disorders in patients who have IBS raises the question of whether IBS can affect other parts of the body as well, rather than being limited to the GI tract.

As discussed in Chapter 2, many physicians think that the symptoms of IBS result from visceral hypersensitivity, that the GI tract of people who have IBS is much more sensitive than a healthy person's GI tract. Stated another way, people who have IBS have a lower threshold for experiencing gastrointestinal pain than do people who do not have IBS. In addition, some people who have IBS experience normal gut sensations and normal gut motility as painful (this subconscious misinterpretation of normal physiology as painful is called allodynia).

The symptoms of the other diseases people who have IBS seem prone to develop include fatigue, headaches, difficulty concentrating, and muscle and joint pain. Pain elsewhere in the body, not affecting the viscera—the hollow organs in the body—is generally referred to as somatic pain. That some people who have IBS have increased somatic pain in addition to the increased visceral pain typical of IBS might support the view that there is a link between IBS and bodily pain in general, a general process producing both heightened visceral pain and heightened somatic pain. Could people who have IBS also have increased sensitivity to pain, or a lower threshold for pain, elsewhere in their body? This question is important to answer because, if true, we would not limit our evaluation and treatment of IBS to just the GI tract but would expand our treatment to the entire body.

The health situation described in the following case story is not unusual among people who have IBS.

Sarah is a 34-year-old woman with a 7-year history of irritable bowel syndrome with constipation. She describes fairly typical symptoms of lower abdominal "cramps and spasms" that occur on a near-daily basis. The abdominal pain or discomfort is always worse just before having a bowel movement. Sarah also has feelings of incomplete evacuation and straining during bowel movements. She frequently feels bloated, and her abdomen is distended. She has struggled with her IBS symptoms and has seen several gastroenterologists. Over the years, all of her test results have been normal (extensive laboratory tests, an abdominal ultrasound, a barium enema, a CT scan of the abdomen and pelvis, and a colonoscopy). She has tried a number of different over-the-counter medications, but they did not improve her symptoms. Until recently, prescription medications hadn't been much help either, but her current gastroenterologist started her on a low dose of a tricyclic antidepressant for her abdominal pain and polyethylene glycol for her constipation (see Chapters 16 and 18 for a comprehensive discussion on the treatment of constipation symptoms and abdominal pain). Although the results have not been perfect, Sarah's IBS symptoms have responded very well to these drugs.

Sarah is having an initial visit with a new internist, Dr. Fine, because her health care plan changed and she was forced to find a new primary care provider. In addition to letting this doctor know about the progress in her IBS treatment, Sarah describes a variety of other symptoms she has been experiencing. She has recurrent headaches with flashing lights and develops a "stabbing" sensation behind her right eye. Her teeth and jaws are often painful and she hears a clicking noise when she chews. She always feels tired and can't seem to get enough rest. Her joints and muscles feel sore and achy, as if she had over-exercised, although she's been so tired that she hasn't been able to exercise routinely for months. Because she has a constant urge to urinate but passes only a small amount of urine on each occasion, she is concerned that she might be developing diabetes.

Dr. Fine listens carefully and asks a lot of questions. She is reassured to learn that Sarah has had all of these symptoms for nearly a year and that they are not getting worse. Sarah has not been losing weight and has not been anemic. No one in Sarah's immediate family has diabetes, celiac disease, inflammatory bowel disease, or any type of cancer. Her previous internist performed extensive blood work just two months ago, all of which produced normal results. She was recently evaluated by a neurologist, who diagnosed her with migraine headaches, which explain the pain and odd sensations in her eyes. Sarah saw her dentist several weeks ago and was told that she has TMJ (temporomandibular joint) syndrome and has been grinding her teeth and clenching her jaw at night. Her dentist recommended the use of a mouth guard at night, to protect her teeth. Sarah asks Dr. Fine if all of these symptoms are connected to her IBS.

Dr. Fine performs a thorough physical examination and finds everything completely normal. She asks Sarah to provide a urine sample to make sure that she does not have a urinary tract infection (she doesn't) or diabetes (she doesn't). Dr. Fine tells Sarah that there are some fairly common medical disorders that often go hand in hand with IBS: migraine headaches, TMJ syndrome, fibromyalgia (which causes pain at certain sites), and interstitial cystitis (a bladder condition). Sarah may have all of these conditions. In addition, Dr. Fine says that the excessive fatigue could be consistent with chronic fatigue syndrome, although Sarah hasn't had the six months of extreme fatigue that would meet the formal definition (discussed below). She questions Sarah more about her sleep and learns that she frequently wakes up and can't get back to sleep. She reassures Sarah that these symptoms are often associated with IBS and are not caused by a new and more serious disease. Dr. Fine says that sleep disorders are commonly associated with IBS, and disordered sleep can worsen IBS symptoms and also contribute to migraine headaches and feelings of fatigue. Sarah seems relieved to hear this. She and Dr. Fine then work out a treatment strategy to address her multiple symptoms.

Let's look at each of the conditions that often arise in people who have IBS. They are not always linked with IBS; not everyone who has IBS will develop any of these disorders, and people who have them will not necessarily have IBS as well.

Chronic Fatigue Syndrome

Chronic fatigue syndrome (CFS) affects approximately 1 person out of 250 (0.4 percent of the population). This is far lower than the prevalence of IBS, which affects approximately 1 in 7 adult Americans. Chronic fatigue syndrome is found in all ethnic groups, all age groups (including children), and all socioeconomic groups. It appears to be slightly more common in women than in men, in people with lower incomes, and in those with lower levels of education. Although it can occur at all ages, it is more likely to be diagnosed in people 30 to 50 years old. Why these groups seem to be more likely to have CFS is not known. Although there are many theories, the exact cause of CFS is unknown.

People who have CFS typically complain of severe, debilitating fatigue that doesn't go away, no matter how much they sleep. This level of fatigue must be present for at least six months and must have had a definite onset (that is, not lifelong) before a diagnosis of CFS can be made. It also must lead to at least a 50 percent reduction in the person's level of daily activities (social, work, school, personal). Additional symptoms include impaired concentration, difficulty sleeping, recurrent headaches, and a worsening, or relapse, of symptoms after exercise. Some patients have symptoms that mimic a viral infection, such as a sore throat, muscle aches (myalgias), joint aches (arthralgias), and a low-grade fever.

Because of the symptoms that seemed viral, many patients and physicians thought that CFS might be caused by a virus. This hypothesis seemed quite reasonable, and a few scientific studies published many years ago appeared to show that the Epstein-Barr virus (EBV), the virus that causes mononucleosis, was associated with the development of CFS. However, other studies have not been able to reproduce this result, and some have provided evidence that directly contradicts this theory. Because of this evidence, most doctors now do *not* believe that EBV causes chronic fatigue syndrome.

One current theory about the etiology (causes) of CFS involves chronic activation of the immune system. The immune system is designed to fight infections using specialized cells and chemicals. If the immune system is in "battle" mode all the time, the chronic exposure to these cells and their specialized chemicals could lead to persistent fatigue in some people. Any of the thousands of viruses that can cause an infection in humans could trigger activation of the immune system, which then persists and becomes chronic in nature. Among the viruses considered likely candidates to cause CFS are the varicella zoster virus (the chicken pox virus), cytomegalovirus (CMV), and some of the herpes viruses (such as human herpes virus 6). The low-grade immune response that develops after any of these viral infections may persist for months or even years in some people and may account for the nonspecific symptoms of CFS.

One other factor that could play a role in CFS is stress. It is well known that stress can adversely affect the immune system. One theory is that, for many people, the stress of having to cope with IBS could significantly disrupt the normal function of the immune system, thereby increasing susceptibility to other conditions and worsening a patient's overall clinical condition.

It is interesting that, as is the case with IBS, the precise etiology of CFS is unknown. Possibly, CFS develops as a result of overlapping causes, which could involve multiple organ systems, including the immune system, the endocrine system (which regulates all kinds of hormones), the musculoskeletal system, and the brain.

As with IBS, the diagnosis of CFS cannot be made if there is an underlying organic problem (for example, an *active* viral infection, a thyroid disorder, etc.). For that reason, a careful history and physical examination and some laboratory tests must be performed. The physical examination will usually yield normal results, although some people who have CFS have slightly enlarged lymph nodes in their neck, which may indicate a previous viral infection. This finding, however, is nonspecific, meaning that many different factors could lead to mild enlargement of the lymph nodes. Lab tests typically include a complete blood count, a thyroid hormone test, electrolytes, and tests to look at kidney function. Because the fatigue of this condition is persistent and severe, and because of the concern that another disease is being overlooked, doctors and patients often pursue an exhaustive workup in their attempt to uncover the cause of the debilitating fatigue. They want to rule out systemic lupus erythematosus (lupus or SLE for short), scleroderma, Lyme disease, and human immunodeficiency virus (HIV). X-ray studies, including bone x-rays and CT scans, are normally done, and it is not uncommon for patients to be referred to specialists, including rheumatologists, infectious disease specialists, psychiatrists, dieticians, and neurologists. If the cause is chronic fatigue syndrome, none of these consultations will provide another diagnosis that explains the symptoms.

The natural history of CFS is that of a chronic disorder. Some people who have CFS are quite fortunate, in that their symptoms slowly resolve with time and they can return to a normal lifestyle. Others note a gradual, slow improvement but never return to their earlier degree of health. For others, unfortunately, this condition becomes a chronic, disabling disorder. A review of current medical studies estimates that approximately 50 percent of people who develop CFS never fully recover from their symptoms. (The Patient Resources section at the back of this book provides a reference for further information.)

Since there is no known cure for CFS at present, treatment focuses on symptom management. People who have CFS are counseled to obtain adequate rest but to not sleep excessively, because excessive sleep may be harmful in the long run. They should start or continue a graded exercise program to maintain overall fitness and prevent deconditioning (deterioration of their muscles from lack of use). Patients are told to follow a healthy diet and to limit stress in their lives. Medications commonly used to treat CFS include antidepressants; as with IBS, the antidepressants may not address the disease itself but may treat the associated depression or anxiety, sleep disturbance, and the like. These medications may help people to cope with CFS. Low-dose anti-inflammatory agents are often prescribed, along with cognitive behavioral therapy (see Chapter 22). Herbal medications and immunotherapy have been touted as "cures" for CFS, although at present there is no good data to support their use in the general population of people who have CFS.

Fibromyalgia

Fibromyalgia is a condition that affects approximately 2 percent (1 in 50) of adult Americans. It is found in all age groups, races, and socioeconomic classes, but it is more common in women than in men, and the majority of those affected are women between the ages of 30 and 50. In the past, this disorder was called fibromyositis, fibrositis, and myofascial pain syndrome. Although many causes have been proposed, the precise etiology of fibromyalgia is unknown.

Typical symptoms include widespread muscle pain at specific spots called "trigger" or "tender" points, which are tender or painful when pressed (see Figure 9.1). To be formally diagnosed with fibromyalgia, a person must have symptoms of widespread pain for at least 3 months and must have tenderness or pain at 11 out of the 18 trigger points. Pain is generally present on both sides of the body and both above and below the waist. People who have fibromyalgia commonly also have other symptoms, which may include chronic headache, difficulty sleeping, and reduced physical endurance. Several studies have shown that someone who has IBS is much more likely to have fibromyalgia than a person of similar age, gender, and race who does not have IBS. In general, approximately one person out of three who has IBS will also have fibromyalgia.

Physical examination of people who have fibromyalgia reveals no irregularities except for the presence of pain at the trigger (tender) points. Laboratory studies (blood count, thyroid tests, erythrocyte sedimentation

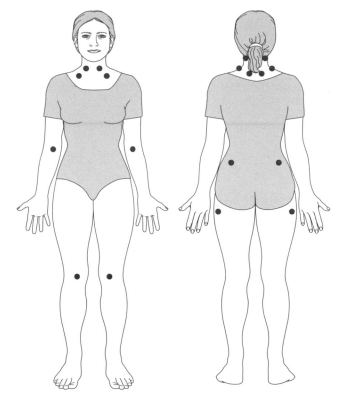

Figure 9.1. Tender Points (Trigger Points) of Fibromyalgia
People who have IBS often also have fibromyalgia. Fibromyalgia is characterized by a variety of symptoms, including muscle pain and tenderness at specific "trigger" points. There are 18 identified trigger points, which are symmetrically located on the neck, forearms, lower back, upper posterior thighs, and knees. The diagnosis of fibromyalgia is made because of tenderness at these trigger points along with the presence of other typical symptoms.

rate) are normal in these patients. X-ray studies, CT scans, and MRIs usually do not need to be performed unless the doctor believes that the patient has an inflammatory condition that affects the joints, such as rheumatoid arthritis, or an unusual connective tissue disorder such as lupus (SLE), Sjogren's syndrome, or polymyalgia rheumatica (PMR).

Treatment of fibromyalgia typically includes rest, heat, an exercise program, the use of anti-inflammatory agents, muscle relaxants, injections of local anesthetics (such as lidocaine) into the trigger point areas, and the use of antidepressants. Pregabalin has been approved by the U.S. Food and Drug Administration for the treatment of fibromyalgia, and many patients find this medication helpful.

Migraine Headaches

Most people have experienced a headache at some point in their life. Headaches are usually a benign but bothersome problem, and they can occur for many reasons. Common causes of headaches include tension (musculoskeletal headaches), eating or drinking icy-cold foods, such as ice cream (these are called ice-pick or ice-cream headaches), and sinus problems.

Migraine headaches differ in distinct ways from most other types of headache. Although symptoms vary dramatically from one person to another, common symptoms include nausea and a stabbing pain behind one eye or on one side of the head. An unusual symptom that may occur is referred to as an *aura*. An aura usually develops before the pain of the headache begins and may include the sensation of seeing flashing lights or of smelling an unusual smell, like rubber or rotten eggs. On rare occasions, the headache can produce a numbness or tingling in the face that can make people think they are having a stroke or a TIA (transient ischemic attack, also called a ministroke). Most migraine headaches last about 4 to 72 hours, and on average, people who have migraines have one or two episodes per month, although around 10 percent have weekly episodes.

Migraines occur more commonly in people who have IBS than in the general population. In the United States, over 28 million people have migraines. Migraine headaches are three times more likely to occur in women than in men. Most people who have migraines develop them during adolescence. They typically persist throughout adulthood, although many women find relief from their migraine headaches after menopause.

Why migraines occur is not completely understood. Studies of the brain using PET scans (positron emission tomography) to measure brain activity have demonstrated that there is increased activity in the brain stem during migraine headaches. In addition, the blood vessels in the brain may swell and some of the sensory nerves may be activated. Interestingly, as with IBS, serotonin may play a role in the development of migraine headaches.

Triggers that may precipitate a migraine headache include the ingestion of caffeine, alcohol (especially red wine), or food additives, such as MSG (monosodium glutamate); lack of sleep; stress; and exposure to perfumes, soaps, detergents, or deodorants. Diagnostic evaluation typically involves a thorough neurologic exam by the primary health care provider. During this examination, vision is checked, the nerves in the head and neck (cranial nerves) are tested, and muscle strength and reflexes are evaluated. The patient's risk factors for stroke (diabetes, high blood pressure, elevated cholesterol) are also assessed.

Treatment commonly involves avoiding precipitating factors; using medications for pain such as aspirin, acetaminophen (Tylenol), or anti-inflammatory agents such as ibuprofen; taking medications (such as Imitrex, Zomig, Amerge, Maxalt or midrin) at the start of a migraine; and taking medications regularly to prevent future attacks (beta blockers, calcium channel blockers, tricyclic antidepressants, valproate).

TMJ Syndrome

The temporomandibular joint (TMJ) is the area where the jaw is attached to the skull by the very strong muscles responsible for chewing. Temporomandibular joint syndrome (TMJ syndrome) affects nearly one in five adult Americans, although only a small proportion of them seek treatment from their primary care physician or their dentist. This condition is more common in middle-aged people than in younger adults, and it is more common in women than in men. Typical symptoms include pain and tenderness in the jaw area, in the muscles of the jaw, in the joint itself, and/or under the ears and an inability to fully open the mouth. The person may also experience headaches, neck pain, or a catch or clicking noise in the joint when chewing. Factors that contribute to the development of TMJ include clenching the jaw or grinding the teeth, other dental problems, poor-fitting dentures, and stress. Diagnostic evaluation includes x-rays of the mouth and jaw, looking for displacement of the joint or evidence of injury to the joint. Treatment includes the application of moist heat to the area; temporary restriction to a soft diet so as to rest the muscles and the joint involved in chewing; anti-inflammatory medications like ibuprofen; muscle relaxants; and use of a mouth guard at night to prevent or reduce the impact of teeth grinding and jaw clenching during sleep. Studies have varied in their reporting of the relationship between TMJ syndrome and IBS; overall, TMJ is present in approximately 20 to 60 percent of people who have IBS.

Chronic Pelvic Pain

Many women who have IBS have problems with recurrent pain in the pelvis or pelvic cavity. The pelvic cavity is the area bounded by the hip bones on each side, the pubic bone in front, and the coccyx (tail bone) in back. Within the pelvic cavity lie the bladder, ureters, and parts of the colon and small intestine; in women also the uterus, cervix, and vagina; and in men also the prostate gland. Patients who have chronic pelvic pain are usually first evaluated by their primary care physicians, although if symptoms persist, they may be referred to any of a variety of specialists— gynecologists, obstetricians, urologists, fertility experts, and/or gastroenterologists. Like IBS, chronic pelvic pain (CPP) is not a narrowly defined disease but a syndrome that can develop for a number of different reasons and involve various organ systems, including the endocrine system (which deals with hormones), the urologic system, the musculoskeletal system, and the reproductive system—hence the variety of specialists to whom one might be referred.

Pelvic pain must be present for at least six months before it is considered chronic in nature. In some patients who have CPP the pain is present on a daily basis, while in others it occurs much less frequently. It may be associated with extremely painful menstrual cycles or painful intercourse (dyspareunia). Sometimes the pain is worse with movement or sitting down. Some of the most common reasons for chronic pelvic pain include endometriosis, "congestion" (swelling) of the veins in the pelvis, scar tissue from previous surgery, bladder problems (such as interstitial cystitis—see below), problems in the muscles that line the pelvic floor, uterine fibroids, a remnant of ovary left despite prior supposed removal of both ovaries, and visceral hypersensitivity. Information gathered from gynecology clinics shows that IBS is frequently also present in women who have painful menstrual cycles, painful intercourse, and CPP.

Treatment of CPP begins with trying to identify the underlying factor that is responsible for the pain. For many patients, this may require a series of visits to different specialists so that specialized testing can be performed. Once the underlying cause is identified, specific treatment can be initiated.

Urinary Problems

Many people who have IBS complain of urinary problems, for instance, increased urinary frequency, increased urination at night, feelings of incomplete urination, spasms or discomfort in the bladder, urinary hesitancy, and inability to completely empty the bladder. Patients who have primary symptoms of urinary urgency and frequency may have an overactive bladder. People who have the symptoms described above who also have pelvic pain and pain partially relieved with urination may have a condition called interstitial cystitis (IC). This is a common condition thought to affect more than 10 million Americans. Typically a chronic condition, it is characterized by symptoms that are very similar to a urinary tract infection (UTI). In fact, many people who have interstitial cystitis have been misdiagnosed as having repeated or recurrent UTIs.

Symptoms of IC include pain or discomfort in the area of the bladder (behind the pubic bone), pain or discomfort with urination, feelings of urinary urgency, and feeling the need to urinate frequently. These symptoms often temporarily improve after urination but then return shortly afterwards. Although less common, some women who have IC complain of bladder pain that awakens them at night or pelvic pain that persists for days after sexual intercourse.

Interstitial cystitis may develop because of inflammation in the bladder wall, recurrent infections in the bladder, or spasms in the bladder wall (which, like the intestinal tract, is made up of smooth muscle). This condition is generally diagnosed with a series of tests, including a urinalysis, urine culture, and tests to measure bladder capacity and bladder emptying ability. Cystoscopy—passing a small lighted instrument into the bladder so that it can be looked at and biopsied if necessary—and distention of the bladder with water (a procedure called hydrodistention) are diagnostic studies commonly used in the evaluation of patients who have symptoms consistent with IC.

Treatment of IC is effective in many patients. As with IBS, effective treatment begins with educating the patient about the condition. Treatment also typically involves changes in diet (avoiding acidic foods, carbonated beverages, alcohol, caffeine), the use of medications to help relax the bladder, anti-inflammatory agents like ibuprofen, tricyclic antidepressants (TCAs), biofeedback, physical therapy, acupuncture, or the use of medications directly instilled into the bladder (such as DMSO, lidocaine, pentosan polysulfate, or heparin). Pentosan polysulfate (Elmiron), a polysaccharide molecule (a long sugar molecule) is the only drug currently approved by the Food and Drug Administration to treat interstitial cystitis. It is thought to improve symptoms by improving healing in the bladder wall, although it may take three to four months before any sustained benefits are noted while on this medication. Some people note a small amount of hair loss while taking pentosan polysulfate; its safety in pregnancy is unknown. In the rare patient who has persistent symptoms, surgery may provide some benefit, and there are preliminary data showing that electrical stimulation of the bladder may help some people who have IC.

Links with IBS?

Pain is a defining symptom of IBS and is the number one reason people who have IBS seek the care of a physician. For many people who have IBS, this pain is limited to the abdomen and pelvis. However, many patients also have somatic pain—pain that involves their bone, muscle, joints, or skin. It is tempting to try to link the pain in the GI tract with the pain elsewhere in the body, especially since so many patients who have IBS experience both. The connection between somatic pain and visceral pain in people who have IBS is not clear-cut, though, for a number of reasons. For example, most patients who have IBS and visceral pain do *not* also have associated somatic pain, so patients who have IBS and both visceral and somatic pain represent a minority of people who have IBS. Also, some who have an overlap of these two pain syndromes experience relief of one type of pain with treatment but no relief of the other type of pain. We would expect that if the pains came from a single underlying problem or precipitating event, then when the pain of one syndrome responded to a particular medication, so would the other. Finally, if two problems were intimately connected, then their natural histories would be similar. In fact, however, it is quite common for somatic pain syndromes to improve while the visceral pain lingers on.

Scientists have proposed several theories in an attempt to link increased visceral pain with increased somatic pain in patients who have IBS. For example, hyperreactive smooth muscle, autonomic nervous system dysfunction, and altered neuroendocrine function are all possible causative factors for both types of pain. At present, however, there is no good scientific data to support any of these theories. Thus, somatic pain and visceral pain, although found together in a subgroup of patients who have IBS, must at this point be considered two separate physiological processes.

One interesting way to connect these two processes would be to look for similarities in how patients react to both kinds of pain. It is well known that people who have IBS are more sensitive to pain in their GI tract. Perhaps people who have TMJ syndrome, migraine headaches, and fibromyalgia are also hypersensitive to pain. This would mean that someone who has both IBS and fibromyalgia would be more sensitive to pain in both the GI tract and in the musculoskeletal system, compared to healthy people. In addition, it is possible that significant stress, anxiety, or depression causes both of these kinds of problems to flare up. Clearly, further research is needed into these questions.

Summary

- Many patients who have IBS also have other types of pain syndromes.
- Some of the most common disorders associated with IBS include chronic fatigue syndrome, fibromyalgia, migraine headaches, TMJ syndrome, and interstitial cystitis.

- It is tempting to try to link these problems with IBS, looking for similar causes (for example, a viral infection), but there are as yet no good scientific data to support such a connection.
- It is possible that these diverse pain syndromes, which can affect many areas of the body, may all be related by an increased sensitivity to pain.

CHAPTER 10

IBS and Diet

The relationship between diet and irritable bowel syndrome symptoms is a topic commonly raised by people being evaluated for IBS. Many patients wonder whether their diet is causing or contributing to their IBS symptoms, and still others worry that their symptoms represent a food allergy. A clinical research study published several years ago found that nearly 80 percent of people who had IBS believed that dietary factors played a role in their symptoms.

The complex relationship between diet and IBS can be broken down into four common questions that people ask their physicians. First, Can eating specific foods make me develop IBS? Second, Can my body's response to certain foods mimic IBS symptoms? Third, Can specific foods make my IBS symptoms worse? And fourth, Do my IBS symptoms represent a food allergy? In this chapter, I address each of these questions and discuss some common food intolerances.

Can Eating Specific Foods Make Me Develop IBS?

No (this is the easiest question about diet and IBS for physicians to answer). The etiology (cause) of IBS is not completely known, and, as discussed in Chapter 3, there are several different reasons why some people develop IBS. Although many physicians believe that people can be genetically predisposed to developing IBS, they also recognize that there are contributing factors, such as surgery, an inflammatory process, an infectious illness, medications, or significant stress. It seems reasonable that diet could be one of these contributing factors, but there are no data available to show that a specific food causes IBS to develop. That is not to say, however, that dietary factors can't contribute or worsen IBS symptoms.

Can My Body's Response to Certain Foods Mimic IBS Symptoms?

Yes. The key word here is "mimic." Patients with lactose intolerance, fructose intolerance, celiac disease, gluten sensitivity, or a diet rich in foods that ferment excessively in the colon may experience symptoms that seem typical of IBS (bloating, excess gas, distention, abdominal discomfort, and diarrhea). If a specific food produces symptoms that mimic IBS, then removal of that food from a person's diet will normally resolve all symptoms. Unfortunately, this rarely happens. What is more common is that a food may contribute to IBS symptoms, but when that specific food is removed from the diet, typical IBS symptoms continue, albeit at a lower level. Here are the common food groups that many people who have IBS are intolerant to:

- Lactose (dairy products)
- Fructose (fruit juices, regular sodas, sports drinks with high-fructose corn syrup, fresh fruits)
- Fructans (onions, peppers, asparagus)
- Galactans (complex carbohydrates found in dried and canned beans)
- Cruciferous vegetables (broccoli, cauliflower, cabbage)
- Gluten (the protein found in bread that gives it a chewy consistency)

Can Specific Foods Make My IBS Symptoms Worse?

In the past, physicians would have rapidly dismissed this question with a quick "no." However, research during the past decade has shown that some foods may contribute (but not cause) IBS symptoms. The relationship between certain foods and IBS symptoms is difficult to define for a number of reasons. One, for the majority of people who have IBS, symptoms wax and wane over time. Symptoms that fluctuate on a day-to-day basis make it difficult to determine whether a single food item is the actual cause. I commonly hear from patients how one specific food seems to cause them problems one day (more bloating, more gas, more diarrhea) but is then well tolerated on other days. This lack of consistency makes it difficult to determine whether a relationship exists between eating certain foods and developing symptoms of IBS. Two, because some foods and beverages may make symptoms of IBS worse, it is often difficult to measure a response when more, or less, of the food is ingested. Thus it is difficult to determine, on a daily basis, the contribution of that specific food to IBS symptoms. Three, people respond differently to different dietary changes. One patient may have great success with a certain diet, whereas another person has no improvement at all. This should not be surprising, because individuals who have IBS are all different from each other in some way. Even if they have similar symptoms, the cause of the symptoms may be quite different. People who have IBS can't be grouped together and treated in an identical manner. In other words, although the underlying mechanisms of IBS are the same (abnormal gut motility, visceral hypersensitivity, heightened brain-gut interactions), symptoms are expressed differently in different patients.

Do My IBS Symptoms Represent a Food Allergy?

Food Allergy versus Food Sensitivity

People who have symptoms of IBS often wonder whether their symptoms represent a food allergy. Although IBS symptoms may be caused by food allergies, food sensitivities, or an intolerance to certain foods, this is a controversial topic with a large amount of misinformation and misperception. Let me first define a few key terms.

People who have IBS and develop gastrointestinal symptoms (bloating, gassiness, abdominal discomfort, and diarrhea) after eating a specific food may be *intolerant* to that food. The concept of food intolerance is simple: some people develop symptoms after ingesting a specific food. The underlying cause of this intolerance may be known in some cases (i.e., lactose intolerance and fructose intolerance—see below) but not in others, although some physicians think that intolerance is an example of normal GI physiology that is just highly exaggerated. Others think that symptoms of food intolerance are yet another example of how the gut is hypersensitive in people who have IBS. Another theory is that these symptoms may represent a mild food allergy.

Some people seem to be overly *sensitive* to different foods. Symptoms of food sensitivity are similar to that of food intolerance, but milder. One example of a food sensitivity is a sensitivity to fat products. Many people, regardless of whether they have IBS, find that they are a little queasy or nauseated after eating a rich, fatty meal. These symptoms may develop because fats slow the normal emptying of the stomach, which can then lead to acid reflux. In addition, the slow emptying of the stomach may make symptoms of bloating and gassiness worse. Other people who are sensitive to fatty foods may develop diarrhea after eating a richer than normal meal. Patients with these symptoms are not allergic to fats and generally can tolerate some amount of fat in their diet; they are just more sensitive to fats than other people. Overall, the area of food sensitivity remains somewhat vague and ill-defined, and the mechanisms that underlie it are still not completely understood.

Whereas some people may be sensitive to or intolerant of certain foods, others develop severe symptoms after eating a specific food. These symptoms may include severe abdominal pain or diarrhea, shortness of breath, development of a rash, or swelling of the mouth, tongue, or throat. Patients with these symptoms are most likely *allergic* to a certain food. One study has shown that 30 percent to 50 percent of individuals who have symptoms of IBS believe that they are allergic to certain foods. However, when tested, only 1 to 5 percent of patients who have IBS are truly allergic to a specific food. This is no different from the general population, where 1 to 3 percent of people are truly food allergic. Food allergies are more common in people who have other "classic" allergic diseases, such as asthma, allergic rhinitis, and atopic dermatitis.

A *true food allergy* is a very specific, immunologically mediated event. The body reacts as though something foreign has been introduced into the body—more specifically, into the GI tract. The body then mounts an immune response and attacks the foreign substance using immunoglobulins released from lymphocytes. Other cells (mast cells) participate as well, and these cells are important in the development of the allergic reaction. During this process, significant inflammation develops throughout the body, including the oropharynx (itching in the mouth or lips; swelling of the tongue, palate, and throat), skin (hives or a rash), pulmonary system (coughing, wheezing, shortness of breath), and the GI tract, which can lead to a variety of symptoms, including abdominal pain, bloating, and diarrhea. True food allergies generally develop within minutes of exposure. Patients with these symptoms should be evaluated by an allergist to identify the specific foods that precipitate such a violent and potentially dangerous reaction. Allergists frequently perform a skin test to identify the specific food that a patient is allergic to, although this is not a perfect test. Patients who have true food allergies are treated with strict dietary avoidance and occasionally with medications. In addition, these patients should always have an emergency epinephrine injection close by (also called an epinephrine pen, or EpiPen). The most common food allergies are shown in Table 10.1.

Common Food Intolerances and Allergies

Lactose Intolerance

Overall, the most common adverse reaction to food occurs with the ingestion of lactose. Using the terms defined above, this is not an allergic reaction but an intolerance. Lactose is the major sugar found in milk products. It is categorized as a disaccharide (di means "two"), since it is made up of two different simple sugars, glucose and galactose. After being ingested, lactose is normally broken down by lactase, an enzyme found in the small intestine. When the milk sugar is not completely digested, the unabsorbed sugar travels through the small intestine and colon. Along the way, the undigested lactose pulls water with it, eventually making the stool looser. In addition, bacteria in the colon ferment the undigested lactose, producing symptoms of gas, bloating, and diarrhea.

The lactase enzyme is found in high levels in newborns and during childhood. This makes sense from an evolutionary point of view, since milk is a vital part of the diet after birth and during early childhood. However, milk becomes a less important part of our diet as we age, since we can obtain calories, protein, and other nutrients from a variety of other foodstuffs. Many people notice that as they get older, they are less able to digest milk and other milk products (cheese, yogurt, ice cream) as well as they did when they were children. This change in digestion oc-

Table 10.1. Common Food Allergies

Peanuts	Eggs	Shellfish
Tree nuts (hazelnuts,	Cow's milk	Soybeans
walnuts, pistachios,	Soy	Wheat
pecans, pine nuts)	Fish	

curs because the ability to produce the enzyme (lactase) that breaks down milk sugar (lactose) slowly decreases over time. Some people may lose all or almost all of their ability to produce the lactase enzyme and thus become completely lactose intolerant. Others lose only a small proportion of their lactase-producing capability and thus are better able to tolerate larger portions of milk products. For most people, lactose intolerance is not an all-or-none phenomenon but rather one of degrees.

Overall, approximately 30 to 35 percent of adult Americans are lactose intolerant at some level. In certain populations (African Americans, Asian Americans), the prevalence of lactose intolerance may be as high as 75 percent. Contrary to popular opinion, lactose intolerance is not more common in people who have IBS compared to the general public. (See Chapter 15 for more information on how to diagnose and treat lactose intolerance.)

Fructose Intolerance

Although lactose is the milk sugar most commonly blamed for aggravating the symptoms of IBS, other sugars may also cause problems in individuals who have IBS. Fructose is the best example. Fructose is a simple sugar (called a monosaccharide) and is commonly added to many foods as a sweetener. Most carbonated beverages, fruit drinks, and energy or sports drinks contain high-fructose corn syrup. A 12-ounce soda typically contains 20 to 30 grams of fructose. Fructose is also present in fruits, berries, peas, onions, and artichokes. Like lactose, some people are fructose intolerant. Symptoms are similar (bloating, gas, loose stools, stomach churning and gurgling) and, as with lactose, people often have a threshold for the amount of fructose they can ingest. One or two soft drinks may be fine during the course of a day, but a large glass of fruit juice at breakfast, two soft drinks at lunch, a sports drink after going to the gym in the afternoon, and one or two sodas in the evening may be just too much for the body to handle. One study of patients who had functional bowel symptoms found that 30 percent developed GI symptoms (gas, bloating, and diarrhea) and had an abnormal breath test with just 25 grams of fructose, whereas 58 percent developed GI symptoms and had an abnormal breath test with 50 grams of fructose. Overall, the frequency of fructose intolerance may not differ significantly when people who have IBS are compared to the general population, but the intensity of symptoms may differ.

Gluten Sensitivity

Many clinicians now recommend a gluten-free diet for patients who have IBS. Although easy to recommend, a true gluten-free diet can be difficult to institute, tricky to follow, and add significant costs to an individual's food budget. Therefore, before adopting a gluten-free diet, you should carefully examine the evidence supporting this diet. To best answer the question of whether a gluten-free diet might improve GI symptoms in people who have IBS, let me first explain what gluten is and review the difference between a true wheat allergy (celiac disease) and gluten sensitivity.

Gluten is a protein found in wheat, barley, and rye. This protein is broken down during the normal digestive process, and the peptides (small pieces of protein) are absorbed. However, in genetically susceptible individuals (those who are human leukocyte antigen [HLA] DQ2 or DQ8 positive), the peptides initiate an immune response mediated by T lymphocytes. A cascade of events then follows, which may include the development of inflammation in the lining of the small intestine, increased permeability of the gut wall, atrophy (wasting away) of the surfaces of the cells that line the small intestine, and consequently the inability to properly absorb necessary nutrients. This is the clinical condition called celiac disease, which represents a true wheat allergy. Celiac disease can be diagnosed using a combination of symptoms, serologic tests (for example, tests for antibodies to tissue transglutaminase [TTG]), and duodenal biopsies. The prevalence of celiac disease in the United States and Canada is estimated at 0.4 to 1 percent (e.g., 4 to 10 people out of 1,000).

Some people who have IBS develop GI symptoms (bloating, gas, distention, and diarrhea) after ingesting products that contain wheat; however, when properly evaluated (e.g., blood tests such as a serum TTG antibody test, a test to look for the necessary genes, or duodenal biopsies at the time of upper endoscopy), they do not meet the criteria for being diagnosed with celiac disease. These patients are considered to have a gluten sensitivity. Although a standardized and precise definition of gluten sensitivity has not been agreed on, a common-sense working definition is that gluten sensitivity is a condition that responds to or improves with the exclusion of gluten from the diet. At present, a favorable response means that dietary avoidance of gluten improves GI symptoms (which vary from person to person). In the future, research studies may show that gluten sensitivity is just one end of a spectrum of gluten-associated disorders.

Gluten Intolerance: Celiac Disease

As noted above, celiac disease is a true food allergy that affects approximately 0.4 to 1 percent of the U.S. population. Celiac disease is not a new disease—it was first described nearly 2,000 years ago, and its presence in children, and their response to a wheat-free diet, was described in the late 1880s by the physician Samuel Gee. In essence, celiac disease is an autoimmune response that occurs in genetically susceptible individuals (they have human leukocyte antigens DQ2 and DQ8). The autoimmune response develops when wheat, barley, or rye (all of which contain gluten) is ingested, creating inflammation in the small intestine, which can cause symptoms of gas, bloating, distention, and diarrhea. In addition, the inflammation can lead to anemia, vitamin deficiencies, osteoporosis, and even nerve injury. It can generally be diagnosed with a blood sample (a serum TTG antibody test) or an upper endoscopy with biopsies of the duodenum. Treatment is avoidance of all grains that contain gluten (wheat, rye, barley). Although this may sound easy, it can be very difficult to avoid all of these food products. Wheat can turn up in all kinds of foods where it does not seem to belong (e.g., salad dressings, cold cuts, ice creams, soy sauce), and it even appears in nonfood items, such as lipstick. When patients are meticulous about avoiding gluten, they generally notice a dramatic improvement in symptoms. Fortunately, more and more stores are now selling gluten-free products, so the diet is much easier to maintain.

High-Fiber Foods

Another group of foods that can mimic or worsen symptoms of IBS are high-fiber foods such as fruits, vegetables, and beans, and over-the-counter fiber products. We are all well aware of the health value of fruits and vegetables. They are low in fat (except avocadoes) and contain essential vitamins and minerals (such as beta-carotene and vitamins E and K). Current recommendations are that all adults consume at least 25 to 30 grams of fiber each day. In general, diets that focus on fruits and vegetables (such as a Mediterranean diet) are thought to increase overall health, well-being, and longevity. Fruits and vegetables, due to the presence of insoluble (not completely digestible) fiber, also add bulk to the stool. The presence of fiber causes retention of water in the stool. Water retention generally leads to increased stool volume, increased stool weight, more rapid passage through the large intestine, and increased ease of evacuation with less straining, which can be helpful for people who experience constipation.

One of the problems with insoluble fiber, however, is that it is not completely digested or broken down within the GI tract. The indigestible and incompletely absorbed products then lead to gas formation within the colon, with increased bloating and distention, which can be uncomfortable. For patients who have IBS and constipation, the addition of fruits and vegetables to their diet is often very effective in relieving symptoms of constipation (stool frequency increases and straining decreases). However, the addition of fiber does not improve the abdominal pain of IBS and for many patients, bloating worsens. Of all the vegetables, the cruciferous vegetables (broccoli, cauliflower, cabbage) are the worst offenders with regard to increased gas production and bloating (see Chapter 15 for the low-FODMAP diet).

Other Foods and Beverages

Other food products that can cause bloating include those that contain sorbitol. Sorbitol is a sugar that is not broken down within the upper gastrointestinal tract. As it passes through the GI tract it is eventually broken down by bacteria in the colon, releasing gas and causing bloating. Sorbitol is commonly used as a sugar substitute and is found in sugar-free candies, gums, and mints. Patients who have significant problems with gas and bloating should review their diet carefully to make sure that they are not taking in sorbitol.

Many other common foods may cause symptoms in people who have IBS, including caffeine, carbonated beverages, onions, and peppers. Caffeine usually does not worsen bloating, but it does act as a stimulant to the GI tract and can increase stool frequency and cause cramps. Some individuals who have IBS and constipation use the side effects of caffeine to their advantage—one or two cups in the morning may help stimulate a bowel movement. Carbonated beverages may cause problems if they are sweetened with high-fructose corn syrup. Additionally, the carbonation bothers some people who have IBS, possibly because the gas bubbles distend or stretch the stomach. Although foods like onions, peppers, chocolate, and other products like alcohol and cigarettes are often blamed by people who have IBS for their symptoms, no research study has ever formally investigated whether these products truly cause worse symptoms in people who have IBS compared to the general population.

A small number of individuals who have severe IBS (frequent symptoms to daily debilitating symptoms) find that they are intolerant to many or nearly all foods. These people may think that they are allergic to almost all foods because everything they eat causes gas, bloating, or abdominal pain or discomfort. However, true food allergies (the most common of which are to peanuts, eggs, and shellfish) occur in only a small percentage of people, and documented allergies to multiple foods are very rare. The following case study describes a woman who believed that she was allergic to all but a few foods.

Jean is a 37-year-old woman who was referred to me because of multiple food allergies. During our first appointment, she told me that food had been "an issue all of my life." She stated that she was allergic to nearly every food and that she currently lived on bottled water, Saltine crackers, lemon pudding, and small amounts of boiled chicken. She had lived that way for several years because "everything" she ate caused bloating, gas, cramps, and abdominal discomfort. She said that sometimes even drinking water caused abdominal pain, gas, and bloating. Jean is 5 feet 7 inches tall. Her physical development and growth were normal during her early childhood and teenage years, and in college her weight ranged from 120 to 145 pounds. She worked in a bookstore after graduating from college and had three children over the next several years. The first two children were healthy; however, the third child was colicky, developed some feeding problems, became very sick during the first few months of life, and after several months in and out of the hospital, died. Jean stayed at home after that and did not return to work. Her weight dropped to 98 pounds and then stabilized at 102 to 103 pounds.

During the decade before I saw Jean, she had tried a variety of diets to improve her symptoms, including low-fat, low-protein, low-carbohydrate, high-carbohydrate, liquid-only, protein-only, all-citrus, Atkins, Mediterranean, and the cabbage soup diet. Symptoms of bloating and abdominal discomfort with altered bowel habits plagued her during all of these diets. She had seen seven or eight gastroenterologists, in addition to two internists, two dieticians, a surgeon, and three allergists. Her weight had been steady at 103 pounds for several years. She had undergone extensive testing, including blood work, several upper endoscopies, abdominal x-rays, CT scans, two colonoscopies, and an x-ray study of her small intestine. All of these tests were normal. A test to measure stomach emptying was also normal, as was a CT scan of her chest and head. Blood work performed several times to look for celiac disease (and duodenal biopsies) were normal. She did not have asthma, seasonal allergies, or atopic dermatitis. Skin testing and specialized blood work to look for allergies were all normal.

In terms of treatment, Jean saw a chiropractor for several sessions but did not experience any relief of her symptoms. She also tried acupuncture without success. Other unsuccessful treatment plans were prescribed by one doctor who treated her with antibiotics for presumed bacterial overgrowth (an uncommon condition in which the small intestine is overpopulated with bacteria) and by a different physician who treated her with several courses of medications for candidiasis (*Candida* is a common yeast). Jean had been scheduled to see a psychiatrist on two different occasions but cancelled those appointments because she didn't want to leave the house. After reviewing her family history, I saw that her family members were all well and that there was no history of food allergies in the family. Jean was somewhat anxious during the interview. She said that she could not get out anymore. Her husband did all of the shopping and ran all of the errands. Except for doctors' visits, she did not leave the house. Her physical examination was normal, except that she was extremely thin. Simple laboratory tests performed on the day of our office visit (blood count, electrolytes, kidney function tests, sedimentation rate, thyroid tests, and liver tests) were all normal.

I had a long discussion with Jean and explained that, although some people can be allergic to some foods, it is rare to be allergic to multiple foods and nearly impossible to be allergic to all foods. Jean's symptoms of bloating, gassiness, and abdominal discomfort after eating a meal were all consistent with IBS. In addition, I explained that her anxiety was probably playing a role in her symptoms and that she had symptoms of agoraphobia (from the Greek—literally, fear of the marketplace—or in more modern terms, fear of leaving the home). I explained that, after eating a severely restricted diet of water, crackers, and chicken for several years, it would take some time for her body to get used to new foods in her diet.

In terms of a treatment plan, I suggested that she gradually introduce new foods into her diet while at the same time initiate treatment for her fear of going out in public and for her anxiety. Jean started taking a daily multivitamin with iron and I prescribed a very low dose of a selective serotonin reuptake inhibitor (SSRI). SSRIs are used to treat a variety of medical problems, including depression, anxiety, obsessive-compulsive disorders, and phobias. Together, we wrote out a schedule so that she would slowly increase the dose of the SSRI every 3 weeks. She was cautioned that she might not notice any improvement in her anxiety or her fear of going out for two to three months. We also discussed her diet at length and wrote out a careful schedule whereby she would introduce a new food into her diet every seven days. I asked Jean to take note of her symptoms during the introduction of the new foods but not to stop them unless severe symptoms developed (such as severe nausea, vomiting, diarrhea). Jean started by adding small amounts of chicken broth during the first week, white rice during the second week, grits and rice cereal during the third week, and egg whites during the fourth week. I asked her to avoid adding wheat products and high fiber foods during the first month. Jean reported back to me via brief phone calls each week, stating that with the introduction of each new food at the start of the week her symptoms were "terrible," although she acknowledged by the end of the week that her symptoms probably weren't that different from her baseline symptoms. At the end of the month, she had gained nearly one pound and (although cautious) seemed somewhat optimistic. During the next several months, with my guidance via frequent office visits and phone calls, she gradually introduced a new food into her diet each week and continued to increase the dose of her SSRI. By the end of the sixth month, she had gained five pounds, had more energy, and felt less anxious. She returned to the care of her local gastroenterologist and internist and over the next 2 years, with careful guidance, frequent visits, and continuation of her medication, she gained another 10 pounds and felt significantly better. She still feels bloating and abdominal discomfort with many foods; however, she now acknowledges that "that's just who I am" and she doesn't eliminate a food from her diet every time she has a brief episode of discomfort or bloatedness.

Elimination and Exclusion Diets

When I first saw Jean, she was essentially already on an elimination diet. Some physicians use an elimination diet to try to sort out the tricky issues of food intolerances, food sensitivities, food allergies, and symptoms of IBS. A strict elimination diet begins by removing virtually all foods from the diet while only ingesting very simple foods that are generally considered well tolerated by all. An example would be to consume only water, white rice, and boiled chicken to start. Then, during the course of weeks to months, different foods are slowly added to the diet, while symptoms are carefully monitored.

Alternatively, some physicians use exclusion diets when they evaluate an individual with suspected food allergies. Exclusion diets start by excluding foods commonly believed to cause GI distress in many people; these foods may include wheat products, coffee, cereals, and dairy products. After two weeks of being on this diet, if no symptoms improve, then it is unlikely that diet plays a role, and practitioners typically instruct patients to return to their original diet. If symptoms improve to some degree, then patients are asked to slowly reintroduce foods, one at a time, to determine whether a food truly causes symptoms. If a symptom recurs, then that food should be eliminated again. Ideally, after waiting several days, the patient should reintroduce that same food into the diet again. This process is called challenge/rechallenge. If the exact same symptoms recur, then it is possible that the patient is intolerant to that food. However, since symptoms of IBS do wax and wane, it is not uncommon for the symptoms to not recur during the rechallenge and the patient to not be truly intolerant to the food. Rather, the typical symptoms of IBS were just confused with the ingestion of that food, and the patient mistook those symptoms of IBS as being related to a food allergy. One study evaluated the use of exclusion diets and found that 50 percent of patients felt that they had some improvement in their symptoms. Note that not all patients improved and that even those who did improve did not have resolution of their symptoms. These study results highlight the difficulty of separating the symptoms of IBS from food intolerance.

People who have IBS commonly have some discomfort or problems after eating specific foods. When visiting a doctor, such patients should provide a thorough history of their symptoms so that physicians can help determine what food, if any, is the cause. Using a symptom diary can be helpful for many people. Although true food allergies are uncommon, people who have severe symptoms should visit an allergist or immunologist for a thorough evaluation. It is important to differentiate the symptoms of food intolerance from the symptoms of IBS—without doing so, individuals may start to avoid all foods.

Summary

- Eating specific foods will not cause you to develop IBS.
- People who have lactose intolerance, fructose intolerance, celiac disease, gluten intolerance, or a diet rich in foods that ferment excessively in the colon may experience symptoms that seem typical of IBS.
- Individuals who have IBS and develop gastrointestinal symptoms after eating a specific food may be *intolerant* to that food. If the symptoms are mild, the person may be considered *sensitive* to that type of

food. If the symptoms are severe, the person is most likely *allergic* to that type of food.

- Lactose is the food substance most likely to cause problems in the GI tract. Nearly 30 to 35 percent of adult Americans are lactose intolerant to some degree. Typical symptoms of lactose intolerance include bloating, gassiness, abdominal distention, and diarrhea.
- Fructose is another sugar that is often difficult to break down in the GI tract. Typical symptoms of fructose intolerance are similar to those of lactose intolerance.
- Gluten sensitivity is when people develop GI symptoms after they ingest products that contain gluten, such as wheat. It is not a true food allergy like celiac disease.
- Celiac disease is a true food allergy (an immune response) that develops due to gluten proteins. It is present in approximately 0.4 to 1 percent of Americans. Treatment consists of avoiding all products that contain gluten.
- Fiber adds bulk to the stool and accelerates transit of stool through the GI tract. However, too much fiber can worsen symptoms of bloating and gas and can even cause diarrhea.
- Sorbitol is often used to sweeten foods and liquids. Since it is not broken down in the upper GI tract, sorbitol may cause gas and bloating when it reaches the colon.
- Some physicians use elimination or exclusion diets to evaluate a patient with suspected food intolerances, sensitivities, or allergies. These diets can be difficult to maintain, and they require time and patience.

CHAPTER 11

IBS and Small Intestine Bacterial Overgrowth (SIBO)

If you asked people who have irritable bowel syndrome what their worst symptoms are, many would say problems with excess intestinal gas and the feeling of being bloated and distended. As discussed in Chapter 6, everyone who eats or drinks anything other than water will produce some gas in the gastrointestinal (GI) tract. Researchers have found that the average adult produces approximately 700 ml of intestinal gas each day. Gas within the GI tract develops from sources other than food and drink, such as swallowed air, diffusion from the bloodstream, and a variety of chemical reactions within the GI tract. The five most common gases found within the GI tract are nitrogen, oxygen, hydrogen, carbon dioxide, and methane. Other gases are present in the GI tract, but they exist only in trace amounts. Nearly all nitrogen and oxygen within the upper GI tract comes from swallowed air. Carbon dioxide may be present from swallowed air, from carbonated beverages, or from chemical reactions that occur in the stomach and upper small intestine (acids and bases are neutralized and form carbon dioxide gas as a byproduct). Most gas production in the GI tract, however, occurs in the colon (large intestine).

Although many of us don't like to think about it, our large intestines are full of bacteria. This extensive population of bacteria is vital to our good health and is often referred to as the gut microflora or microbiota or gut microbiome. The average individual has anywhere from five hundred to one thousand different species of bacteria living in the colon at any one time. The total number of bacteria in the colon is estimated at approximately 10^{13} to 10^{14} (ten to the thirteenth or fourteenth power)—to put this in perspective, you have more living bacterial cells in your colon (approximately 3–4 pounds worth at any one time) than you do living cells in all other organs in your body combined. These bacteria have a variety of jobs: they are critical to maintaining the health of the large intestine, they play an important role in the immune system of the gastrointestinal tract, they help metabolize (break down) medications, they produce essential fatty acids and vitamins, and they serve in digestion and nutrient absorption.

Gut microflora typically reside only in the large intestine. However, in some people who have IBS, the bacteria migrate from the colon into the small intestine (see Figure 6.1 for a review of the anatomy of the GI tract). When abnormal amounts of colonic bacteria migrate from the colon into the small intestine, a condition called small intestine bacterial overgrowth (SIBO) develops. SIBO may be caused by an infection in the gastrointestinal tract, surgery to the small or large intestine, altered motility of the intestinal tract, diverticula (abnormal sacs or pouches) in the small intestine, low levels of acid in the stomach (stomach acid helps to prevent bacterial overgrowth), various medications, changes in the immune function of the GI tract, or other unknown causes. No matter why SIBO develops, when these colonic bacteria colonize the small intestine, the physiology of the small intestine changes.

Symptoms of SIBO

Major symptoms of SIBO include excessive gas and bloating. As the colonic bacteria in the small intestine digest and ferment food products that are much larger and more complex than normal, they produce excess gas. If you have ever made bread at home, you know that bread rises when yeast is added. Rising occurs due to gas production (carbon dioxide) when yeast is exposed to food (sugar or starch). A similar process occurs when too many bacteria are present in the upper small intestine—they ferment food products too vigorously and produce excess gas. Excess gas is not dangerous, but it can certainly be uncomfortable. In people who have long-standing SIBO, colonic bacteria in the small intestine may also lead to changes in vitamin levels (such as low vitamin B12 and vitamin D levels or high folate levels) and cause chronic diarrhea.

Diagnosing SIBO

Studies during the past decade have shown that some, but not all, people who have IBS also have SIBO. Because nearly all patients who have IBS have symptoms of gas and bloating, how can health care providers determine if the gas and bloating are a direct result of SIBO? In other words, because symptoms of gas are nonspecific—making it extremely difficult to tell if the excess bloating is from SIBO or not—testing may be necessary. There are two main methods of accurately diagnosing SIBO. The first is upper endoscopy (see Chapter 8), in which a physician carefully passes a sterile catheter into the proximal jejunum and takes a sample of the fluid (called an aspirate) to send to the lab. Laboratory technicians count the number of bacteria present and also culture the bacteria (they attempt to grow the bacteria on a Petri dish to identify the exact type of bacteria present). Although this method of diagnosis may sound simple, there are multiple problems with this approach. One, although upper endoscopy is generally safe, it is invasive, expensive, and does involve some small risks. Two, it is very difficult to obtain a sample of small intestine fluid without contaminating it with fluid from adjacent organs, especially the oropharynx. Three, many labs do not have the expertise or technical capabilities to culture small intestine fluid. For these reasons, most health care providers now attempt to diagnose SIBO with noninvasive measures, such as a breath test.

Breath testing is based on the principle that bacteria (whether in the small intestine or in the colon) produce hydrogen and methane gas in response to nonabsorbable carbohydrates; hydrogen gas produced within the intestinal tract can then diffuse across the wall of the intestinal tract and into the bloodstream, where it travels to the lungs and is exhaled. During a breath test, a patient ingests a carbohydrate "meal" (typically either a premeasured dose of lactulose or glucose) after an overnight fast, and then samples of his or her exhaled breaths are analyzed at routine intervals (usually every 15 minutes for 3 to 4 hours). In a healthy individual, a breath test would show a sharp rise in breath hydrogen (and/ or methane) after the carbohydrate "meal" passes through the ileocecal valve into the colon (see Figure 11.1). In a patient who has IBS and bacterial overgrowth, the "ideal" positive breath test would show an early peak (within 60 to 90 minutes) of hydrogen or methane, due to the test meal being metabolized by small intestine bacteria, and then a second peak as the carbohydrate reaches the colon. If the test is positive, meaning that there is evidence of excess hydrogen or methane production, then the patient is diagnosed with SIBO and treatment can be initiated (see Chapters 17 and 19).

Different laboratories use different carbohydrate test "meals." The most commonly ordered breath test is the lactulose breath test. Lactulose is a nonabsorbable sugar that passes through the stomach and small intestine without being broken down. When it passes into the colon, colonic bacteria digest it and produce gas (hydrogen) as a byproduct. Advantages of the lactulose breath test include ease of use, well-defined standards, and ability to compare data from one lab to another (because of its widespread use). Other labs use glucose as the test meal; some believe that this is a slightly better test, although it is used less commonly. At present, there are no large comparisons of the lactulose and glucose breath tests, so whichever test is offered to you by your health care provider is a reasonable option.

As discussed earlier in this chapter, because bloating is a nonspecific symptom that may be caused by many different pathophysiological (abnormal physiological) processes, it cannot reliably be used to diagnose SIBO. For that reason, some members of the medical community recommend testing *all* people who have IBS with symptoms of bloating for bacterial overgrowth and then treating them only if the test is positive. Treatment usually involves antibiotics, which are expensive and are associated with some risk, so the practice of testing for bacterial overgrowth helps ensure that antibiotics are given only to those patients who have SIBO. However, testing *all* people who have IBS with symptoms of bloating for bacterial overgrowth is a difficult strategy to implement, as that would mean testing 15 percent of the U.S. adult population. In the current economic and health care climate, such a strategy is impractical and financially untenable. Other practitioners recommend empiric therapy, which means that if they think the symptoms of gas and bloating are due to SIBO, treatment is initiated because of those symptoms, without any specialized testing. The following case study illustrates many of the issues

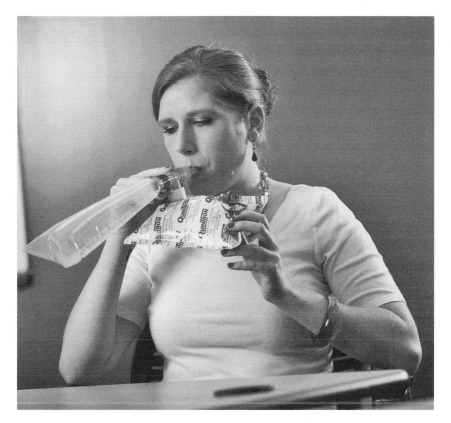

Figure 11.1. Patient blowing into the sample bag as part of the hydrogen breath test
Courtesy of Mark Washburn/Dartmouth-Hitchcock.

that patients encounter when faced with persistent symptoms of gas and bloating and the question of SIBO.

Susan is a 27-year-old woman referred for further evaluation due to persistent symptoms of lower abdominal discomfort, bloating, gassiness, and occasional loose, nonbloody stools accompanied by a sensation of urgency. These symptoms appeared approximately five years ago, after Susan developed a presumed viral gastroenteritis while traveling in Mexico. She initially had severe watery diarrhea, which slowly improved with time. Her major symptom now is feeling gassy and bloated. She states that sometimes she looks "five months pregnant" due to the bloating and that some days it is so severe that it is uncomfortable to wear skirts or tight pants. Susan is single; she works full-time as a copyright editor, does not use tobacco products, and has two to three glasses of wine per weekend. No one in her family has a history of celiac disease or inflammatory bowel disease. Her weight has remained stable over the past five years, and she is not allergic to any medications. She takes a daily oral contraceptive and occasional acetaminophen for headaches. Susan's past medical history is unremarkable—her only surgery was an appendectomy as a child.

On physical examination, she does not appear distended and is not tympanic (meaning that when the abdomen is tapped [also called percussed] by the examining health care provider, it sounds like a drum). Previous medical providers performed many different tests on Susan, including stool samples to look for a bacterial or parasitic infection, several sets of blood work with a CBC (complete blood count), tests for celiac disease (serumTTG antibody and serum IgA), a colonoscopy with random biopsies, an x-ray study of the small intestine, and an upper endoscopy with small bowel biopsies. All of these tests were completely normal. Because Susan read somewhere that bloating could be a sign of ovarian cancer, she also had a pelvic ultrasound (which showed normal results).

Susan tried many different methods of appeasing her symptoms. Although loperamide improved her diarrhea, it did not help her bloating. She avoided all dairy products for two weeks without improvement. She took all fructose-containing products out of her diet for one month, also without benefit. She lowered her fiber intake to less than 10 grams per day, which helped her diarrhea a little bit but did not improve her bloating. She even went on a gluten-free diet for two months, but this did not seem to help (and it was expensive and hard to maintain). She tried two different over-the-counter probiotics, each for approximately six weeks, without any benefit.

After discussing Susan's symptoms with her, I diagnosed her as having postinfectious IBS from the GI tract infection she developed during her trip to Mexico (see Chapter 3). Although the original infection had long since resolved, it may have injured the nerves to the GI tract (the enteric nervous system) and may also have changed her colonic micro-flora or caused her to develop SIBO. We had a long discussion about her symptoms and the medication and dietary restrictions she had tried thus far (and how they had failed to improve her symptoms). We also discussed the fact that symptoms of gas and bloating are nonspecific, meaning that they can develop for a multitude of reasons. Finally, we discussed empiric treatment (antibiotics) versus objective breath testing. Susan said that she really wanted to understand why she had these symptoms, especially because all of her tests had been normal to date. In addition, as a teenager and young adult she had had some problems with antibiotics (GI upset, diarrhea, yeast infections) and wanted to avoid these problems if possible. For these reasons, we decided to have Susan undergo a breath hydrogen test. The test showed clear evidence of SIBO—probably a result of her prior gastrointestinal infection. I prescribed a course of nonabsorbable antibiotics (rifaximin). Susan called 2 weeks after finishing the 10-day course of antibiotics to say that her bloating and loose, urgent stools had resolved and that her lower abdominal pain had improved. She hadn't suffered any side effects from the antibiotic and was very pleased with the results.

Treatment of SIBO

I generally recommend performing a breath test for SIBO only after patients have failed a thorough trial of dietary changes. These dietary changes typically include sequential weeks of eliminating dairy, fructose, fiber, and gluten; going on a strict elimination diet for at least 10 days (the classic elimination diet includes only water, broth, white rice, boiled chicken, and egg whites); or using the low-FODMAP diet for at least 1 month (see Chapter 15).

Although some providers recommend empiric treatment with antibiotics, which eliminates unnecessary breath tests, a positive response to the antibiotic does not provide any insight into the underlying cause of the symptoms. Patients who respond to antibiotics may really have had SIBO, or their results might have been due to a change in colonic bacteria (or were simply a placebo response). For many people who have IBS and excessive gas and bloating, it does not matter why their symptoms improved—they just want to feel better. Other treatments for gas and bloating are discussed in Chapter 19.

Summary

- Small intestine bacterial overgrowth (SIBO) occurs when abnormal amounts of colonic bacteria migrate from the colon into the small intestine.
- SIBO can cause significant problems with gas, bloating, distention, and diarrhea.
- SIBO is present in some, but not all, people who have IBS.
- SIBO cannot be diagnosed by x-rays, upper endoscopies, CT scans, blood work, or colonoscopies. It is most commonly diagnosed using a breath hydrogen test.
- Treatment of SIBO typically involves a nonabsorbable antibiotic.

CHAPTER 12

IBS versus IBD

Many people who have irritable bowel syndrome are concerned that they have been misdiagnosed; they believe that they have inflammatory bowel disease (IBD), not IBS. Perhaps they think they have been misdiagnosed because the names of the two disorders are similar or maybe because IBS is sometimes mistakenly called "colitis." Many people who have IBS have heard about complications associated with IBD, and they worry that they will need surgery. Other people mistakenly believe that IBS is a precursor to IBD, meaning that if they have IBS, they will eventually develop IBD. A clinical research study designed to measure attitudes and concerns of people who have IBS found that 30 percent of the study population believed that IBS turns into IBD.

Chapters 3 and 5 of this book discuss how IBS can develop for many different reasons, how its symptoms can be bothersome and intrusive, and how the symptoms can be chronic for many people. These chapters also state that IBS never turns into anything dangerous or life threatening, such as IBD or colon cancer. The following case study describes a patient who was concerned that his symptoms were consistent with IBD and not IBS. Later on in this chapter, I'll summarize information about the two most common inflammatory bowel diseases: Crohn's disease and ulcerative colitis.

Christopher is a 23-year-old graduate student whose physician sent him for a second opinion in gastroenterology due to concerns that he had IBD. Christopher first noticed symptoms during college. He often had episodes of urgent diarrhea in association with lower abdominal cramps. He reported that sometimes he had the urge to have a bowel movement but only passed mucus. He felt tired and wasn't sleeping well. He was concerned because his second cousin had similar symptoms and had been diagnosed with Crohn's disease.

Christopher went to his university's student health center, where he underwent a careful physical examination that did not show anything abnormal. The physician noted that Christopher's weight was stable and, focusing on his concerns about possible Crohn's disease, she did a careful examination of his eyes, mouth, joints, and skin. She did not find any evidence of extra-intestinal Crohn's disease (see definition later in this chapter). Blood work (CBC and erythrocyte sedimentation rate [ESR]) came back normal, showing no evidence of an infection, inflammation, or anemia. Stool studies from one of Christopher's episodes of diarrhea all came back normal as well. The student health center physician told Christopher that many of his symptoms were consistent with IBS and that it was possible that stress was precipitating some of his episodes. She suggested some dietary changes and the as-needed use of loperamide.

Christopher took these suggestions to heart but was still concerned that his symptoms represented something other than IBS. The health center physician referred him to a gastroenterologist at the university hospital, who reviewed his medical history, carefully examined his family's medical history, studied his diet for foods that can prompt symptoms mimicking IBS, and investigated alternative diagnoses such as celiac disease. Christopher's physical examination was again normal, and the gastroenterologist stated that he did not believe that Christopher had Crohn's disease or the other common inflammatory bowel disease, ulcerative colitis, but that the only way to be certain was to perform more blood work and a colonoscopy.

Because Christopher had done more Internet research and had learned that Crohn's disease was most common in young adults and could be hard to diagnose, he decided to undergo further testing. His blood work (a repeat CBC and ESR) and colonoscopy of the entire colon and lower small intestine (terminal ileum), including random biopsies of the lower small intestine and colon, were normal. Although this news seemed to reassure Christopher, during the next two years, he continued to have intermittent symptoms of lower abdominal cramps, spasms, pain, urgency, loose stools, and the passage of mucus. He discussed his symptoms with his parents, who told him that his mother's aunt had "colitis," although they weren't sure of the exact type. This news made Christopher nervous, and he sought out the advice of another gastroenterologist.

Dr. Schneider went over Christopher's medical history, questioning him about other family members, his stress levels, and his diet. She reviewed his previous diagnostic tests and medical treatments and noted that he had gained weight during the past two years. Dr. Schneider and Christopher discussed how he did not have GI symptoms and felt well when he was on vacation or during long holidays. She acknowledged his concerns about Crohn's disease and spent time with him reviewing the prevalence rates of Crohn's disease (uncommon) compared to IBS (common). In addition, she reviewed his test results with him and showed him the data indicating that having very distant relatives with IBD did not increase his risk of having IBD.

When Dr. Schneider asked Christopher about his concerns and fears, he reiterated that he was sure that he had Crohn's disease and speculated that maybe it had not yet been detected because it was Crohn's disease of the small intestine. Dr. Schneider acknowledged that approximately one-third of people who have Crohn's disease have only small bowel disease, and that it could have been missed during Christopher's colonoscopy (which only examined the colon and the lowermost part of the small intestine, the terminal ileum). The two discussed the risks and benefits of different tests and medications. Christopher stated that he didn't want to take any more medications (although the loperamide did help his symptoms of diarrhea) but that he did want to be sure of the diagnosis. They agreed to repeat the blood count and to perform another test to look for inflammation in the bloodstream (C-reactive protein) as well as to have Christopher get an x-ray test of his small intestine (upper GI series with small bowel follow-through). All test results were normal.

Christopher now felt more relieved knowing that, over the course of three years, he had not developed any additional symptoms, his blood count had remained normal, and all of his test results were normal (three separate tests to look for inflammation, stool studies, and specialized tests to evaluate the colon and small intestine). He recognized that Crohn's disease is uncommon compared to IBS, and he learned that having very distant relatives who have IBD probably does not increase his risk of developing IBD (although having a first-degree relative who has IBD does). With this information in mind, Christopher focused on a stress reduction program involving exercise, a more regular schedule, yoga, and visits to a social worker to discuss proactive methods to reduce stress. He followed up with the student health center physician and, several months later, he noted a significant improvement in his symptoms with only the occasional use of loperamide.

What Is the Difference between IBS and IBD?

In contrast to IBS, inflammatory bowel diseases are not very common. In the United States, approximately 7 out of 100,000 people have Crohn's disease and 80 out of 100,000 have ulcerative colitis (UC). IBS affects approximately 15,000 out of every 100,000 people.

Crohn's disease and UC are often characterized as autoimmune disorders, which means that they develop because the body starts to attack itself, causing inflammation in the GI tract. With people who have Crohn's disease or UC, it is unclear whether their bodies are trying to attack a foreign pathogen or antigen (an appropriate response) or whether their bodies get confused and attack themselves for unknown reasons (an inappropriate response). Regardless of the type of response, this autoimmune process distinguishes Crohn's disease and UC from IBS, which is not an autoimmune disorder.

Also unlike IBS, Crohn's disease and UC are characterized by inflammation in the GI tract. People who have Crohn's disease may have ulcers and inflammation anywhere from the mouth to the anus, whereas inflammation is limited to the colon and anorectal area in people who have UC. In both cases, the inflammation is usually easy to see during a colonoscopy. (Although the colon of a person who has IBS may not function normally, it appears normal when inspected during a colonoscopy.)

A final difference between IBS and IBD is that the majority of patients with Crohn's disease, and many patients with UC, eventually require surgery. Individuals who have IBS never require surgery specifically for their IBS symptoms. With these key differences in mind, let's review the two most common forms of IBD: Crohn's disease and ulcerative colitis.

Crohn's Disease

Crohn's disease was formally recognized as a disease in 1932, although medical reports from the mid-1700s describe patients with similar symptoms. Crohn's disease is not common—it affects only 7 to 10 out of every 100,000 people. Although it is most frequently diagnosed in people ages 15 to 30, research studies have shown a small second "peak" in the age of diagnoses, meaning that a substantial number of people are diagnosed with Crohn's disease for the first time in their seventies. In terms of sex, slightly more women are diagnosed with Crohn's disease than men.

Unfortunately, similar to the case with IBS, the exact cause of Crohn's disease is unknown. Clearly, a genetic predisposition exists for the development of Crohn's disease. If you have a first-degree relative with the disease, your risk of developing it is 14 to 15 times higher than the general population (recognizing, of course, that Crohn's disease is uncommon, so your risk may increase from 7 to 10 out of 100,000 to 100 to 150 out of 100,000—still fairly low odds). Genetic susceptibility has also been demonstrated in twin studies, in which an identical (monozygotic) twin had Crohn's disease and her or his twin sibling had nearly a 2 in 3 chance of developing it as well. For reasons not completely known, Ashkenazi Jews are more likely to develop Crohn's than non-Jews (genetic testing has identified an area on chromosome 16 that may be involved).

Other theories about the cause of Crohn's disease include previous viral or bacterial infections, stress, and smoking (Crohn's disease is more prevalent among smokers). However, many experts believe that Crohn's disease may be triggered by a simple virus or bacterium that combines with a food substance or normal colonic bacteria. This combination is detected by the immune system as "foreign," initiating an immune response leading to inflammation in the GI tract.

No matter the cause, Crohn's disease is a persistent immune response in which the body attacks itself and causes inflammation in the GI tract (anywhere from the mouth to the anorectum). Although one of the defining characteristics of Crohn's disease is a small superficial ulcer (called an apthous ulcer), over time, Crohn's disease can affect the entire thickness of the intestinal tract, which can lead to significant scarring and the formation of strictures (narrowing of the GI tract). The inflammation can be so severe that it goes through the lining of the GI tract and affects adjacent organs, such as the bladder, uterus, vagina, and even the skin (inflammation that goes from the GI tract to another organ is called a fistula).

Symptoms of Crohn's disease depend on the section of the GI tract involved and the extent of involvement. Half of all people who have Crohn's disease have disease of the small intestine and colon. Approximately one-third have Crohn's disease limited to just the small intestine. A few people have only colonic involvement, and the rare person has Crohn's disease of the esophagus or stomach. Abdominal pain (often in the area around the umbilicus [belly button], but it can be anywhere in the abdomen) is the most common symptom of Crohn's disease. Patients may have loose stools and occasional low-grade fevers, and they may lose weight. In addition, many patients have extra-intestinal manifestations of Crohn's disease, such as inflammation in the eyes (episcleritis and uveitis), arthritis, back pain, ulcers in the mouth, and skin ulcers.

Physicians use a mixture of different tests to diagnose a person with Crohn's disease. A combination of appropriate symptoms and typical findings (e.g., ulcers in the mouth and on the shin and inflammation in the eyes) on physical examination is the first step to diagnosis. Blood work may show evidence of anemia; unlike with people who have IBS, blood tests that identify inflammation in the body (such as ESR and CRP) are usually elevated in people who have Crohn's disease. Stool studies may show evidence of blood and inflammatory cells in the stool (these are both absent in stool studies of people who have IBS). Finally, most patients who have suspected Crohn's disease undergo a colonoscopy and an x-ray study of the small intestine, and these two tests usually show evidence of ulceration and inflammation in the GI tract.

Treatment for Crohn's disease is complicated and depends on the patient. Unlike treatment for IBS, steroids are frequently used, as are very potent drugs called immunomodulators, which are designed to suppress the immune system and hopefully stop or minimize the autoimmune response. Finally, people who have Crohn's disease are at an increased risk of developing cancer of the small intestine and colon, and up to 70 percent will eventually require some type of surgery for their disease. Again, this is in stark contrast to the treatment of people who have IBS, who will never require surgery specifically for their IBS symptoms.

Ulcerative Colitis

Ulcerative colitis, the most common inflammatory bowel disease, was formally recognized as a disease in 1859. Approximately 80 to 120 of every 100,000 people have UC, and it appears to affect men and women equally. Although people of any age group may have ulcerative colitis, it is most common in people between the ages of 20 and 40. Similar to Crohn's disease, Ashkenazi Jews are more likely to have UC than non-Jews. Genetic predisposition to UC is likely although less common than in people who have Crohn's disease (approximately 10 percent of people who have UC have a first-degree relative with the disease). Twin studies support a genetic component to UC, although once again, much less so than twin studies of Crohn's disease. For example, if an identical twin has UC, the other twin has a 30 percent chance of having it (if this was purely a genetic disorder, the identical twin's risk of UC would be 100 percent).

As with IBS and Crohn's disease, the cause of UC is unknown. Most experts believe that for a person with a certain genetic background, an infection, an inflammatory process, or an abnormal response to a normal component of the GI tract (such as normal gut microflora) could trigger an autoimmune response and the development of severe inflammation. Strangely enough, smokers seem to be protected from UC (several studies have shown that nonsmokers are more likely to get UC than smokers). Researchers do not know why smoking might be protective for people who have ulcerative colitis but harmful for people who have Crohn's disease.

Ulcerative colitis generally begins in the rectum and then extends to varying degrees into the colon. Unlike Crohn's disease, it does not have the potential to affect the mouth, esophagus, stomach, or small intestine. In approximately 50 percent of people who have UC, it is limited to the rectum and sigmoid colon. Thirty percent have inflammation that begins in the rectum and extends past the sigmoid colon but does not reach all the way around the colon to the cecum. Approximately 20 percent of people who have UC have an inflammatory process that affects their entire colon, which is called pancolitis. Ulcerative colitis is different from Crohn's disease because it only affects the surface of the colon; it does not burrow through the many layers of the bowel wall and thus can't directly affect other organs.

The main symptoms of UC are diarrhea, bloody stools, abdominal pain, and the passage of mucus. Although these symptoms may appear similar to those of IBS, people who have UC usually notice blood mixed with their stool, or they only evacuate blood clots or bright red blood. Many people who have UC mistakenly think that the bleeding is due to hemorrhoids. No matter what the cause is, the presence of blood in the stool should always prompt a person to seek medical attention. When patients who have UC undergo flexible sigmoidoscopy or colonoscopy, it is clear that the blood loss is due to inflammation of the colon and not hemorrhoids. Similar to the case with Crohn's disease, people who have UC can have other problems outside of the colon, meaning that they may develop ulcers in their mouth or on their legs and arms, they may have inflammation in their eyes, or they may develop back pain or joint problems.

The diagnosis of UC is made because of a patient's history, stool samples, blood work, and examination of the colon with either sigmoid-oscopy or colonoscopy (see Chapter 8). A history of abdominal pain with diarrhea and evidence of bleeding warrants immediate blood work (CBC), to check for anemia and to rule out an infection, as well as stool studies to rule out an infection of the colon. Many patients who have UC are mildly anemic due to blood loss from the chronically inflamed colon. Stool studies are used to rule out an infection as the cause of the bleeding, because some GI infections (*Salmonella, Shigella, Campylobacter,* and *Yersinia*) cause bloody diarrhea. Although stool studies from patients who have UC usually show evidence of inflammation and red blood cells, they do not normally show evidence of an active bacterial or amoebic infection. Endoscopic examination of the colon shows inflammation in a person who has UC (inflammation is not seen in people who have IBS).

Endoscopy helps determine if the patient has UC limited to the anorectal area or lower colon or whether it involves the entire colon.

The treatment of UC includes either topical or oral medications that are designed to minimize inflammation and suppress the immune system. The type of medication depends on whether the disease is located only in the lower colon or the entire colon. For patients who have UC located only in the anorectal area and/or sigmoid colon, medicated enemas may be all that is required. For individuals who have inflammation throughout their entire colon, treatment will include oral medications.

Unlike people who have IBS, people who have UC are at higher risk for colon cancer than the general population (the level of risk depends on the number of years with the disease). Some patients who have UC with persistent bleeding or severe inflammation of the colon may require surgery to remove the colon.

Summary

- IBS is frequently confused with IBD, even though these two disorders are completely different.
- The two most common types of inflammatory bowel disease (IBD) are Crohn's disease and ulcerative colitis (UC).
- Both Crohn's disease and UC involve inflammation in the colon, which can easily be seen by a physician during a colonoscopy. This inflammation is not present in people who have IBS.
- Both Crohn's disease and UC are treated with medications designed to stop the inflammation that occurs in the GI tract. These medications are quite different from those used to treat IBS.
- Many individuals who have Crohn's disease and UC eventually require surgery. In contrast, surgery is never needed to treat IBS symptoms.

PART III

Treating Irritable Bowel Syndrome

CHAPTER 13

Treatment Basics

When people consult a health care provider about symptoms they are experiencing, the provider tries to find the underlying cause (etiology) of the symptoms. A cardinal rule in medicine is that the most effective treatment for any medical condition treats the underlying cause rather than just the symptoms. If the originating condition (the etiology) is successfully treated, the disease will normally be cured and the symptoms resolve.

Unfortunately, the cause of irritable bowel syndrome remains unknown, so treatment cannot take this ideal approach but instead must focus on improving symptoms. This is a critical concept to understand, since at present we are not able to cure patients of IBS. While research on the causes of IBS continues, health care providers must concentrate their efforts on treating symptoms and improving patients' quality of life and ability to cope with a chronic medical problem.

Getting Started

How should treatment for IBS be initiated? Some general rules apply to all patients who have irritable bowel syndrome. First, successful management of the disease requires that the treating physician be well educated in the etiology, pathophysiology, and treatment of people who have IBS. Although this seems obvious, many people receive treatment from health care providers who do not actually know a great deal about IBS. It is important that patients find a provider who is intimately familiar with this disorder and has up-to-date information. New medical information becomes available every day, and it is difficult for any physician to remain current in every medical condition. If you are working with a physician who still believes that depression or anxiety is the cause of IBS or that the symptoms you are experiencing are "all in your head," then you would do well to search for a health care provider whose knowledge and understanding of IBS are more current.

Second, find a health care provider who is interested in treating patients who have IBS. Again, this seems an obvious point to make, but physicians are no different from anybody else. They have likes and dislikes. Some providers enjoy treating patients who have migraine headaches, while others do not. Some enjoy treating patients who have diabetes, while others do not. To maximize the likelihood of obtaining relief of your IBS symptoms, it is important to find a provider who not only has a current working knowledge of this problem but who also enjoys working with individuals who have IBS.

Specifically, find a health care provider who recognizes that, for most patients, IBS is a chronic disorder. Some physicians feel more comfortable treating people who have conditions that are acute and short lived rather than chronic in nature. Because IBS is a chronic disorder, both patient and physician need to accept the fact that they will be working together to manage the disease over the long term. If your provider is used to treating conditions that are short lived, then he or she may try to employ "quick fixes" that may not be helpful to you in the long run. You may want to ask friends, coworkers, and relatives about physicians they know who are experienced at treating this disorder (remember, since more than one in seven adults have IBS, it's fairly easy to find someone who has similar symptoms).

The treatment of IBS begins with the first interview and physical examination, which will usually establish a relationship of mutual interest and confidence between the patient and the physician. During this time, the physician should take a thorough history, paying special attention to the details of all contributing factors. These factors include diet, exercise, current and past medical history, surgical history, family history of medical problems, allergies and adverse drug reactions, medications, drug and alcohol use, emotional health, professional and interpersonal relationships, and the fears and concerns of the patient. Getting a thorough history is a big step toward determining whether the symptoms are caused by an organic problem or are all due to IBS. In addition, a thorough history is often reassuring to the patient, because it indicates that the doctor is taking the complaints seriously.

After taking an exhaustive history, the physician should perform a thorough physical examination. As discussed in Chapter 7, this part of the initial evaluation clarifies that there is not an organic cause for the symptoms, such as an ulcer, an infection, or a cancer in the colon or rectum. Many patients are reassured if no evidence of an organic disease is found during the physical exam.

If it looks likely that IBS is causing the symptoms, the health care provider should then explain to the patient the mechanisms that produce symptoms of IBS. This is a good time for an exchange of concerns and ideas between patient and physician. Questions can be answered and information verified. Although time in the initial appointment may have run out and a follow-up visit may need to be scheduled, the provider should next explain to the patient what to expect in the upcoming weeks and what to anticipate in the future, describing the natural history of IBS (see Chapter 5). The patient and physician should discuss the patient's hopes and expectations. The treatment goals of people who have IBS vary dramatically, depending on which symptoms bother them most. For example, some patients want to focus their treatment on constipation, while other patients are most eager for relief of bloating. This discussion should also include expectations about diagnostic testing, the benefits and side effects of medications, the possible need for referral to other physicians, and the timing of follow-up visits and phone calls.

Treating IBS is not a straightforward matter. Many patients and physicians mistakenly believe that there is a single therapy usable by all patients who have IBS. There are several reasons why no single treatment plan or medication can be used. First, there are three well-recognized subtypes of IBS (diarrhea predominant, constipation predominant, and IBS with mixed symptoms of alternating diarrhea and constipation). Each of these subtypes needs to be treated differently. Also, individual symptoms within each type vary widely. In a large group of people who have IBS and diarrhea, the frequency of diarrhea will vary significantly. Therefore, some patients may require only changes in diet, while others may require a combination of changes in diet and the use of several medications. The tremendous differences in patients' goals for therapy are another reason a single treatment can't apply to everyone. Finally, people differ in their response to specific therapies. While one patient may respond very well to a particular medication, another with virtually identical symptoms may not respond at all. Thus, the patient and physician must work together to find the best treatment for that individual's symptoms.

That being said, as with the treatment for other common diseases, the physician should still adhere to several common principles of treatment: patient education, providing guidelines on diet and exercise, and instituting medical (medicine) therapy, if appropriate. Along the way, the doctor should try to work with the patient to identify specific goals, so that an individualized treatment plan can be developed for that patient. Unlike some other medical problems, surgery is never a treatment for IBS symptoms. Finally, any treatment plan should include routine follow-up appointments. These scheduled follow-up appointments are critical in the treatment of IBS, because they allow both the patient and the physician time to carefully review the response to the current therapy, make changes in the treatment program if necessary, and identify further goals and endpoints. In addition, because advances continue to be made in the field of IBS treatment, routine follow-up appointments allow your health care provider to keep you up to date on research efforts involving diet, behavioral therapy, medications, and complementary and alternative therapies.

Probably, before you get around to consulting a health care provider about your symptoms, you will have received treatment suggestions from friends, family, coworkers, or even your pharmacist. You may also have read about treatment of IBS on the Internet or in magazines and books. Some of this information may be dated or incorrect, or it may not apply to you. Bring this information with you to your first appointment, along with a list of questions and concerns, so you can make your visit efficient and worthwhile (for more on this topic, see Chapter 23). Another approach that is useful to many people is keeping a diary of symptoms and daily routines to share with their physician. Diary entries can sometimes pinpoint precipitating (causal) or worsening factors (see Table 13.1 for a sample diary entry).

Table 13.1. Excerpt from an IBS Diary

Day	Pain	Bloating?	Bowel Habits	Notes
Mon. 8/14	OK— 1 brief episode	None	4 bowel movements before work	Late getting to work because of prolonged bathroom time.
Tues. 8/15	Bad—6 long episodes	Bad	6 bowel movements; nearly had an accident	Meeting at work; presentation in front of lots of people I didn't know; hamburger didn't agree.
Wed. 8/16	Bad—7 episodes	Feels like I'm pregnant	7; loose; lots of urgency	Getting ready to get major report in at work; lots of meetings; stressed.
Thurs. 8/17	Bad most of the day	Some	3 bowel movements in the morning	Report turned in; boss liked it.
Fri. 8/18	Great—no pain	None	None	Went to the movies; dinner out (hamburger and French fries); did great.
Sat. 8/19	Great—no pain	None	None	Went to the park; did some shopping; ate pizza.
Sun. 8/20	Mild—2 episodes	Lots—all after lunch	2 bowel movements after lunch	Visited friends; salad and soup for lunch; big ice cream sundae for dessert.
Mon. 8/21	Good	Less than yesterday	4 bowel movements before going to work	Okay once I got to work, but late getting there.
Tues. 8/22	Okay	Lots	3 loose bowel movements after lunch	Had salad and milkshake for lunch— tasted great.

(continued)

Table 13.1. *(continued)*

Day	Pain	Bloating?	Bowel Habits	Notes
Wed. 8/23	Terrible— worst ever	Severe	6 bowel movements	Bad day at work. We lost one of our major clients; didn't eat all day. Took 6 Imodium.
Thurs. 8/24	Terrible	Severe— very distended	8 bowel movements	Stayed home. Can't go to work because of the diarrhea. Took 6 Imodium.
Fri. 8/25	Bad	Bad	4 bowel movements	On rice and toast diet; stayed home; 8 Imodium.
Sat. 8/26	Good	Mild	None. Great day.	Went to the zoo; good day; ate pizza.
Sun. 8/27	Good	Lots after lunch	2 loose bowel movements after lunch	Visited a friend. Pizza for lunch and then some great ice cream for dessert.
Mon. 8/28	Okay	Mild	4 in the morning before work	Late for work again; in the bathroom a lot.

Keeping an IBS Diary

A characteristic of IBS is that the symptoms tend to occur in patterns. Some people have extremely good powers of recall and can accurately report their symptom patterns and bowel patterns to their physician. Other people have more difficulty recalling activities, meals, and symptoms, especially if they occurred more than a few days ago. Even people with the best of memories, however, can benefit from keeping a record of symptoms, ideally on a daily basis, during the course of a month. Although a month seems like a long time to write down all of this information, a shorter diary may not be as helpful or as accurate, because symptoms of IBS typically wax and wane over the course of about a month. Patients should record abdominal pain (location, intensity, and length of each painful episode), constipation, bloating, and/or diarrhea. Pain can be rated on a 0-to-10-point scale, with 0 being the absence of pain and 10 being the worst pain ever experienced. The number of bowel movements per day should be noted, along with their consistency. All of this information is important, and reporting it all to your doctor would be impossible without a written record. Many of us can't remember what we had for dinner two nights before a doctor's appointment, so it's unrealistic to try to recall the amount of bloating or the number of bowel movements from a month ago. Along with symptoms, individuals should also record significant occurrences of the day, such as stressful events at home, school, or work (meetings, presentations, financial discussions). Other information to record would be exercise, travel, diet, and responses to medication.

The information recorded in an IBS diary, in addition to being very useful to the treating physician, can help a patient uncover clues about what might be triggering symptoms. Clare's experience, and a week from her diary, illustrate how this works.

Clare is a 28-year-old woman who has had symptoms of irritable bowel syndrome for nearly 5 years. Her symptoms are mostly frequent, watery bowel movements with significant feelings of urgency before them. She has intermittent lower abdominal discomfort on most days. The discomfort increases to pain before an episode of diarrhea and generally eases afterwards. On some occasions, the sense of urgency has come on so suddenly that she has had to leave a meeting or social event and rush to the bathroom. She has been concerned that she might even have an accident. She had tried over-the-counter medications, including fiber products and Pepto-Bismol, without relief. She has used Imodium intermittently, and this seems to help to some degree. One of her friends told her that she probably had a wheat allergy, so she stopped using all wheat products for several weeks, but this did not seem to improve her symptoms.

Clare went to see Dr. Englar, her new primary care physician, who recorded a thorough history and performed a physical examination. Because Clare's symptoms had generally been stable for so long, she had not lost weight, and no one in her immediate family had a history of colorectal cancer, inflammatory bowel disease, or celiac disease, Dr.

Englar told Clare that she probably had IBS with diarrhea. She suggested that they continue the evaluation by having some simple lab tests (CBC, TSH, and ESR) done on a sample of Clare's blood. Stool cultures seemed unnecessary; it was unlikely that this was a viral, bacterial, or parasitic infection, since the symptoms had lasted for five years and Clare used only city water or bottled water, did not camp, and had not traveled outside of the country recently. They discussed starting a medication for IBS with diarrhea, but Clare wanted to avoid medications, if possible.

Clare raised the issue of whether stress could be playing a role in the symptoms and also asked about the effect of diet. Dr. Englar suggested that a good way to identify whether stress or diet was playing a role in Clare's symptoms would be to keep a daily diary for a month and then return for a follow-up visit to review the behavior of Clare's symptoms. Clare agreed that this was a reasonable approach. A sample of Clare's diary is shown as Table 13.1.

When Clare returned for her follow-up appointment, she and Dr. Englar carefully reviewed the diary. Two points came to light almost immediately. It seemed that Clare consistently had more frequent or looser bowel movements after consuming dairy products. Also, the amount of milk product she took in seemed to make a difference. If she ate just a small amount (like one slice of pizza), then she did fine. However, if she ate large amounts or multiple dairy products (pizza and ice cream), diarrhea always followed. Dr. Englar felt that this was pretty good evidence that Clare also had some degree of lactose intolerance (discussed in Chapter 10).

The diary also revealed that Clare's symptoms were always worse on Mondays and on days when things were especially hectic at work. It was also interesting that Clare's symptoms were consistently better on weekends. Dr. Englar asked Clare how her symptoms were when she was on vacation, and Clare realized that her symptoms were always the least troublesome during vacations. Clare admitted that she found her job stressful, and she could see from the diary that her symptoms always got worse during times of stress.

Clare and Dr. Englar discussed these two findings and formulated a plan that focused on dietary changes and stress management. Clare agreed to keep a diary for another two months while following the plan and then to review the diary together and see if these strategies improved her symptoms.

This case story highlights the value of keeping a diary. It allowed Clare to readily pinpoint two contributing factors to her IBS symptoms—stress and excess lactose intake. Not every individual will so easily identify precipitating factors or events, and many people find keeping a daily diary to be a nuisance or outright burdensome. However, this safe, easy, and cheap method produces positive results for many people.

Summary

- The focus of treating patients who have IBS is to improve symptoms and quality of life. Caring for the patient is the preeminent goal, since we can't cure the disorder at present.
- Find a health care provider who is both interested in treating patients who have IBS and knowledgeable about the disorder.
- All people who have IBS are unique. Thus, different treatment strategies need to be employed for different patients. There is no single pathway that can be used to treat all individuals who have IBS.
- Use a symptom diary to track symptoms to try and identify factors or events that might precipitate or worsen symptoms.

CHAPTER 14

Lifestyle Modifications

How Useful Are Lifestyle Modifications?

These days, people are better informed about health matters than at any other time in history. Many people know the risks and benefits of medications and have opinions on the usefulness of specialized tests, and nearly everyone knows about the importance of diet and exercise. Physicians, as well as family members, coworkers, and friends will commonly recommend exercise and lifestyle modifications to each other for a variety of medical conditions. These modifications (losing weight, decreasing fat intake, increasing dietary intake of fresh fruits and vegetables, cutting back on red meat intake) are known to improve a variety of disease symptoms, positively influence mood and emotional health, and prolong life. Certainly, they have benefits for people who have diabetes, hypertension, arthritis, and heart disease. Do similar recommendations apply to people who have irritable bowel syndrome? Are there data to support the use of exercise and lifestyle modifications for people who have IBS?

The role of lifestyle modifications in the treatment of IBS has not been well studied, for reasons that are easy to appreciate. First of all, patients and physicians all have different definitions of "lifestyle modifications." You can't test the effect of something that is undefined. For example, if we were designing a study to test whether adopting a less stressful lifestyle improved the health of people who have IBS with diarrhea, how would we define "less stressful lifestyle"? It would be different for each participant. How would we *measure* responses to lifestyle modifications? Should we use only objective measures, such as the number of days with constipation or the number of days with diarrhea, or should we try to quantify subjective measures, such as sensations of abdominal pain or bloating after changes in diet or medication? If we used these subjective measures of symptoms, what rating scale would help us tabulate the results?

There is little information in the scientific literature about the effects of lifestyle modifications on people who have IBS. One well-designed scientific study described a small group of patients who were enrolled in a structured program that included lectures on diet, exercise, and different approaches to tackling the symptoms of IBS in a positive, constructive manner. According to the report, patients who completed the course felt that their abdominal pain lessened overall, but no significant improvements were observed with other symptoms.

Despite the lack of scientific data, physicians treating people who have IBS have learned from their patients about some lifestyle factors that can worsen IBS symptoms and some elements of daily life that, if addressed proactively, can improve IBS symptoms. These components include exercise, sleep, and stress reduction.

Exercise

Because a routine exercise program has been shown to positively influence the natural history of diabetes, hypertension, and cardiovascular disease, the benefits of exercise automatically apply to other diseases, such as IBS. Although little data in the past supported the role of exercise in the treatment of IBS, now three small research studies are worth mentioning.

A survey study that gathered information from a group of women, some of whom had IBS, found that the women who had IBS were generally less likely to be physically active than other women. However, the women who had IBS and were physically active were less likely to be bothered by some of their IBS symptoms than were women who had IBS but were less active. Another small study performed at the Mayo Clinic evaluated the effects of exercise as part of a multicomponent IBS treatment program. Patients who had IBS were enrolled in exercise classes and other classes that covered diet and stress reduction. Six months after completing the treatment program, some of these patients noted an improvement in their level of abdominal pain.

Although both of these studies lend some support to the notion that exercise may improve IBS symptoms, it is hard to know how much benefit patients can expect and whether all patients will improve if they embark on an exercise program. In an attempt to address some of these shortcomings, in a recently published study, researchers randomly assigned men and women who had IBS to either a treatment group, in which physical activity was encouraged during a 12-week period, or to a control group, in which patients were asked to maintain their typical lifestyle (not very active). The people who had IBS in the physical activity group were given advice by a physiotherapist to try to slowly increase their activity so that they were eventually participating in 3 to 5 sessions per week (of a variety of exercises) that would last 20 to 60 minutes per session. A variety of measurements and questionnaires were performed at the beginning and at the end of the study, and the groups were evenly matched with regard to age, sex, race, educational level, employment status, type of IBS, and severity of IBS. The researchers reported that patients who participated in the 12-week exercise program had a significant reduction in the severity of their IBS symptoms. Individuals in the exercise group also noted some improvement in their overall quality of life (through a validated scoring system). This study provides good evidence that physical activity improves IBS symptoms.

Although the precise mechanism by which physical activity improves IBS symptoms is unknown, it may be related to a reduction in stress, an improvement in constipation symptoms, or an improvement in the transit of intestinal gas, which may lead to an improvement in bloating. Further research is needed to confirm these results, but exercise is now something I routinely recommend to my patients who have IBS.

Sleep

Sleep disturbances (often referred to as disordered sleep) are common in the general population. Disordered sleep includes not being able to fall asleep, awakening too early and not being able to go back to sleep, having fragmented sleep (a pattern of falling asleep and then awakening that occurs repeatedly throughout the night), waking up not feeling refreshed, and having very shallow (or light) sleep. Other than the obvious problems of feeling exhausted and having difficulty concentrating or performing tasks the day after a poor night's sleep, disordered sleep can contribute to other health problems, such as cardiovascular disease, obesity, and mood disorders. Some researchers estimate that nearly 50 percent of the general population experiences some symptoms of insomnia each week.

Although more research needs to be done regarding sleep and IBS, disordered sleep may worsen IBS symptoms in some people. Nearly 25 years ago, a study showed that 30 percent of people who had IBS experienced poor sleep, compared to just 5 percent of a control group who did not have IBS (note that this number is much lower than the 50 percent mentioned above because the researchers from the earlier study used a very strict definition of poor sleep). Several years later, a small prospective study showed that 74 percent of people who had IBS characterized themselves as being "poor sleepers." These people also reported that more severe IBS symptoms in the morning correlated with poor sleep the night before (a finding that was confirmed several years later in a study of women who had IBS).

Symptoms of IBS undoubtedly reduce a person's quality of life. The term "quality of life" refers to a general measure of a patient's daily well-being and is meant to include physical and mental (psychological) symptoms. Multiple studies have clearly demonstrated that IBS symptoms detract from the daily home, professional, and social life of a patient. One IBS research study determined that poor sleep was another independent factor that contributes to the reduced quality of life for people who have IBS. This finding emphasizes that treatment for IBS can't rely on just one component (such as only treating bloating). Rather, an effective treatment plan needs to address the many different factors that contribute to the development of IBS symptoms, and disordered sleep is one of those factors.

Because such a large number of people who have IBS also experience disordered sleep, researchers have logically questioned whether IBS causes poor sleep or whether poor sleep causes IBS. The answer is probably a combination of both. Symptoms of bloating, intestinal gas, and abdominal pain could definitely prevent falling asleep or cause disrupted sleep. The following day, poor sleep may worsen IBS symptoms, creating a vicious cycle. Although not yet studied in individuals who have IBS, there is evidence from sleep studies that poor sleep decreases a person's pain thresholds. This means that pain is more easily sensed after a night of poor sleep than after a night of good sleep. Many people feel a little bit more irritable or "edgy" after a poor night's sleep. For a person who has IBS and is already more sensitive to gut stimulation than other individuals, a night of disrupted sleep is likely to worsen IBS symptoms.

The treatment for disordered sleep is very individualized. Similar to the treatment for IBS, one size does not fit all. I usually recommend these simple steps:

- Routine bedtime and routine awakening time is helpful. Don't allow your sleep schedule to change every day. The body generally likes routines, so try to go to bed at approximately the same time each night and get up at the same time each morning (this includes weekends and holidays).
- Your bedroom should be cool and dark. An overly hot bedroom disrupts sleep.
- Get into a routine before going to bed. This may mean a warm shower or bath 30 to 60 minutes before bedtime (but not overly hot), reading for 30 minutes, or watching a little bit of TV.
- Consider having "background" noise in the bedroom. This can mean a fan on low speed, "white noise," or soft, soothing music.
- Think of your bedroom as your "retreat." Don't use your bedroom as your TV room, playroom, or office. The idea is to trick your brain into thinking that once in the bedroom, it's time for sleep.
- Naps can backfire. If necessary, a brief nap after lunch or in the very early afternoon is okay, but nothing longer than 20 to 30 minutes.

- Don't go to bed overly hungry or overly full. If you missed dinner, consider having a light snack one to two hours before bed (for example, a piece of fruit and a few crackers). Don't eat a large meal and go right to bed—you might have severe acid reflux, which will keep you up. Also, monitor the volume of fluids that you drink in the evening. You don't want to have an overly full bladder that awakens you.
- Avoid caffeine after lunch (or at least no caffeine-containing product of any kind six hours before bedtime).
- Try to exercise each day to reduce IBS symptoms and to improve sleep. But don't exercise three to four hours before bed, because this may make falling asleep more difficult.
- Don't use alcohol as a method of falling asleep. It is okay to have a glass of wine or a drink with dinner; however, three to four drinks right before bed may make you fall asleep faster but will disrupt your sleep overall, making you more tired and edgy (and, of course, drinking so much alcohol will ultimately injure your liver).
- If you awaken and cannot fall back asleep within 15 to 20 minutes, don't stay in bed for hours tossing and turning. Get up, leave the bedroom, and sit in another room to read, knit, or watch TV until you are sleepy. Then, return to bed.

If these suggestions do not work after a trial period of two to three weeks, then you should talk to your doctor about over-the-counter or prescription sleep medications. Keep in mind that some sleep medications can become habit-forming, meaning that you will constantly require them to get any sleep, you may have more sleep problems if you stop them, and you may need ever-increasing doses to get some sleep. In addition, although sleep medications may help you sleep, they may cause grogginess the next morning or a feeling of being "hung over."

Over-the-Counter Medications

Melatonin. A natural hormone, it is found in the body and is involved in the normal sleep-wake cycle. Melatonin is commonly used to prevent or minimize jet lag. It is sold at most pharmacies and health food stores and is reasonably priced. Melatonin is generally considered quite safe, although some people report feeling a little dizzy or fatigued the day after taking it. It has the potential to interfere or interact with blood-thinning medications (such as Coumadin) and oral contraceptives, so you should check with your doctor before taking it. A good starting dose is 1 mg taken approximately 1 hour before bedtime. If your sleep does not improve after 1 week, then increase to 2 mg each night (again, 1 hour before bedtime). If it still isn't helping with your sleep problem, add an additional 1 mg dose every 7 to 10 days, until you are taking 8 mg a night total. At that point, if you are still having sleep problems, then melatonin is probably not the medication for you, and you should slowly cut back on the dose (decrease by 1 mg every 3 to 4 days) until you are completely off the medication. Stopping melatonin all at once isn't thought to be dangerous, but you may notice a temporary worsening of your insomnia. Long-term trials evaluating melatonin's safety and efficacy are not available; for that reason, most physicians recommend that it only be used for short-term relief (two months or less).

Valerian. A plant supplement available at most health food stores, valerian has not been well tested. Although it is unknown exactly how valerian helps people with their sleep problems, many people who prefer to use alternative medications believe it is helpful. Some people report that it causes mild abdominal distress or a feeling of irritability. Doses vary based on how it was manufactured—you will want to speak to the owner of the health food store to get reliable information about its use.

Diphenhydramine (Benadryl). An antihistamine, diphenhydramine is traditionally used to treat mild seasonal allergies or allergic reactions. A side effect of this medication is that it causes fatigue and sleepiness in some individuals. It is generally considered safe, but it can cause a dry mouth, fatigue the following day, and a feeling of grogginess. In the rare patient it can cause blurry vision, memory problems, or urinary retention (difficulty emptying the bladder). You should not take diphenhydramine if you have glaucoma or if you drink alcohol. It is sold in different doses and forms; usually 12.5 mg taken 1 hour before bedtime is a good place to start (some people require 25 mg each night).

Doxylamine. This is another antihistamine with the same potential side effects as diphenhydramine (Benadryl).

Other agents. A variety of other over-the-counter (OTC) agents are available. One example is "I Sleep Soundly." Keep in mind that many of these OTC agents are sold as supplements and thus are not regulated or tested by the FDA.

Prescription Medications

Many sleep medications are now available by prescription. The number of choices available highlights how common sleep disorders are in the general population and also points out that no single medication is right for all people with disordered sleep. Currently available medications include eszopiclone (Lunesta), zolpidem (Ambien), ramelteon (Rozerem), and zaleplon (Sonata). All of these medications have side effects, and all require a careful discussion with your health care provider to review risks and benefits of the medication, especially if you are taking other prescription or over-the-counter medications, to prevent dangerous drug interactions.

Stress Reduction

We live in a stressful world, and most of us encounter stress every day. Stress is different for different people. For some people, stress may be due to work or relationships. For others, stress may be related to health issues or financial issues. Some people are able to deal with stress at work but have a very difficult time dealing with financial stress. Others find that dealing with stress from difficult family situations is easy, but dealing with stress from a chronic medical or psychological illness is nearly insurmountable. Because stress comes in so many forms, a "one-size-fits-all" treatment program won't work. Here is a list of suggestions on how to reduce stress that you may want to think about incorporating into your daily routine:

- Exercise. In addition to helping with sleep, daily exercise has been shown to reduce stress. This does not mean that you have to spend thousands of dollars on work-out equipment or a gym membership. Daily exercise can easily be incorporated into your routine by taking a walk at lunch, biking on weekends or in the evenings, and climbing extra stairs.

- Make a list. Stress can develop from a sense of being overwhelmed by life's multiple daily activities. Sit down every night after dinner and make a list of things to accomplish the next day. Make sure that the list is reasonable—don't set out such a massive agenda that you fail, which will only worsen your stress.
- Meditation. Finding time to sit quietly and relax and reflect on the day, or the day yet to come, can help relieve stress.
- Deep breathing. As simple as it seems, standing or sitting quietly and taking several long deep breaths (and holding them) during a 3- to 5-minute period can greatly reduce stress and provide an immediate sense of calm. Doing this in a quiet, dark area is even better.
- Laugh. Many medical studies have shown that people who have fun, laugh, and play are less likely to suffer from stress, high blood pressure, and heart disease than those who do not. So, have fun with your friends, tell a joke, and laugh about old times.
- Socialize with friends. Work can consume people and create stress. Make sure that you take time each week to socialize with friends, family, and neighbors. Do not be a loner. Make the extra effort, if necessary, to connect with someone at work, at church, or in your neighborhood.
- Get a pet. The health benefits of having a pet are well known. Pets reduce stress, improve mood, and help reduce blood pressure.
- Volunteer. If you are feeling overwhelmed and stressed due to demands at home and at work, it can be hard to imagine finding time to donate to others. However, volunteering at a food bank, shelter, church, local school, or civic center can greatly improve your stress level. Giving to others will improve your negative feelings and may help put the chaos of everyday life into perspective.

Summary

- Although we have limited data about the effects of lifestyle changes on IBS symptoms, routine exercise appears to improve IBS symptoms.
- Poor sleep is common in people who have IBS and may change pain thresholds. Improving sleep will usually improve IBS symptoms.

- People can reduce their stress in a variety of ways. If one approach does not work, don't give up—just try another.
- Most physicians who specialize in treating people who have IBS believe that routines are important. The GI tract in individuals who have IBS seems to function better on a set schedule. Meals, exercise time, sleep, and trips to the bathroom should fit into a schedule that is maintained throughout the week, including weekends.

CHAPTER 15

Diet Modifications

As discussed in Chapter 10, significant controversy exists regarding the role of diet in the treatment of irritable bowel syndrome. This controversy continues because of the diversity of IBS symptoms, the variety of ways individuals respond to certain foods, the difficulty of determining which food is causing the symptoms, and the overlap between IBS, food intolerances, food sensitivities, and food allergies.

For the majority of people who have IBS, symptoms wax and wane over time. Symptoms can fluctuate daily, making it difficult to tell whether a particular food has affected a person's symptoms. Many people who have IBS say that a specific food seems to cause problems one day (more bloating, more gas, more diarrhea) but be well tolerated on other days. This lack of consistency makes it hard to determine the relationship between eating certain foods and the occurrence of symptoms. Keeping an IBS diary, as described in Chapter 13, is helpful when making such a determination.

People respond differently to particular foods and to specific dietary changes. One person who has IBS may react with severe cramping and diarrhea to a food that presents no problem to another person who also has IBS with diarrhea. One patient may obtain great success with a certain diet, whereas another person experiences no improvement at all. Irritable bowel syndrome is a complex disorder. Even if patients have similar symptoms, the triggers for those symptoms may be quite different, so they can't all be treated in an identical manner.

In some individuals who have IBS, there is a direct relationship between consuming a certain food and experiencing symptoms shortly thereafter. Such people may be tempted to think that avoiding that food will cure their IBS. Although certain foods may trigger or worsen IBS symptoms, they are not the cause of the syndrome. The underlying mechanisms of IBS include abnormal gut motility, visceral hypersensitivity, prior infections, changes in colonic flora, and heightened brain-gut interactions (see Chapter 3). IBS symptoms are expressed differently among patients, and some people have food triggers that others do not. Avoidance of a problem food may lead to an improvement in some symptoms but will not produce complete resolution of all IBS symptoms.

Clinicians, researchers, and patients now have more information about specific foods, or food groups, that seem to worsen IBS symptoms for some people. Lactose intolerance, fructose intolerance, and sensitivity to fermentable foods, gluten, and carbohydrates appear to be the most bothersome conditions for people who have IBS. Diet modifications for each of these conditions are described below.

Avoiding Lactose

For people who have symptoms of IBS, a period of abstinence from dairy products is usually helpful to determine which symptoms, and the proportion of those symptoms, are due to lactose intolerance as opposed to IBS. I usually recommend 7 to 10 days of absolutely no dairy products as a reasonable trial. During this time, the patient is asked to maintain a diary of GI symptoms. If symptoms improve during this time period, then the patient probably has some degree of lactose intolerance. Milk products are then slowly reintroduced into the diet, typically by adding 2 to 3 ounces every day in any form the patient desires. This gradual reintroduction allows the individual to determine where her or his threshold is and make appropriate dietary adjustments.

If people find it difficult to withhold milk products from their diet or to follow symptoms closely while reintroducing them, a milk challenge test can be easily performed at home. This test is simpler and speedier but less detailed and more uncomfortable than the milk cessation trial. In this method of determining whether lactose intolerance is present, the person is asked to drink two pints (32 oz) of low-fat milk in one sitting.

Anyone who can drink this quantity of milk and not develop any symptoms of gas, bloating, abdominal distention, or diarrhea is not lactose intolerant.

Lactose intolerance can also be assessed in the laboratory. After fasting overnight, the patient drinks a predetermined quantity of lactose, usually 25 to 50 gm, dissolved in water. The patient is then asked to blow into a tube every 15 minutes for approximately 3 hours. The level of hydrogen gas in each exhalation is measured (this is similar to the breath hydrogen test to look for evidence of small intestine bacterial overgrowth, described in Chapter 11). Patients who are not lactose intolerant will have consistent levels of breath hydrogen during the three-hour study period, because the lactose is broken down slowly in the small intestine and absorbed by the body. Patients who are lactose intolerant, however, will have an increase in the amount of breath hydrogen in 1½ to 2½ hours, approximately the time it takes for the lactose to travel through the small intestine and reach the beginning of the colon, where it encounters the colonic bacteria, producing a sharp rise in breath hydrogen. I do not recommend the breath hydrogen test for the vast majority of patients who may be lactose intolerant, because it is somewhat expensive to perform and may not offer any more information than a simple milk challenge test (which costs the price of a quart of milk) or the milk abstinence trial. It can be helpful, however, for those individuals with confusing symptoms, those who seem to be intolerant to even small portions of milk products, and those who continue to have symptoms despite avoiding milk or using a lactase supplement.

Identifying lactose intolerance is important for people who have IBS because it may lead to a significant reduction in some symptoms. (Obviously, if all symptoms disappear, then the true diagnosis for the patient was *only* lactose intolerance, not IBS *and* lactose intolerance.) Many individuals who have lactose intolerance are unaware that they are intolerant to milk, which complicates treatment, because medications designed to treat IBS won't help the symptoms caused by lactose intolerance. Sorting this issue out allows the patient and the physician to better understand which symptoms occur because of dietary problems and which symptoms occur due to IBS and to appropriately treat both.

For treating lactose intolerance, pills containing lactase are available over the counter at most grocery stores and pharmacies. People who have lactose intolerance should take one or more pills before they consume a milk product (the dose depends on the level of lactose intolerance and the size of the serving of dairy food). Lactase-supplemented milk products are sold under the brand name Lactaid. Patients who are strongly lactose intolerant are advised to use soy milk, rice milk, almond milk, or lactaid-100 milk (in which 100 percent of the lactose is already broken down). Lactose-free cheeses and other products (for instance, ice cream made from rice or soy) are also available.

Some people note that they can tolerate a serving of dairy if ingested with a meal (such as drinking a glass of milk with dinner). Taking the dairy product with a meal causes the dairy product to move more slowly through the GI tract, allowing for increased absorption of calcium and Vitamin D and decreased symptoms of gas and bloating. Other patients are able to tolerate dairy products more easily if they slowly add a small amount of dairy to their daily routine over the course of several months. Because nearly all of the milk sugar has been broken down during its production, yogurt can be a good way to take in protein, calcium, and Vitamin D. Very hard cheeses (extra sharp cheddar, parmesan) have little lactose remaining and can also be well tolerated in small servings.

Finally, note that there are some clinical consequences to avoiding dairy products. Vitamin D and calcium are found in dairy products, and avoiding all dairy products may lead to Vitamin D deficiency and low levels of calcium, which can contribute to osteoporosis and possibly even hypertension. If necessary, both Vitamin D and calcium can be replaced with over-the-counter or prescription medications.

Avoiding Fructose

A simple way to determine whether some of your symptoms are the result of fructose intolerance rather than IBS is simply to avoid all fructose-containing liquids and foods—all carbonated drinks, all fruit juices, all types of sports drinks, and those fruits and vegetables that contain fructose (such as pears, apples, mangos, peaches, Mandarin oranges, watermelon, and pineapple). Continue this test for 7 to 10 days. If, during this trial, your symptoms of gassiness, bloating, and diarrhea improve, you are probably fructose intolerant to some degree. You can then gradually reintroduce small amounts of fructose-containing foods and liquids in an attempt to determine your threshold of tolerance (a reasonable goal is less than 25 gm of fructose per day). Alternatively, your doctor can schedule you for a fructose tolerance test. This test is similar to the breath hydrogen test used to diagnose lactose intolerance.

The Low-FODMAP Diet

The acronym FODMAP stands for Fermentable Oligo-, Di-, and Mono-saccharides and Polyols. This term is meant to group a variety of food products that are more likely to cause gas, bloating, and distention. These symptoms may develop because some of these food substances (such as fructose) are poorly absorbed in the small intestine and thus pass undigested into the colon, where they are broken down by colonic bacteria. Symptoms may also develop because many of these food substances are very small in size and, as such, draw water into the intestinal tract (making stool loose and watery). Finally, many of these food products are rapidly fermented by bacteria. The rate of fermentation of food products in the colon is determined by the length of the carbohydrate chain. The short-chain carbohydrates that should be avoided on the low-FODMAP diet are more rapidly fermented in the colon, and therefore they quickly cause distention and discomfort.

The low-FODMAP diet has received a lot of attention from the media and the medical community for a number of reasons. One, it is a diet and not a medication and thus, theoretically, it will usually not cause any adverse side effects. Two, since it is not a medication, it will normally not be expensive (however, there are always costs associated with changing your diet; some of these costs may be monetary, and other costs may include an investment of time). Three, since it is a diet, many patients and health care providers believe that it will be easy to institute and follow (not necessarily true—see the guidelines below). Finally, the low-FODMAP diet puts the patient in control and allows the patient to monitor his or her own symptoms.

If the goal of the low-FODMAP diet is to avoid foods that either can rapidly pass through the GI tract into the colon undigested or are more likely to ferment in the colon (and thereby to improve symptoms of gas, bloating, and diarrhea), then how should a person who has IBS modify his or her diet accordingly?

Foods to Avoid on the Low-FODMAP Diet

- Foods with excess fructose. This means fruits such as apples, cherries, mango, pears, peaches, canned fruits in their natural fruit juice, watermelon, and large quantities of fruit juice or dried fruit. Vegetables to be avoided include asparagus, artichokes, and sugar snap peas. Honey and products with high-fructose corn syrup (juices, regular soft drinks, sports/energy drinks) should also be avoided.
- Fructans (fructo-oligosaccharides). These are made up of short chains of fructose with a glucose molecule on the end. These include grains (rye, wheat bread, crackers, biscuits, wheat pasta, couscous); fruits such as peaches, persimmons, plums, and watermelon; and vegetables such as onions, peppers, artichokes, brussels sprouts, broccoli, cabbages, fennel, garlic, okra, leeks, and legumes (beans, peas, lentils).
- Galactans (galacto-oligosaccharides). These are short chains of sucrose with galactose (similar to the fructans list above).
- Polyols (also called sugar alcohols). These include low-calorie sweeteners such as sucralose as well as sorbitol, mannitol, xylitol, and malitol (which are often used in sugar-free candies, gums, and mints). Fruits that contain sorbitol include apples, apricots, pears, blackberries, nectarines, and plums. Vegetables that contain mannitol include cauliflower, mushrooms, and snow peas.

Note that avoiding lactose is not considered a part of the low-FODMAP diet. However, if a person is lactase deficient, then lactose cannot be broken down, and it acts similarly to fructans and galactans in producing gastrointestinal distress.

Foods That Fit within the Low-FODMAP Diet

- Gluten-free or spelt toast
- Corn or rice cereals
- Eggs

- Lean proteins (chicken, turkey, fish, lean pork, lean lamb, lean red meat)
- Cheeses with no/low lactose (typically the hard cheeses)
- Rice cakes
- Quinoa
- Select fruits (smaller volumes of bananas, grapefruit, grapes, kiwi, honeydew melons, tangelos, oranges, strawberries, lemons, limes, and blueberries)
- Select vegetables (bamboo shoots, bok choy, carrots, eggplant, green beans, lettuce, tomato)

What Data Support This Diet for Patients Who Have IBS?

As described in a recently published study, 82 patients who had IBS and attended a dietetic outpatient clinic found that, compared to a standard diet, the low-FODMAP diet significantly improved their symptoms of bloating, abdominal pain, and flatulence. Overall compliance with the diet was high in this study (the participants were counseled by dieticians). The average time to improvement of symptoms of gas and bloating was 3½ weeks—a sign that people who have IBS should not expect all of their symptoms to improve quickly with this diet. Note that, if followed very carefully, the low-FODMAP diet may create some problems with constipation in individuals who have IBS with mixed or alternating diarrhea and constipation and will probably worsen constipation symptoms in people who have IBS with constipation. I generally recommend at least four weeks on the low-FODMAP diet to see if there is any improvement or change in symptoms.

A Gluten-Free Diet

Until recently, other than anecdotal reports, there were no good data to show that a gluten-free diet might improve symptoms of IBS. In 2011, researchers evaluated the benefits of a gluten-free diet in a study of 34 patients (30 women and 4 men) who met specific criteria for the diagnosis of IBS. All 34 patients were carefully tested to make sure that they did not have celiac disease. Patients were then randomized to either a diet containing gluten or a gluten-free diet for six weeks (food was prepared for them so that it appeared identical, regardless of whether it contained gluten or not). Symptoms were monitored throughout the six weeks and serum, urine, and blood samples were checked at the beginning and the end of the study period. The authors reported that patients who had IBS and ingested gluten were more likely to report typical symptoms of IBS, compared to those patients who had IBS and ingested foods without gluten. Specifically, symptoms of abdominal pain, bloating, and tiredness were all worse in the gluten group compared to the gluten-free group.

This study was not designed to understand the mechanism of how gluten might cause symptoms of IBS, but its results are intriguing in that they appear to show gluten as a trigger for a variety of GI symptoms in people who have IBS. Although a gluten-free diet can be difficult to follow, for those who have persistent symptoms of IBS and who wish to use only dietary treatment measures, a gluten-free diet is safe and certainly worth trying.

A Low-Carbohydrate Diet

Another diet modification that can improve symptoms of gas and bloating is decreasing or eliminating carbohydrates. The theory is that carbohydrates contain starches and sugars, and these are the substances that are likely to ferment while being broken down in the colon (large intestine). If carbohydrates are removed from the diet, then (again, theoretically) there is less material to ferment in the colon, with less production of gas, which leads to an improvement in symptoms of bloating, distention, and diarrhea. A small clinical trial tested this theory with people who had IBS with diarrhea (IBS-D) by placing some patients on a very low-carbohydrate diet (only 4 percent of daily calories were from carbohydrates) and comparing their symptoms to that of patients who had IBS-D and were maintained on a normal carbohydrate diet (55 percent of daily calories). All meals were prepared by a commercial kitchen, and the calorie content was balanced so that patients did not lose or gain weight. During this four-week study, patients who had IBS-D and were placed on a very low-carbohydrate diet felt better, had reduced stool frequency, and had an improvement in stool consistency (loose stools became more formed) and abdominal pain. Overall, patients tolerated the diet well. However, the study was only four weeks long and the meals were prepared for the patients, which made the diet easy to follow (and less costly). The downsides to the low-carbohydrate diet followed by the patients who had IBS-D included the following: (1) 51 percent of the calories consumed were from fat, which is detrimental to long-term health; (2) 45 percent of the calories consumed were from protein, which can be expensive, potentially detrimental to health over the long run, and not necessarily sustainable; (3) essentially no fruits or vegetables were allowed in the diet, which may be detrimental to a patient's long-term nutritional status. Additional studies are needed to confirm these results. However, if a person who has IBS is going through a particularly difficult time with gas, bloating, and diarrhea, a diet that focuses on lean proteins and much smaller servings of carbohydrates (with an emphasis on simple carbohydrates such as white rice and white potatoes) may help.

General Eating Habits

Despite the fact that IBS is so common and causes so many debilitating symptoms, little research has been performed on the effect of diet on people with functional bowel disorders. However, most experienced clinicians offer the following advice. One, avoid fad diets and diets that emphasize extremes (for example, the all-grapefruit diet). These are rarely helpful and in the long run rarely healthful. Two, don't become food phobic. Use the food diary described in Chapter 13 to track your symptoms, and enjoy the foods you tolerate well. Three, for many people who have IBS, it is not what they eat but rather the act of eating that often causes symptoms. If you have a hypersensitive gut, a smaller-portioned meal will usually be less challenging to your GI tract and better tolerated than a large meal. This is especially important for patients who have IBS and diarrhea and who frequently have very urgent diarrhea during or shortly after a meal. A large meal will trigger a stronger gastrocolic reflex, resulting in more urgent diarrhea, whereas a smaller meal won't elicit such a powerful response. Finally, having a set routine, especially for the timing of meals, can be helpful to all people who have IBS, whether they have diarrhea or constipation or alternate between the two. It may take a little time and recording of symptoms and events to discover what works best for your gut, but most people's GI tracts respond well to the rhythm of predictable routine.

Summary

- For people who have symptoms of IBS, a period of abstinence from dairy products is usually helpful to determine which symptoms, and the proportion of those symptoms, are due to lactose intolerance as opposed to IBS.
- To determine whether symptoms are the result of fructose intolerance rather than IBS, avoid all fructose-containing liquids and foods—all carbonated drinks, all fruit juices, all types of sports drinks, and those fruits and vegetables that contain fructose (such as pears, apples, mangos, peaches, Mandarin oranges, watermelon, and pineapple).
- The low-FODMAP diet has been shown to improve symptoms of gas and bloating in some people who have IBS.
- Avoiding gluten may improve symptoms in some individuals who have IBS, even if they don't have a wheat allergy.
- An eating regimen that features smaller, more-frequent meals and emphasizes regular routine will be less likely to trigger IBS symptoms.

CHAPTER 16

Treatment Options for IBS with Constipation

Of all the people who suffer from IBS, approximately one-third have problems with constipation. The term *constipation* means different things to different people. When some people say that they are constipated, they mean that they have infrequent bowel movements, maybe every 3 to 4 days. Other people use the term to refer to excessive straining in order to have a bowel movement or to pain or discomfort with the passage of stool. Still others mean that they do not feel as if they have completely emptied all the stool from their rectum (this is called "incomplete evacuation"). These different meanings are important to point out, because when you see your physician and tell him or her that you are constipated, your doctor may infer that you mean one of these definitions when in fact you mean another. Both patients and physicians need to be specific about these details for the most appropriate treatments to be chosen.

Lifestyle Changes

The first line of treatment for people who have mild symptoms of IBS and constipation generally focuses on lifestyle modifications, changes in diet, and the use of fiber supplements. During the initial patient evaluation in our clinic, we review the amount of fluid that the person takes in each day, determine the amount of dietary fiber consumed, and discuss whether the patient exercises regularly and the type of exercise. We also carefully review what treatments the patient has tried in the past, including over-the-counter products, prescription medications, natural medicines, homeopathic medicines, and any other alternative treatment.

Fluid Intake

There are very few scientific data to support the idea that drinking more water will lead to a significant improvement in constipation. The body has an amazing ability to absorb large amounts of fluid from both the small intestine and the colon (the small intestine can absorb up to 14 liters of water per day, and the colon can absorb up to 4 to 5 liters of water per day). Thus, it is difficult to drink so much fluid that the fluid intake alone will increase the frequency of stools or make them softer and looser.

Although for years we have been told that we should drink at least 8 glasses of water (64 ounces total) per day, it hasn't been scientifically established that this specific amount is vital to good health. We all need to drink adequate amounts of fluid in order to remain hydrated and maintain a normal amount of fluid in our bloodstream. With a normal fluid balance, the kidneys, heart, skin, central nervous system, and muscles all function more efficiently and remain healthier. Your body will let you know when you have not had enough fluid, because you will feel a little more tired than usual, your mouth may feel dry, or your urine may be darker (more concentrated) than usual. Water is a healthy way to maintain normal hydration, because it avoids the extra sugar and calories incorporated in fruit juices and sports drinks and the gas found in carbonated drinks. Fluids should be available at each meal and throughout the day. Common sense dictates that if you are thirsty, you should drink. If you take certain medications, the accompanying instructions or your physician may tell you to take in more fluid than usual or to take each dose with a full glass of water. In particular, if you take fiber supplements (discussed below), you will need to take in enough fluid, because the fiber products work by becoming hydrated. If they are taken without sufficient fluid, they may actually worsen constipation. Overall, increasing fluid intake by itself leads to an improvement in constipation only in people who were truly dehydrated.

Diet

When physicians discuss constipation with patients, we generally focus on two aspects of diet: volume and fiber content. Although it is an often-neglected subject, the quantity of food you eat plays an important role in bowel health. Stool is largely material that cannot be broken down and absorbed by the GI tract (plus dead cells and lots of bacteria from the colon). People who go on a strict diet or severely limit their caloric intake quite often become constipated. An extreme example is anorexics, who typically suffer from constipation because they eat so little. If you need to lose weight, it is easy, with the right kind of diet, to take in plenty of volume and fiber without overdoing the calories. For a discussion of fiber, see the section just below.

Fiber

Current dietary recommendations are that everybody should take in 25 to 30 grams of natural fiber each day. Natural fiber can be found in many different foodstuffs, including fresh fruits, fresh vegetables, and whole-grain breads and cereals (see Table 16.1). Fiber comes in two different forms—soluble and insoluble. Examples of foods that contain soluble fiber are potatoes and oatmeal, while commercial products that contain soluble fiber include Metamucil (psyllium), Citrucel (methylcellulose), and Benefiber (guar gum). Examples of foods that contain large amounts of insoluble fiber are bran flakes, kidney beans, and pears.

Soluble fiber can be broken down and digested by the GI tract, while insoluble fiber cannot. What are the advantages and disadvantages of using more of one kind of fiber than another? Because soluble fiber products can be broken down in the GI tract, they typically cause less gas and bloating. However, soluble fiber, because it is broken down and split by bacteria, does not absorb as much water as insoluble fiber. Thus soluble fiber may be less helpful in treating constipation than insoluble fiber.

Fiber generally has two major mechanisms of action. It increases stool volume, and it helps to speed up the transit of material through the GI tract. In addition, by providing bulk to the stool, fiber often increases the ease of evacuation and decreases straining. When it is difficult for people to take in adequate amounts of fiber through their diet, fiber

Table 16.1. Fiber Content of Selected Foods

	Serving size	Total soluble and insoluble (in grams)
Vegetables (cooked)		
Artichoke	1 globe	6.5
Asparagus	½ cup	1.8
Beans, green	½ cup	1.3
Beans, kidney	½ cup	5.7
Beans, lima	½ cup	6.1
Broccoli	½ cup	2.8
Cabbage, green	½ cup	2.1
Carrots	½ cup	2.6
Cauliflower	½ cup	2.0
Celery (raw)	½ cup	1.0
Corn	½ cup	2.0
Cucumber (raw)	½ cup	0.4
Eggplant	½ cup	1.2
Lettuce, iceberg (raw)	½ cup	0.4
Peas, green	½ cup	4.4
Potato, baked (with skin)	½ cup	1.5
Potato, sweet	½ cup	3.8
Spinach	½ cup	2.7
Squash, acorn	½ cup	4.0
Tomato (raw)	½ cup	1.0
Zucchini	½ cup	1.3
Fruits (uncooked)		
Apple (with peel)	1 medium	3.7
Apricots	1 cup	3.7
Banana	1 medium	2.7
Blackberries	1 cup	7.2
Blueberries	1 cup	3.9
Boysenberries	1 cup	7.2
Cantaloupe	1 wedge	1.3
Grapefruit	1 medium	2.8
Grapes	1 cup	1.6
Orange	1 medium	3.1
Pear (with peel)	1 medium	4.0
Pineapple	1 cup	1.9
Plums	1 medium	1.0
Prunes	½ cup	5.7

(continued)

Table 16.1. (continued)

	Serving size	Total soluble and insoluble (in grams)
Raspberries	1 cup	8.4
Strawberries	1 cup	3.4
Watermelon	1 slice	0.8
Grain Products and Nuts		
Bread		
Rye	1 slice	1.6
White	1 slice	0.6
Whole wheat	1 slice	2.0
Cereal		
Bran	1 ounce	9.7
Corn flakes	1 ounce	1.0
Oat bran (uncooked)	1 ounce	4.3
Oatmeal (uncooked)	1 ounce	3.0
Shredded wheat	1 ounce	2.8
Pasta	2 ounces	2.1
Popcorn	1 cup (popped)	1.0
Rice		
Brown (cooked)	½ cup	1.8
White (cooked)	½ cup	0.3
Almonds (roasted)	½ cup	6.4
Peanuts (roasted)	½ cup	6.1

supplements (methylcellulose, psyllium, polycarbophil, coarse bran, or ispaghula husk) can be used. Fiber supplements act as hydrophilic agents, meaning that they absorb water. By absorbing significant amounts of water, fiber adds bulk to the stool, preventing excessive dehydration of the stool as it passes through the colon and leading to more rapid transit of the stool through the intestinal tract.

In the past, treatment for IBS encouraged a *low*-fiber diet. The concern, before about 1970, was that additional fiber would "irritate" the GI tract and make symptoms of IBS worse. During the last 30 years, however, fiber has become a mainstay of therapy in the treatment of IBS. Especially in this era of "managed care," in which insurance companies and health care plans try to carefully control the use of prescription medications, fiber products represent a safe, inexpensive dietary supplement that provides relief of constipation for some people. Despite its widespread use, however, the data do not agree about the effectiveness of fiber treatment in people who have IBS and constipation. Let's begin by reviewing some of the research studies that have evaluated the potential benefits of fiber therapy.

One study, published in 1977, found that 14 patients who had IBS and were treated with a high-wheat-fiber diet noted an improvement in abdominal pain and bowel complaints, compared to 12 patients who had IBS and were placed on a low-wheat-fiber diet. Another study, published in 1980, followed a small group of patients who had IBS as they progressed from a "normal" diet (low in fiber) to a fiber-added diet (moderate in fiber) and then to a high-fiber diet. All patients noted an improvement in the transit of materials through the colon as fiber was added to the diet. Other small studies have also shown that fiber products (ispaghula husk, calcium polycarbophil [Equalactin], psyllium [Metamucil], methylcellulose [Citrucel]) have improved symptoms of constipation in patients who have IBS. In addition, when the results of many studies that had investigated the effects of fiber in people who have IBS and constipation were analyzed as a group (a type of research called meta-analysis), there was a consistent improvement in colonic transit time and an increase in stool output for patients treated with fiber.

These results seem encouraging, and in fact, many patients who have IBS do note an improvement in their constipation symptoms when treated with fiber supplements. However, improvement in transit time through the GI tract and an increase in stool weight do not always translate into an improvement in the other clinical symptoms of IBS. In fact, most of these studies did *not* show any improvement in the chronic abdominal pain and discomfort that characterize IBS. In addition, at least 30 percent of patients noted a significant worsening of bloating and abdominal distention with these agents (especially with insoluble fiber products). One study found that as many as 55 percent of patients who had IBS and were treated with bran fiber experienced significant aggravation of abdominal pain and distention.

In summary, adding fiber to the diet is a reasonable treatment for people who have constipation and may improve symptoms of constipation in some individuals who have IBS. If you decide to start a fiber supplement, begin slowly. If you start at the maximum dose on the first day, you are virtually guaranteed to feel worse, not better, due to problems with gas, bloating, and abdominal discomfort. I generally ask patients to begin with a small amount of fiber each day (a half teaspoon of psyllium, or half of a fiber tablet), taken before the evening meal with a large glass of water. Every five to seven days the patient slowly increases the dose, so that by the end of the month, the person is on the maximum recommended dose. This gives the GI tract time to adjust to the added volume of fiber, minimizes side effects, and allows the patient time to make other changes in daily routine that might be needed because of changes in bowel behavior.

If a person who has IBS is already on a high-fiber diet, adding more fiber will *not* improve symptoms of constipation, although the additional fiber will undoubtedly worsen complaints of bloating, gas, and distention. Research studies have consistently shown that fiber products do not improve abdominal pain and, in fact, may actually worsen it, because they can cause more bloating and distention.

Exercise

Physicians often recommend exercise to their patients as a matter of course during a routine check-up or office visit. Certainly, exercise has been shown to improve many health conditions, including high blood pressure, diabetes, osteopenia (mild bone loss) and osteoporosis, obesity, and a variety of heart conditions. In addition, routine exercise can reduce stress, tension, and anxiety, improve mental health, and possibly lead to an improvement in the immune system. Limited data support the view that regular exercise improves motility in the GI tract. Patients who routinely exercise (jogging, walking, playing tennis, biking) often find that when they get out of their regular exercise pattern, they become constipated. This may reflect a direct effect of exercise on the GI tract, or the increase in constipation may be due to the change in daily routine or an accompanying change in diet. Because many patients find that some exercise seems to alleviate constipation, we often recommend that exercise be incorporated into a person's weekly routine. Many people find that a brisk walk after breakfast or after dinner seems to stimulate the colon and ease evacuation of stool, especially when coupled with routine, scheduled bathroom time (see "Bowel Training" below). No large scientific study has evaluated the effects of exercise on IBS and constipation, however.

Bowel Training

Having a bowel movement is normally an easy task routinely accomplished. As mentioned previously, there is a wide range of what can be considered normal bowel habits. Many people simply fall out of their natural habits, for a variety of reasons, and so become constipated. One of the most common reasons is ignoring the urge to have a bowel movement. In many people this urge occurs when awakening, and in others it typically occurs after eating. People who ignore this urge (sometimes described as a "crampy" sensation or a sensation of "pressure" or "fullness" in the rectum) can quickly become constipated. For example, office workers, teachers, truck drivers, or operating room nurses may get up, have breakfast and their morning cup of coffee or tea, and then go to work. They may then develop the urge to have a bowel movement, but the phone begins ringing, the fax machine has to be attended to, classes begin, the truck is on the highway, or the surgical case takes longer than expected. The urge to have a bowel movement is then ignored or actively suppressed. This urge may then disappear until the next day, when the same activities again prevent going to the bathroom to evacuate stool. All of a sudden, people who used to routinely have a bowel movement each morning are now doing so once each weekend.

Normally, the GI tract is very quiet at night but "wakes up" each morning with a wave of peristaltic activity at approximately four or five o'clock in the morning. This is one reason why some people have a bowel movement first thing in the morning. Eating food or drinking warm liquids stimulates the stomach and sets up a reflex with the colon, called the gastrocolic (or gastrocolonic) reflex. In many people, 15 to 45 minutes after food stimulates their stomach, they will feel the urge to have a bowel movement. (This is the same reflex that is so highly exaggerated in patients who have IBS and diarrhea that they can barely finish a meal before they are running to the bathroom.) This is an important reflex that should be taken advantage of by patients with constipation.

When we talk about bowel training, we basically mean listening to the normal signals that the body sends us every day and trying to accommodate them. The gut loves routines. This means getting up at approximately the same time each day, having breakfast (to help initiate the gastrocolic reflex), possibly drinking a large mug of caffeinated coffee or tea or taking a walk (to further stimulate the GI tract), and then setting aside time to use the bathroom at a scheduled time each day, typically 30 to 45 minutes after the morning meal. Ideally, this should be the same time each day. This simple routine, easy to incorporate in most people's daily schedule, is a safe and very effective approach to improving constipation. Finally, some people find that it is easier to have a bowel movement if they place their feet on a small stool; this technique changes the shape of the pelvic floor (it helps widen the anorectal angle—see Chapter 6) and makes it easier to evacuate.

Medications

When patients first see a physician for treatment of IBS symptoms, they often have tried various medicines without adequate relief. As part of history taking, we review not only which medications have been tried and the dose of each (in milligrams, number of pills per dose, number of times per day), but also how the medication was taken (liquid, tablet, capsule; by mouth, suppository, injection), and for how long it was tried. Table 16.2 lists many of the medications, both prescription and nonprescription, that are used to treat constipation.

As we introduce new medications in a treatment program, I generally recommend that each be tried for a minimum of four weeks, so that the results can be properly evaluated (unless a side effect or adverse drug reaction occurs, requiring earlier cessation of use). Since many patients who have IBS have symptoms that have lasted for months or years, it is unfair to judge the value of any single medication after a trial of only a few days or a week.

We are all aware that medications are a two-edged sword. They can certainly improve the symptoms of medical conditions, whether the

Table 16.2. Medications Used to Treat Constipation

Chloride channel activators

  Lubiprostone (Amitiza)

Combination agents

  Docusate sodium and sennoside (Senokot-S)
  Docusate sodium and casanthrol (Peri-Colace)

Fiber

  Methylcellulose (Citrucel)
  Psyllium (Metamucil)
  Calcium polycarbophil (Equalactin, FiberCon)
  Guar gum, partially hydrolyzed (Benefiber)
  Coarse bran or ispaghula husk

Guanylate cyclase C activators

  Linaclotide (Linzess)

Herbal agents

  Aloe vera (*Aloe barbadensis*)
  Buckthorn (*Rhamnus catharticus*)
  Cascara sagrada (*Rhamnus purshianus*)
  Chinese rhubarb (*Rheum palmatum*)
  Frangula (*Rhamnus frangula*)
  Manna (*Fraxinus ornus*)
  Senna (*Cassia senna*)

Miscellaneous

  Mineral oil
  Colchicine
  Misoprostol (Cytotec)

Osmotic agents and unabsorbed sugars

  Magnesium hydroxide (Phillips Milk of Magnesia, Freelax)
  Magnesium citrate
  Polyethylene glycol (Miralax)
  Lactulose (Chronulac, Kristalose)
  Lactitol
  Sorbitol

Stimulant laxatives

  Bisacodyl (Dulcolax, Gentlax)
  Senna, sennosides (Senokot, Ex-Lax, Swiss-Kriss)
  Aloe
  Cascara

Stool softeners

  Docusate sodium (Colace)

symptoms are acute or chronic in nature. However, all medicinal preparations have the potential for causing side effects—responses that are not the intended effect, are usually unwanted, and can be either benign or harmful. These potential side effects do not come only with prescription medications; they may be caused by over-the-counter products, dietary supplements (recall the controversy with ephedra in weight loss supplements), and complementary and alternative medications, including herbal preparations. Some medications can cause constipation or make it worse. Table 16.3 lists several of these substances. If you are taking one of these medications, at your next visit with your physician you may want to discuss whether the medicine is really needed or whether there is an alternative medication that would not be constipating.

Over-the-Counter Medications

Stool softeners. Stool softeners are considered emollients because they act to soften and lubricate the stool, to a small degree. Docusate sodium (one brand name is Colace) is the best known of this type of medication. In usual doses, docusate (one pill twice a day) may increase the fluid content of stool by 3 to 5 percent, thereby softening the stool and allowing easier evacuation. No research study has demonstrated that stool softeners are any better than a placebo at treating symptoms of constipation. So, although stool softeners are safe and relatively inexpensive, they are rarely helpful for people who have constipation.

Osmotic agents. Osmotic agents act by drawing water into the intestinal tract. The increased fluid load in the GI tract helps to accelerate the movement of materials through the GI tract and helps to soften stool. Osmotic agents function differently from the stool softeners described above. Many agents in this class are sold over the counter. They are sometimes described as "salts" because they typically contain large amounts of magnesium or sulfate. Use of these agents for longer than two weeks can lead to elevated levels of magnesium in the bloodstream, which can be dangerous, especially in people with kidney problems such as renal insufficiency or renal failure. Typical osmotic agents are magnesium hydroxide (milk of magnesia), magnesium sulfate, or magnesium citrate. These medications are best used only intermittently to treat mild cases of

Table 16.3. Medications That May Cause Constipation

Anticholinergic agents (hyoscyamine, dicyclomine, Detrol)
Anticonvulsants (phenytoin, phenobarbital)
Antidiarrheal agents (Imodium, Lomotil)
Antihistamines (either alone or in cold remedies)
Anti-Parkinsonian agents (L-Dopa)
Antipsychotics (thorazine)
Calcium channel blockers (diltiazem)
Cholestyramine (Questran)
Diuretics (lasix)
Fiber, if not taken with adequate fluids
Narcotics (oxycodone, Percocet, Vicodin)
Nonsteroidal anti-inflammatory agents (ibuprofen, Motrin, Aleve)
Sucralfate (Carafate)
Tricyclic antidepressants (Elavil, Norpramin)

constipation. They generally do not cause abdominal bloating or distention but may cause abdominal cramps and spasms.

Sugars that cannot be absorbed within the GI tract may also act as
osmotic agents. These large sugar molecules draw water into the GI tract,
thus stimulating gut transit. A good example is sorbitol, commonly used
to sweeten gums, candies, and mints. Products containing sorbitol are often labeled "dietetic" or "sugar free," since, not being absorbed, sorbitol
does not contribute to caloric intake.

Polyethylene glycol (PEG) is another type of osmotic agent, but its
chemical structure is quite different from the over-the-counter osmotic
agents described above. PEG is a large, inert molecule that is not absorbed in the GI tract. PEG preparations are commonly used to help
prepare patients for colonoscopy or flexible sigmoidoscopy. These agents
are now sold in prescription form as well as over the counter with a variety
of trade names (Miralax, Nu-Lytely) and generically as glycolax. In smaller
doses, PEG can be used daily or intermittently to treat constipation. At
present, the FDA has not approved PEG for long-term use. Although
several small studies of its efficacy have shown that patients often note
an improvement in symptoms of constipation, PEG preparations do not
improve abdominal pain or bloating associated with IBS.

Stimulant laxatives. Products in this group (for instance, Dulcolax) contain senna, cascara, aloe, or bisacodyl. Many of these ingredients are derived from plants. All stimulant laxatives have two major mechanisms of action. They increase colonic contractions and they stimulate the intestinal tract to secrete water, which hastens the movement of materials through the GI tract. Small research studies have shown that senna both increases stool frequency and improves stool consistency in people who have constipation. At present, there are no randomized, controlled studies evaluating any of these agents in people who have IBS and constipation. In general, these medications are recommended for intermittent use only. However, contrary to popular opinion, long-term use of stimulant laxatives does not cause people to become dependent on them.

Long-term utilization of these medications may lead to discoloration of the colon, a condition called melanosis coli. This discoloration of the lining of the colon (ranging from black to dark yellow) occurs because these laxatives appear to cause premature death of some of the cells that line the colon. These dead cells are then ingested by other cells (macrophages), which break down dead cells. The break-down products are deeply pigmented, leading to the discoloration of the colonic mucosa. This condition is not dangerous and will slowly resolve once the person stops taking the laxative.

Side effects are fairly common with all of these agents and include cramps, abdominal pain, and diarrhea. Stimulant agents are found in widely-used products sold at supermarkets, health food stores, and nutrition centers. Note that laxatives containing phenolphthalein are no longer sold, because of concerns about their safety after reports of allergic reactions came to light.

Enemas and suppositories. Some people with constipation occasionally use either enemas or suppositories to treat their problem. Enemas work by softening stool and by stimulating the colon to contract. When an enema is used, the liquid can travel as high up as the descending colon (see Figure 6.1 for a diagram of the intestinal tract). The descending and sigmoid colon are where stool is normally stored until it is an appropriate time to have a bowel movement. The enema solution softens the stool that is stored there, which may improve the ease of evacuation. In addition, insertion of the tip of the enema bottle or tube into the rectum stimulates sensory receptors in the rectum and initiates reflexive contractions of both the sigmoid colon and rectum, further assisting the evacuation of stool.

Although a variety of enemas are sold over the counter, there are no studies comparing the effectiveness of one versus the other. Warm water enemas (using a hot water bottle and the correct tubing and tip) are obviously the cheapest and are usually just as effective as commercial products. In the case of warm water enemas, the water should be only warm, not hot, and should be slowly instilled, *not* forced into the rectum at high pressure by vigorously squeezing the bag. The tip of the enema bottle or tube should be lubricated with K-Y Jelly and inserted gently into the rectum. Forcing the tip or inserting it too deep can lead to serious injury. Although rare, there are cases where people have perforated (poked a hole in) their rectum by forcing the tip of the enema bottle in too forcefully or too deep. Enemas typically work best if the liquid can remain in place for 30 to 45 minutes, preferably while the patient is lying on his or her left side. The liquid should then be evacuated and is expected to carry the softened stool with it.

Some commercial enemas contain a large amount of phosphate. People who have kidney problems should avoid these agents, because the phosphate can be absorbed from the colon, leading to dangerously high levels in the blood. Lastly, some enemas can cause the mucosal lining to become significantly irritated and inflamed or even bleed. If this occurs, the enema should be immediately stopped and no further ones attempted until the reaction has been evaluated and has healed. This will require a visit to your health care provider, but the examination will probably be quick. Enemas can help some patients but are appropriate only for short-term, intermittent use.

Suppositories (glycerin is the type most commonly used) work in a similar manner to enemas. Inserting the suppository stimulates sensory receptors in the rectum, which then causes the rectum to contract. The glycerin may lubricate the rectum and add a small amount of moisture. Bisacodyl (Dulcolax) suppositories stimulate muscular contractions in the colon using a direct irritative effect that may lead to more forceful contractions of the colon but also to more pain, cramping, and spasms.

Neither of these types of treatment for constipation has been evaluated in large-scale trials. Overall, they are considered safe if used appropriately, but they do not affect the underlying causes of chronic constipation.

Other agents. One old-fashioned remedy for constipation is taking mineral oil or castor oil. In theory, the oil will soften the stool and lead to easier evacuation. However, taking these oils rarely helps constipation, and the oils pass through the GI tract without being absorbed and may seep out of the rectum, staining the clothes. Although an uncommon side effect, inflammation in the liver (hepatitis) may result from taking mineral oil, and chronic use has the potential to deplete the body of critical fat-soluble vitamins (vitamins A, D, K, and E). In addition, mineral oil should never be used by older people, because if it is inadvertently inhaled (aspirated), it can cause a life-threatening pneumonia.

Prescription Medications

Osmotic agents. Polyethylene glycol (PEG) is described above. It is now most commonly used in the over-the-counter form, although some insurance companies still pay for this medication if it is required for long-term use and is prescribed by a physician.

Unabsorbed sugars. Another class of prescription medication often used to treat patients who have IBS and constipation is unabsorbed sugars. These agents, which are sold under a variety of trade names, include lactulose, lactitol, mannitol, and sorbitol. We'll look at lactulose as an example. Lactulose is made up of two sugar molecules (galactose and fructose) joined together. It is taken in the form of a sugary-sweet syrup that cannot be broken down and digested by the small intestine and instead passes into the colon, where it is broken down by the bacteria there. Because the sugar is not absorbed, it acts like an osmotic laxative, similar to milk of magnesia (see above), causing increased stool frequency and a softening of stool consistency. Because the sugars are not absorbed, they generally do not cause elevated blood sugar levels. Several small studies have shown that lactulose improves symptoms of constipation, but it has not been tested specifically in patients who have IBS and constipation.

A major side effect of the unabsorbed sugars is that they all have the potential to cause or worsen symptoms of gassiness, bloating, and distention, because they ferment in the colon, producing hydrogen gas and carbon dioxide. Although these products may improve constipation (increased frequency and softer stools), many patients find that the side effects far outweigh the benefits of these drugs. In my experience, these agents are not usually helpful for patients who have severe constipation.

Note that sorbitol is a common additive used by the food industry as a sweetener in sugar-free products. People who consume large amounts of sugar-free candies, gums, or mints that contain sorbitol often notice an increase in bloating, distention, and occasionally diarrhea.

Lubiprostone. Lubiprostone was approved by the FDA in 2008 for the treatment of IBS with constipation in women. It is sold under the brand name Amitiza. The recommended dose of lubiprostone is 8 micrograms (mcg) twice daily, although some patients who have IBS with constipation (IBS-C) just need 8 mcg once daily.

Lubiprostone is categorized as a chloride channel activator and works differently from all of the products described above. After being swallowed, lubiprostone stimulates the cells lining the small intestine and colon to secrete (release) small amounts of chloride followed by small amounts of sodium. The secretion of chloride and sodium (in effect, small amounts of salt) in turn causes water to enter the GI tract. The addition of water to the GI tract can help loosen stool and make it easier to pass. This active secretion of chloride followed by small amounts of water may stimulate the muscles and nerves of the GI tract, which can improve peristalsis.

Several large research studies have proven the effectiveness of lubiprostone in treating symptoms of IBS-C. One of the largest studies involved nearly twelve hundred men and women who had IBS-C. Patients in this study received either lubiprostone or a placebo for a 12-week period. Before and during the study, researchers measured the patients' symptoms of IBS (abdominal pain, bloating, and constipation) so that the effectiveness and safety of lubiprostone could be determined. To be categorized as having responded to the treatment with lubiprostone, patients had to have most or all of their IBS-C symptoms improve for the majority of the 12-week study period. None of the medications described earlier in this chapter (over-the-counter or prescription) have been subjected to such a long study period or to such strict criteria. The results of this study showed that patients treated with lubiprostone were nearly twice as likely to have their IBS symptoms improve or resolve as compared to those patients who were given a placebo. Lubiprostone was also found to be very safe, without any significant side effects (other than mild nausea in some patients and diarrhea in others).

More recently, a similar study evaluated the long-term safety and efficacy of lubiprostone during a 48-week trial period. Lubiprostone remained both effective and safe during this prolonged period of use, which is important for patients who have IBS and typically have persistent symptoms that last months or years, thus requiring chronic medical therapy.

So why is lubiprostone currently approved only for women who have IBS and constipation, and not men? Although men were included in the research studies, there were far more women in the studies. The FDA did not have enough information to confidently state that men who have IBS and constipation would respond favorably to this medication. However, the FDA did approve lubiprostone for the treatment of chronic constipation in both men and women. This approval should be reassuring to men who have IBS and constipation, because symptoms of chronic constipation and IBS with constipation are similar, and because the underlying pathophysiology is often the same.

With regard to safety, lubiprostone has been proven safe to use in patients 65 years old and older who have symptoms of constipation. It has not yet been approved by the FDA in the pediatric population (younger than 18 years old), although studies to evaluate the safety and effectiveness of this medication for children and adolescents are ongoing. Even though less than 1 percent of lubiprostone is absorbed by a patient's GI tract (this is one of the reasons it is so safe), it is always appropriate to be extra cautious with women who might become pregnant or who are breast-feeding. Thus, the FDA has recommended that this medication not be used for women who are breast-feeding or pregnant. But this recommendation does not apply just to lubiprostone—the vast majority of medications on the market should not be used by women who are pregnant or breast-feeding.

Linaclotide. Linaclotide is a new medication that was recently approved (August 30, 2012) by the FDA for the treatment of symptoms of IBS and constipation. It is sold under the trade name Linzess. Linaclotide, a small chemical that consists of only 14 amino acids, acts differently from all other available over-the-counter agents and prescription medications because it mimics the action of a natural chemical in the body. When ingested, linaclotide stimulates the production of a chemical called cGMP. When the level of this chemical is increased in the cells that line the GI tract, a series of reactions occur that ultimately result in an increased flow of electrolytes (bicarbonate and chloride) and water into the GI tract. Similar to lubiprostone, this increased flow accelerates movement of materials through the GI tract, which can improve symptoms of constipation.

The efficacy and safety of linaclotide has been proven in studies that included adult men and women with typical symptoms of IBS-C (lower abdominal pain and discomfort, bloating, and constipation). During the 12-week studies, patients were randomly placed into groups to receive either the study drug (linaclotide) or a placebo. Symptoms were measured at the beginning, middle, and end of the study to assess the effectiveness of linaclotide at improving symptoms of IBS and constipation. The studies clearly show that linaclotide improves symptoms of IBS-C, including symptoms of hard stool, straining, incomplete evacuation, and lower abdominal pain and bloating. Patients in the study tolerated linaclotide well; no serious side effects were identified. Some patients had symptoms of diarrhea (as with lubiprostone), although this may be more a sign of efficacy than a side effect of the medication. Linaclotide appears to be safe for long-term use. In a study of more than 800 patients for 26 weeks, linaclotide was effective at improving symptoms of IBS-C and was not found to have any serious side effects. Data on the use of linaclotide in elderly or pediatric populations are not yet available.

New and Upcoming Treatment Options

Medicine is constantly evolving, and researchers and clinicians are always searching for new medications and therapies to improve patients' symptoms. Below is a brief list of medications that may become available in the future to help treat symptoms of IBS with constipation.

Prucalopride

This medication helps stimulate serotonin receptors in the GI tract. It is approved for use in the European Union for the treatment of chronic constipation and has been shown to be safe and effective in both women and men. Its success at treating symptoms of chronic constipation means it probably also could improve symptoms in people who have IBS and constipation.

Velusetrag

This medication also stimulates serotonin receptors in the GI tract. Preliminary studies have shown that it improves symptoms of constipation in both men and women. Additional studies are required to determine its efficacy and safety in people who have IBS.

A3309

This is a novel medication that is currently being developed. It acts differently from all the other agents described in this chapter by preventing the absorption of bile in the lower small intestine (ileum). If bile is not absorbed in the small intestine, more bile enters the colon, which acts to accelerate movement of materials through the colon. Preliminary studies have shown benefits for patients who have constipation. Additional trials are needed with patients who have IBS and constipation to determine its efficacy and safety.

Summary

- Contrary to popular opinion, simply drinking more water will rarely improve symptoms of constipation.
- Adding more natural or supplemental fiber to your diet will help with constipation *if* you are fiber deficient and if you take in enough fluid to hydrate the fiber supplement.
- Fiber does not treat the abdominal pain that characterizes IBS, and fiber can worsen symptoms of bloating.
- Osmotic agents (for example, milk of magnesia) and stimulant laxatives may temporarily improve constipation, but they usually are not effective for long-term use. In addition, these agents may worsen abdominal cramps, spasms, and pain, and they do not treat bloating.
- Lubiprostone (Amitiza) has been approved by the FDA for the treat-

ment of IBS with constipation in women and for chronic constipation in both women and men.

- Linaclotide (Linzess), recently approved by the FDA, appears to be safe and effective at treating IBS-C symptoms.
- Other agents are currently under development for the treatment of IBS with constipation.

CHAPTER 17

Treatment Options for IBS with Diarrhea

One-third of people who have irritable bowel syndrome have significant problems with diarrhea. Diarrhea can describe many different characteristics—too rapid stools or too loose stools, for instance—but most physicians define the condition as more than three bowel movements per day. People who have IBS and the predominant complaint of diarrhea do not all have identical bowel patterns. Some are troubled by frequent loose bowel movements throughout the day, while others have them only after eating a meal. Patients may have 3 to 4 movements per day or be overwhelmed by 12 to 15 per day. Some individuals who have IBS feel that they are able to control their episodes of diarrhea, no matter how frequent; others are frustrated by the significant urgency associated with their diarrhea and fear having an accident.

As discussed in Chapter 6, for people who have IBS and diarrhea, food travels more rapidly through either the small intestine or the colon or both. Despite the accelerated transit through the intestinal tract and despite the frequent bowel movements, most patients have normal stool weights, that is, they do not produce more stool than people who do not have IBS. In addition, and contrary to what one might expect, people who have IBS and diarrhea do not typically become dehydrated, nor do they lose weight or become malnourished from failure to absorb sufficient nutrients.

Because people who have IBS and diarrhea experience more rapid transit of material through their gastrointestinal system, most therapies used to treat them focus on slowing down the GI tract, using either over-the-counter or prescription medications, both discussed below. The initial evaluation of patients who have IBS with diarrhea will include a careful review of the patient's diet, and there are some dietary adjustments, described below, that may help relieve symptoms. In contrast to patients who have IBS and constipation, for whom changes in fluid intake and exercise may lead to some improvement, these interventions are not effective for people who have IBS and diarrhea.

Diet

Unrecognized dietary indiscretions often contribute to the chronic diarrhea that characterizes IBS. If you are a person who has symptoms of IBS, it is important during your initial evaluation to review your diet carefully with your physician, in order to determine whether dietary factors are adversely affecting your bowel habits. This dietary review should include both your main meals and any snacking and on-the-run eating. All liquids that you drink should be noted, along with nutritional supplements, vitamins, natural medications, fiber supplements, and herbal supplements. Keeping a careful food diary for the week prior to your appointment will not only help you give a correct accounting of your daily intake of foods and liquids but also may help identify any foods or liquids that are triggering symptoms.

As discussed in Chapter 10, lactose and fructose are two food elements that have the most potential to worsen symptoms in patients who have IBS and diarrhea, although fibrous foods, fiber supplements, and caffeine are also frequent offenders. Your physician will be interested in your intake of dairy foods, not only milk, but also cheese, ice cream, cottage cheese, and yogurt (recognizing that most lactose is broken down during the fermentation process of making yogurt). He or she might suggest a one-week trial of abstaining from *all* dairy products as a good way to determine whether milk and other dairy products play a role in your symptoms.

Fructose occurs naturally in many fruits and is used as a sweetener in a variety of foods and liquids, usually in the form of high-fructose corn syrup. Soft drinks, fruit drinks, sports drinks, "energy drinks," and many nutritional supplements derive a large percentage of their calories from high-fructose corn syrup. Some people routinely drink one or two glasses of juice at breakfast, have two or three soft drinks during the day, and then consume a sports drink after exercising. All of these drinks contain large amounts of fructose, and this amount of fructose can easily over-whelm the absorptive capacity of the GI tract and cause diarrhea, even in healthy people who do not have IBS.

Clinicians have long recognized that patients who have IBS and diar-rhea seem to be more sensitive to fructose than other people, but the reason was not known. Research has now shown that up to 50 percent of patients who have IBS and diarrhea may not be able to break down and absorb fructose normally. Unabsorbed fructose acts like an osmotic agent, drawing extra water into the intestinal tract, thereby accelerating intestinal transit. In addition, when unabsorbed fructose enters the co-lon, it is broken down by bacteria during the process of fermentation. This produces gas (hydrogen and carbon dioxide), which can further worsen symptoms of bloating and distention. The same process occurs with unabsorbed lactose.

Many patients find that completely avoiding all fructose-containing foods for an entire week dramatically improves (but does not eliminate) their symptoms. They can then slowly add back small portions of fructose-containing foods and liquids, to determine how tolerant or intolerant they are to specific products. They may be able to tolerate two cans of soda or one soft drink and one glass of juice with minimal or no symptoms, while an intake of three servings per day produces significant symptoms of gas, bloating, distention, and diarrhea.

Another dietary factor that can worsen symptoms in individuals who have diarrhea is fiber. For years, we've all been told that eating a lot of fiber is good for us. In many ways, this is true, as diets high in fiber can aid in weight loss, lower blood pressure, lower cholesterol, and help maintain bowel health in people who do not have diarrhea. However, too much fiber can overwhelm the GI tract and worsen many of the symptoms for a person who has IBS. Specifically, too much fiber can accelerate intestinal transit, leading to diarrhea. In addition, fiber that is not broken down will pass into the colon and, when broken down by bacteria there, pro-duce gas, exacerbating bloating and distention.

People who have IBS and diarrhea are often mistakenly told that adding more fiber to their diet will improve their symptoms. This advice is given in the belief that additional fiber will absorb excess water and thus improve stool consistency. For the occasional patient who has IBS, additional fiber does seem to improve stool consistency to some degree, making it less loose. But for most people who have IBS and diarrhea, fiber only seems to make symptoms worse. So, the first step for most individuals who have IBS and diarrhea is to eliminate any fiber supplements from their diet, especially over-the-counter products and nutritional supplements. This simple step generally leads to a significant improvement in symptoms. When further improvement is needed, following a diet that is *low* in fiber usually produces further improvement. Such a diet emphasizes lean proteins and small to moderate portions of carbohydrates, with a small amount of natural fiber for nutritional balance. As discussed in Chapter 15, the low-FODMAP diet can also improve symptoms in many patients who have IBS and diarrhea.

Caffeine is greatly enjoyed by most adults in coffee, tea, and soft drinks. However, caffeine can stimulate the GI tract. For many people, that cup or two of morning coffee predictably stimulates a bowel movement. For people who have constipation, this characteristic of coffee can be used to their advantage. However, for those who have diarrhea, caffeine may worsen diarrhea and cause cramps and spasms. Since caffeine is addictive, if you take in a lot of caffeine each day you should not eliminate caffeine all at once, as you may suffer from mild withdrawal symptoms. These symptoms include headaches, restlessness, agitation, anxiety, disturbed sleep, and moodiness. When asked to keep track of their caffeine intake, some people are surprised by the amount they consume each day. Two cups of coffee in the morning, one cup of coffee for a mid-morning and mid-afternoon break, and two or three soft drinks during the day add up to a significant dietary load of caffeine. A slow withdrawal from caffeine usually leads to some improvement in diarrhea and feelings of bowel urgency; this can be done by slowly decreasing the number of servings each day or by gradually substituting decaffeinated coffee and soft drinks.

Medications

As noted in the case study presented in Chapter 14, many medications are available over the counter or by prescription and may provide significant relief of symptoms, but they can also cause side effects. Finding the correct medication for you—one that alleviates your symptoms without intolerable side effects—may take some trial and error. The process begins by listing any medications (for any condition) and any supplements or herbal preparations that you are currently using and all the treatments for diarrhea that you have tried in the past. Many of the medications used in treating diarrhea are listed in Table 17.1. The way they work and their side effects are described below.

Over-the-Counter Medications

Loperamide. Loperamide (Imodium) is now the first choice for treating intermittent diarrhea. It first became available over the counter in liquid form in 1988 and in caplet form a year later. Loperamide is a very mild opiate (a type of narcotic). However, because only a small portion of it enters the brain, because the dose is small, and because the drug is rapidly broken down by the liver, the common side effects of narcotics (sedation, mental clouding, confusion, euphoria, respiratory depression, and addiction) are rarely encountered.

Loperamide slows the transit of materials through the intestinal tract, thereby allowing more fluid to be absorbed. It also slightly increases muscle tone in the anal canal, which can be helpful to people experiencing fecal soiling or fecal incontinence. Each caplet contains 2 mg of loperamide, and each teaspoonful (5 ml) of the liquid preparation contains 1 mg. A typical starting dose is 2 mg; for severe diarrhea, patients can take up to 8 pills a day for brief periods of time. Care should be taken to discontinue loperamide as soon as diarrhea is controlled, to avoid inducing constipation, especially in people who have IBS and are prone to alternating constipation and diarrhea.

Loperamide is not recommended for people who have inflammatory bowel disease (ulcerative colitis or Crohn's disease), because it may cause a condition called toxic megacolon. Loperamide should not be taken

Table 17.1. Medications Used to Treat Diarrhea

Bulk-forming agents (fiber products)
 Psyllium (Metamucil)
 Methylcellulose (Citrucel)
 Calcium polycarbophil (Equalactin, FiberCon)

5-HT3 antagonists
 Alosetron (Lotronex)

Bismuth products
 Bismuth subsalicylate (Pepto-Bismol)

Opiates
 Loperamide (Imodium)
 Diphenoxylate-atropine (Lomotil)
 DTO (deodorized tincture of opium)

Anticholinergic agents
 Atropine
 Dicyclomine (Bentyl)
 Hyoscyamine (Levsin, LevBid, NuLev)
 Scopolamine

Resin-binding agents
 Cholestyramine (Questran)

Tricyclic antidepressants
 Amitriptyline (Elavil)
 Nortriptyline (Pamelor)
 Desipramine (Norpramin)
 Imipramine (Tofranil)

Herbal preparations
 Agrimony (*Agrimonia eupatoria*)
 Bilberry (*Vaccinium myrtillus*)
 Blackberry (*Rubus fruticosus*)
 Cinquefoil (*Potentilla erecta*)
 Jambolan (*Syzygium cumini*)
 Lady's mantle (*Alchemilla vulgaris*)
 Uzara (*Xysmalobium undulatum*)

during the early stages of an *infectious* diarrhea. Diarrhea is one way the body eliminates toxins so, although diarrhea is unpleasant, during the initial stages of an infectious diarrhea it is important *not* to slow down the GI tract, since this would delay the evacuation of the infection from the body.

Many individuals who have IBS and diarrhea use loperamide prophylactically, to prevent episodes of fecal incontinence or minimize the risk of having diarrhea while traveling. This strategy can be especially helpful for people who have IBS and diarrhea who suffer from severe fecal urgency. In these patients, 1 to 2 mg of loperamide 45 minutes before a meal can significantly improve the heightened gastrocolic reflex that leads to the feelings of urgency after eating a meal. This prophylactic dosing should be done only when bowel patterns are well known, when the person's response to the medication has been established, and after discussions between patient and physician.

Although loperamide is widely used by people who have IBS and diarrhea and has been well tested in the general population, no large research studies have evaluated its benefits for the IBS population. Finally, while loperamide may improve diarrhea, it does not help the bloating and abdominal pain that typify IBS.

Pepto-Bismol. This inexpensive pink liquid has been around since 1901 and is a favorite of many people for treating mild cases of GI upset (indigestion, heartburn, fullness in the upper abdomen, nausea, or diarrhea). The active ingredient in Pepto-Bismol is bismuth subsalicylate. Although the exact mechanism of action of bismuth subsalicylate is unknown, it may have both mild anti-inflammatory properties and antimicrobial (antibacterial) activities. In addition, Pepto-Bismol contains a small amount of claylike particles (silicon dioxide), and it is possible that these bind to toxins in the GI tract and keep them from stimulating or inflaming the GI tract. For some people, Pepto-Bismol improves pain, fullness, and bloating in the upper GI tract as it coats the lining of the stomach. It is available in both liquid form (262 mg of bismuth subsalicylate per tablespoon [15 ml]) and tablet form (262 mg per tablet).

Although large-scale studies have not been performed to evaluate the efficacy of Pepto-Bismol for people who have IBS, several small double-blinded (when neither the patients nor the practitioners know until the end of the study who is receiving the medication versus the placebo), placebo-controlled studies have shown that it does relieve diarrhea in a general population of people with that symptom. This medication is generally considered safe for short-term use. Long-term use is not recommended, because it has the potential to cause several dangerous conditions (among them, salicylate toxicity, encephalopathy), especially in patients who have abnormal kidney function. Pepto-Bismol can turn the stool dark, which is often distressing to patients, especially since very dark stool can be a sign of internal bleeding, but this side effect is harmless.

Probiotics. You can barely open a newspaper now or turn on the television without seeing or hearing something new about probiotics. Although these agents are now widely used (and also misused) for a variety of ailments and conditions, a lot of misinformation about probiotics remains. Probiotics are live microorganisms which, when administered in an adequate amount, are intended to confer a health benefit to the host (the patient). There are a number of probiotics now available to consumers. Most are sold over the counter, although some are available only by prescription. Some of the most commonly used probiotics include strains (types) of lactic acid bacilli (e.g., *Lactobacillus, Bifidobacterium,* and *Lactococcus*). Other commercially available probiotics include strains of the bacteria *E. coli Nissle* 1917, *Clostridium butyricum, Streptococcus thermophilus, Streptococcus salivarius, Bacillus coagulans,* and *Enterococcus faecium.* Finally, some probiotics are nonpathogenic (not dangerous to the host) strains of yeast (e.g., *Saccharomyces boulardii* and *Saccharomyces cerevisiae*).

Although the discussion about the use of probiotics for the treatment of IBS symptoms is fairly new, the concept of using "good" microbes to improve intestinal health, and possibly even general well-being, has been around for quite some time. More than one hundred years ago, the Nobel Prize winner Elie Metchnikoff hypothesized that the consumption of yogurt, which contained the bacteria (the probiotic) *Lactobacillus,* was responsible for the increased longevity of eastern Europeans.

Probiotics are available in many different forms. They may be found naturally in food products such as yogurts and fermented milk, and they are now added to food bars, cereals, and even some baby formulas. Probiotics are also readily available over the counter in the form of capsules, pills, and powders. The amount of the probiotic bacteria is usually lower in naturally probiotic foods than in prescribed and over-the-counter probiotic products.

One question that patients commonly ask is, "How do probiotics work?" The honest answer is that no one really knows at present. Many different theories exist, and it is quite possible that probiotics work differently in different people (which may explain why probiotics seem to work so well for some people who have IBS but not for others). Probiotics may improve gastrointestinal symptoms by improving the immune system of the GI tract; suppressing the growth of harmful bacteria; improving the absorption of important vitamins and minerals; and/or producing products that maintain the health of the cells that line the colon. Although it may seem odd to recommend a product to a patient without knowing exactly how it works, there are good data to show that probiotics do work (see below), and this lack of knowledge shouldn't stop physicians from recommending something that can improve individuals' symptoms of IBS.

A good example of a patient who might benefit from a probiotic is someone who develops IBS symptoms after a viral gastroenteritis (such as postinfectious IBS). If you recall from our discussion in Chapter 3, some patients develop IBS symptoms after an infectious illness. In these people, the infection may have changed the normal composition of the gut flora (the bacteria that normally reside in the large intestine). The theory is that a "good" bacteria (such as a probiotic) can be added back to the GI tract to slowly restore the natural balance of bacteria in the large intestine. In support of this theory, some data show that the composition of the intestinal flora is different in patients who have IBS compared to those who don't. Unfortunately, we are not yet able to precisely measure the type and content of bacteria in everyone's colon. It is possible that in the future we will be able to measure colonic bacteria accurately enough that we can diagnose an individual with a specific deficiency of one gut bacteria or another and then make a specific recommendation about a probiotic that contains the missing bacteria.

As you read labels of probiotic products, remember that although many different probiotics have been recommended for patients who have IBS, *most* have not been specifically tested in such patients. Many probiotics make strong claims with little if any real data to support those claims. Because probiotics are currently considered food and dietary supplements, they are not strictly regulated by the FDA. In contrast to medications that have been FDA approved for the treatment of IBS, probiotics do not have to undergo rigorous testing or evaluation in clinical trials to assess their efficacy and safety.

Despite the lack of FDA regulation, two types of probiotics are worth mentioning here. *Bifidobacterium infantis* 35624, sold over the counter as Align, has been tested in two large placebo-controlled trials with patients who have IBS. Patients treated with Align showed a significant improvement in IBS symptoms of bloating, diarrhea, and pain, compared to those treated with a placebo. Align should be used once daily for at least 90 days to determine whether it can improve IBS and diarrhea symptoms. In addition, the product VSL#3 (which contains eight different strains of bacteria) appears to slow movement of materials through the large intestine and may improve symptoms of diarrhea and bloating in patients who have IBS and diarrhea. (See Chapter 20 for a discussion of the limitations and safety of probiotics.)

Prescription Medications

Antibiotics. One of the most interesting areas of research in the field of IBS during the last few years has been that of antibiotics for the treatment of IBS. This type of treatment is somewhat unusual, because patients who have IBS do not have an active infection in their GI tract that is the cause of their symptoms. However, as described earlier, one hypothesis about the development of IBS symptoms is that the normal gut flora (the normal content of bacteria in the large intestine) has been changed, possibly by an infection that has long since resolved. The treatment theory is that a course of antibiotics may again alter the balance or content of bacteria within the colon, thereby improving IBS symptoms. Alternatively, some researchers and clinicians believe that IBS symptoms develop due to the condition called SIBO (small intestine bacterial overgrowth; see Chapter 11). If this hypothesis is correct, then using antibiotics to treat the bacteria that inappropriately reside within the small intestine makes sense.

The best-studied antibiotic for the treatment of IBS with diarrhea is rifaximin. Rifaximin is a unique antibiotic because nearly all of it stays within the GI tract. In fact, less than 0.4 percent is absorbed from the GI tract, which makes it very safe. In addition, rifaximin is known to act on many of the bacteria that inhabit the large intestine (these are grouped under the categories of gram negative rods and anaerobes). Although the exact mechanism for why rifaximin improves IBS with diarrhea symptoms is unknown (Does it treat SIBO? Does it change colonic flora? Does it temporarily lower the bacterial content of the colon?), the results of five large, well-designed research studies have shown that patients who had IBS and were treated with rifaximin felt significantly better than patients who had IBS and were treated with a placebo pill. For the treated individuals, symptoms of bloating improved, as did symptoms of abdominal pain and diarrhea. Based on these five studies, the ideal IBS population for rifaximin treatment is composed of patients who have IBS with diarrhea or patients who have IBS with mixed symptoms of diarrhea and constipation. Occasionally, treatment with rifaximin can cause constipation in some patients; therefore, this medication is not recommended for people who have IBS and constipation.

According to the research, the most appropriate dosage of rifaximin is 550 mg taken 3 times daily for 14 days. Patients who have a positive response to rifaximin may expect an improvement in IBS symptoms for three to six months. Rifaximin is the first medication used to treat IBS (of any type) in which a patient only needs to be treated for a short time (just two weeks) but will still be experiencing benefits three to six months later. Although rifaximin has not yet been approved by the FDA for the treatment of IBS, a large multicenter study is currently under way. If the study results are positive, physicians are hopeful that rifaximin will be approved and available for patients who have IBS.

Other Agents

All of the medicines described below slow down the gastrointestinal tract by some means, so they should be used with care and close physician consultation by people who have IBS and alternate between diarrhea and constipation.

Lomotil. Lomotil is a brand name prescription medication consisting of diphenoxylate hydrochloride and atropine. Diphenoxylate is similar to loperamide in that it is a mild narcotic and works by slowing down the GI tract. When the GI tract is slowed down, more water can be absorbed, which leads to less frequent and more formed bowel movements. In addition, diphenoxylate may decrease the secretion of fluid into the GI tract. Atropine is classified as an anticholinergic agent (see below). It works throughout the GI tract to slow motility and also blunts the strong contractions of the colon and small bowel that are perceived as spasms and cramps.

Some patients find that Lomotil works better than Imodium to treat their diarrhea, especially if they suffer from persistent abdominal cramps and spasms. Lomotil, like Imodium, will not help with bloating due to IBS. However, in contrast to loperamide, a slight potential for becoming addicted to the diphenoxylate component exists. Also, because of the anticholinergic effects (the atropine component), loperamide can cause some people to suffer from a dry mouth and to develop a rapid heart rate (tachycardia).

DTO (deodorized tincture of opium). Tincture of opium is essentially a liquid preparation of opium (along with a small amount of deodorant to help disguise the unpleasant taste). Since it is a narcotic, DTO, like loperamide and diphenoxylate-atropine, slows the GI tract and promotes fluid absorption from the colon. Because it is more addictive, this prescription medication is generally reserved for patients who fail to get relief from maximum doses of loperamide or diphenoxylate-atropine. The typical starting dose is one or two drops each morning in a small amount of water or juice. Patients then monitor their symptoms and, if necessary, may slowly increase the dose by an additional drop or two each morning. Patients report that DTO does not help with the pain, gassiness, or bloating of IBS.

Anticholinergic agents. This term encompasses a large group of fairly similarly acting prescription medications; some of the most common are atropine, scopolamine, and dicyclomine. Anticholinergic agents block the actions of acetylcholine, a neurotransmitter involved in gut motility. More specifically, acetylcholine is one of the major chemicals that initiate and maintain smooth-muscle contraction in the GI tract. When the actions of acetylcholine are blocked, the smooth muscle of the GI tract relaxes and quiets down. This leads to a slowing of gut motility and increased fluid absorption from the GI tract.

Unlike with opiates, there is no potential for addiction with anticholinergic agents. However, because these medications act throughout the entire body, not just in the GI tract, side effects can develop, especially with larger doses. These side effects include dry mouth, dry eyes, changes in vision, difficulty urinating, fatigue, sleepiness, and, rarely, constipation.

Cholestyramine. This prescription medication, classified as a resin-binding agent, functions very differently from all of the substances discussed above. It acts by binding to bile acids, which are important to the digestive process because they help absorb fats. Bile acids are formed in the liver, pass through the bile duct, and are emptied into the small intestine, where they help to absorb fats. In some patients, bile acids can cause diarrhea, if they irritate the lining of the colon and stimulate colonic motility.

Cholestyramine is generally started at a small dose once or twice a day and then gradually increased to four times a day, if necessary. It is available in both individual-dose packets and in a large can; the brand name is Questran. Although cholestyramine has never been studied with a large group of people who have IBS, it has been proven to help people who have other types of chronic diarrhea. Cholestyramine is considered safe, although if used for long periods of time or at high doses, cholestyramine has the potential to bind to certain medications and vitamins, causing them to be excreted from the body without being properly absorbed.

Tricyclic antidepressants (TCAs). This class of prescription medications was used for many years to treat depression, although in retrospect, they were not very effective at treating symptoms of depression in most people. Newer agents (the SSRIs—see Chapter 22) have nearly completely replaced TCAs in the treatment of depression. However, TCAs are often very effective in relieving some of the symptoms of IBS and diarrhea, if carefully used at low to moderate doses. TCAs tend to slow colonic transit to some degree and thus decrease the frequency of bowel movements. In addition, these agents seem to blunt or block some of the strong contractions in the GI tract of people who have IBS and diarrhea. Thus, many patients find a significant improvement in bowel urgency, spasms, pain, cramps, and diarrhea when treated with TCAs.

The relief of IBS symptoms is itself a side effect of TCAs, for that was not their intended function, but they also have a number of undesirable side effects, especially if used at the high doses typically required for patients who have severe IBS symptoms. These side effects, which include constipation, sedation, dry mouth, dry eyes, and urine retention, are all related to their anticholinergic action (see above), and they make taking the drug unpleasant for many patients. Some of the TCAs most commonly prescribed for relief of IBS symptoms are listed in Table 17.1.

Alosetron. Alosetron (sold as Lotronex) is a 5-HT3 antagonist. Alosetron works by blocking the action of serotonin at specific receptors in the GI tract. Excess serotonin can lead to overstimulation of the GI tract, causing rapid transit of material through the intestines and the generation of strong muscular contractions in both the colon and small intestine. Serotonin receptors are located throughout the GI tract. The concept of blocking a specific receptor is based on the "lock and key" model: if a specific receptor site (the lock) is physically blocked by an antagonist molecule (such as a medication), then the neurotransmitter molecule (the key) that normally fits into the lock cannot attach, and the receptor cannot receive its message and be activated. In this case, serotonin cannot attach to its specific receptor, because the receptor site is blocked by alosetron. If serotonin cannot bind to its receptors, then it cannot speed up gut motility and initiate strong muscular contractions, a process important in the development of symptoms of IBS with diarrhea.

For women who have diarrhea-predominant IBS, alosetron has been shown to be effective at treating many of the common symptoms of IBS. (Too few men participated in the original studies for the reports to make scientifically sound statements about the drug's effectiveness in men.) Women treated with this prescription drug noted a significant improvement in their diarrhea, a reduction in their level of abdominal pain, and an improvement in the sense of urgency associated with having a bowel movement. These results were demonstrated in four large, randomized, double-blind, placebo-controlled studies involving thousands of patients. A panel of experts from the American College of Gastroenterology (a professional organization composed of nearly ten thousand gastroenterologists and researchers) noted that alosetron provided a significant reduction in all the symptoms of diarrhea, abdominal pain, and bloating in patients who have IBS and diarrhea. Many women who had tried and not been helped by traditional therapies noted a dramatic improvement in their IBS symptoms while taking alosetron.

Alosetron is currently available for use under an RMP (Risk Management Program). Approximately 280 medications on the market are available under an RMP. This program requires that if your doctor prescribes alosetron to you, you sign a form saying that she or he reviewed the risks and benefits of this medication with you (please note that the risks and benefits of every medication should always be explained to you, not just for alosetron). Alosetron is part of an RMP because a few study individuals who had IBS and diarrhea became very constipated or possibly developed an uncommon condition called ischemic colitis after taking alosetron. Ischemic colitis is a condition in which there is a reduction in blood flow to the colon, which can lead to pain and bloody diarrhea. The risk of developing ischemic colitis while taking alosetron is quite low—about one in one thousand. Approximately one thousand people who have IBS and diarrhea would need to be treated with alosetron before one of those patients developed ischemic colitis. When ischemic colitis does occur (either in a patient who has IBS or in any other patient), it generally resolves on its own without any long-term effects after the patient stops taking alosetron. Research has shown that, in general, people who have IBS are at increased risk for ischemic colitis—it is not solely associated with those people who have IBS and are taking alosetron.

If your doctor decides that alosetron may be the right medication for you, then you can become a part of the prescribing program for Lotronex. You will need to sign a consent form and stay in contact with your doctor. Since this program was instituted, there have not been any major adverse reactions to alosetron. This highlights the fact that, when a knowledgeable health care provider prescribes this medication for an appropriate patient (such as a woman who has IBS and diarrhea), it is quite safe.

Herbal agents. A number of herbal preparations for the treatment of diarrhea are currently on the market (see Table 17.1). None of these herbal remedies has been subjected to double-blind, placebo-controlled trials for any large group of people who have diarrhea, and none has been tested in a research setting by patients who have IBS and diarrhea. However, they are now frequently used by people who have IBS. If you decide to try an herbal remedy, you should buy it from a reputable source and make sure that it is in a pure form, rather than mixed with a variety of other agents. In addition, you should talk to the owner or manager of the health food store or pharmacy where you purchase these agents, to evaluate that person's professional knowledge of the use of the medication. If you have friends who have used the product, you should talk to them about their experience. Follow the printed directions carefully, and start at the lowest dose you can, slowly increasing the amount without exceeding the dosage on the instructions. Let your primary care doctor know that you are going to try the product, and contact him or her if you notice any change in your health. It is possible that one of these agents will improve your diarrhea, but given the absence of research on these substances, and given the complicated nature of IBS, don't be surprised if these agents do not improve other symptoms of IBS, like abdominal pain, bloating, and distention, even if they do ease the diarrhea.

Summary

- Diet can play a significant role in IBS with diarrhea.
- Patients who have IBS and diarrhea should carefully review their intake of caffeine, lactose, fructose, sorbitol, and fiber, because these can all worsen diarrhea.
- The medical treatment for diarrhea focuses on slowing transit through the GI tract. This allows better absorption of water, the formation of more-solid stool, and less frequent bowel movements.
- Loperamide (Imodium) and diphenoxylate-atropine (Lomotil) are both very mild narcotics that can improve diarrhea by slowing the GI tract. They are usually not effective at treating the abdominal pain or bloating frequently experienced by patients who have IBS and diarrhea.
- Probiotics are being extensively studied with patients who have IBS. The probiotic Align has been shown to improve IBS and diarrhea symptoms in two large, well-designed studies.
- Antibiotics may help some patients who have IBS and diarrhea, but they need to be chosen carefully, because many antibiotics can worsen IBS and diarrhea symptoms.
- Alosetron is the only medication currently approved by the FDA for the treatment of IBS with diarrhea. It has been shown to be safe and effective for many patients who have IBS and diarrhea.

CHAPTER 18

Medications for Abdominal Pain Associated with IBS

Treating the chronic abdominal pain felt by people who have irritable bowel syndrome can be frustrating to both patients and physicians. If the diagnosis of IBS has not yet been made, it is frustrating that diagnostic studies and tests repeatedly turn up normal or "negative" instead of providing a clear reason for the symptoms. Chronic abdominal pain can be quite difficult to treat, and in people who have IBS, the abdominal pain tends to be persistent or recurring. In addition, it is bothersome that even if the altered bowel habits of IBS are eased, the abdominal pain can persist. These problems are well illustrated by the case of Maria, a patient who has IBS and chronic abdominal pain.

When Maria was 32, she visited a new internist for a third opinion about her long history of abdominal pain and altered bowel habits. Her pain had begun during her senior year of high school after she was robbed. Although she was not injured physically, she was severely traumatized emotionally. She cancelled her plans to go to college and instead took on a part-time job. She moved in with her boyfriend, but that relationship soured and she lived on her own for the next several years. She worked at a variety of jobs during that time, but they usually ended up with her quitting or being fired. Maria dated several men during the next few years, but each relationship was fairly short lived.

In her mid-twenties Maria developed problems with lower abdominal pain and intermittent diarrhea. At first the diarrhea and pain occurred once or twice a week, usually as she was getting ready to go to work. She saw her primary care physician, who told her that the abdominal pain was probably just a spasm of her GI tract and that avoiding milk products and minimizing fiber would relieve her symptoms. These changes did not help her pain and, in fact, her symptoms worsened. At the time of her follow-up visit her doctor ordered some laboratory tests and an ultrasound of her abdomen. Both tests yielded normal results. Maria was relieved to hear that the tests were normal, but she wondered why she was still having the pain, which was occurring even more frequently. Maria's doctor prescribed hyoscyamine, a medication designed to relax the smooth muscle of the GI tract. It seemed to work only intermittently.

Maria's symptoms intensified over the next several years, becoming significantly worse after her mother died of ovarian cancer. She became depressed and withdrew from family and friends. Maria did some reading at the library and some research on the Internet and became convinced that her symptoms meant that she, too, had ovarian cancer. Her doctor listened carefully, performed a thorough physical examination, and made an appointment for her to see a gynecologist for a complete pelvic examination. This exam was normal, but the gynecologist ordered some specialized blood tests and a CT scan of the abdomen and pelvis to eliminate any possibility of cancer and, she hoped, to reassure Maria. Fortunately, these tests all came back normal.

Maria noted a further worsening of her pain, however, and she was next referred to a gastroenterologist. A colonoscopy was scheduled, because of her chronic diarrhea. The colonoscopy, including biopsies (samples of tissue) of the colon, revealed no abnormalities. Again Maria was pleased by the test results but wondered why she still had pain every day. The gastroenterologist gave her a prescription for dicyclomine (another medication to relax the smooth muscle of the GI tract) and told her to use the medication regularly for her abdominal pain. He also prescribed Lomotil, for her diarrhea. On this regimen, Maria's diarrhea improved, but her abdominal pain worsened. She stopped going to work because she said it hurt too much to work. She lost her job and filed for medical disability. During the next 6 months, Maria gained over 45 pounds, which made her even more depressed. She saw a second gastroenterologist, who performed an upper endoscopy (also called an EGD); this test was also normal. Blood work was ordered to measure the function of her thyroid, liver, and pancreas, and all results were normal.

Maria went to see another internist. This doctor recognized Maria's depression and gave her a prescription for an antidepressant; however, Maria did not fill the prescription. Shortly thereafter, because of severe abdominal pain, Maria went to the emergency room late one winter evening. The emergency room was extremely busy, because several automobile accidents had occurred at once. A young doctor there reviewed her records, performed a brief examination, and gave her six tablets of Percocet (a type of narcotic). As she took one Percocet tablet twice a day for the next three days, Maria finally obtained some relief from her chronic abdominal pain. However, after the medication ran out, her pain reappeared. She went back to see her most recent internist and requested a renewal of the Percocet. The doctor refused, stating that she did not prescribe narcotics for the treatment of chronic abdominal pain.

Out of frustration, and because of continued pain, Maria made an appointment with a surgeon, who ordered an ultrasound of her gallbladder and a test to measure how well the gallbladder emptied bile into the small intestine. Although the ultrasound looked normal, he said that the pain might be due to the gallbladder emptying bile a little more slowly than normal. He recommended that she have her gallbladder out. She agreed, convinced that this would cure her pain. After her gallbladder was removed, Maria noted an improvement in her pain for about a week, while she was on postsurgical pain medication, but then all of her symptoms returned and her diarrhea worsened. She then consulted a third gastroenterologist, who repeated some of the blood tests and ordered another CT scan of her abdomen and pelvis. These tests were once again normal. This doctor prescribed Donnatal (another medication to help the smooth muscle of the GI tract relax) twice a day with Lomotil four times a day. This combination of medications helped her diarrhea, but her daily abdominal pain continued. She then made an appointment to see a third internist, to discuss her abdominal pain.

Although Maria's case may seem complex and drawn out, her story is not all that uncommon. Chronic abdominal pain can persist for years and often leads to extensive and sometimes unnecessary testing, repeated and expensive doctor visits, and even unnecessary surgery. In fact, several good research studies have shown that women who have IBS are two to three times more likely than women who do not have IBS to have unnecessary surgery, including unnecessary removal of the gallbladder, appendix, and uterus.

The section below reviews current concepts about why abdominal pain occurs in people who have IBS and discusses the treatment options that are available. The chapter concludes with a look at the possibility of treating the totality of symptoms of IBS, by definition a multisymptom condition. Identifying one medication that is best for *all* patients who have IBS is not possible. Within a given class of drug, most of these medications are not significantly better or worse than the others. Finding the right one or ones for an individual person is often a matter of trial and error, to determine which medication provides the best relief of symptoms with the fewest side effects in that patient.

Abdominal Pain

Persistent, intractable, or recurrent abdominal pain is the most common reason why people who have IBS make an appointment to see a physician. Many people who have IBS learn to cope with their constipation or diarrhea, no matter how inconvenient or disabling these symptoms may be. They use over-the-counter medications to minimize symptoms, they adapt to their symptoms by adjusting work or travel schedules, and they just generally learn to live with their bowel patterns. But abdominal pain is a different matter. Over-the-counter remedies (aspirin, acetaminophen, and anti-inflammatory agents like Motrin or Advil) are rarely effective in the treatment of IBS.

Chronic abdominal pain can significantly impede daily function and is obviously unpleasant. No one likes to suffer from pain, whether it's from a migraine headache, a twisted ankle, or chronic abdominal pain from IBS. It can disrupt school and work and can significantly diminish the quality of daily life on multiple levels—physical, emotional, and mental. In addition, chronic pain can be exhausting, both mentally and physically; persistent pain, of any sort, wears people down. It may lead to anger, pessimism, hopelessness, and even depression. Finally, the fact that relief cannot be obtained with simple over-the-counter remedies often causes people to worry that something serious "must be going on" inside of their body, and they fear that the pain is due to cancer.

For some people who have IBS, the abdominal pain is just an intermittent annoyance, while for others it may be excruciating and disabling. Some patients describe the pain as a dull ache or discomfort; others call it crampy or like a spasm. Still others describe their pain as twisting, burning, or stabbing in nature. Most patients who have IBS have pain in the lower left quadrant or in the lower central pelvis, above the pubic bone. These are the areas, respectively, of the descending colon, sigmoid colon, and rectum. However, IBS pain may occur anywhere throughout the abdomen. Most individuals who have IBS have a pattern of pain that is typical for them and does not change over time. The pain may change in intensity, but the character of the pain tends to remain the same.

Abdominal pain is experienced by people who have IBS for four main reasons. One, extraordinarily strong contractions can occur in the smooth muscle that lines the colon and small intestine. Two, it appears that people who have IBS are more sensitive to stimulation in the GI tract (heightened visceral sensitivity). Three, patients who have IBS appear to perceive pain differently in their brain. The ability to "block out" or ignore painful sensations from the gut is lower in patients who have IBS than in people who do not have IBS; thus, a greater proportion of painful sensations from the gut are sensed. Four, distention of the colon or small intestine from gas may cause pain or discomfort for some patients (this is discussed in Chapter 3).

Medications currently available to treat chronic abdominal pain are listed in Table 18.1 and discussed below.

Over-the-Counter Analgesics

Medications that relieve pain are classified as analgesics (*an* means "without"; *algesia* means "pain"). Many over-the-counter analgesic agents are now available. They fall into one of three main categories. One category is products that contain aspirin (Bufferin, Excedrin, etc.). Aspirin, derived from the bark of the willow tree, has been used to treat pain since at least the 1700s. Aspirin was formally introduced in 1899, and it is

Table 18.1. Medications Used to Treat Abdominal Pain

Smooth-muscle antispasmodics

    Hyoscyamine (Levsin)

    Dicyclomine (Bentyl)

    Librax (chlordiazepoxide + clidinium)

    Donnatal (phenobarbital + atropine + hyoscyamine + scopolamine)

    Glycopyrrolate (Robinul)

Anticholinergic agents

    Atropine

    Glycopyrrolate (Robinul)

    Hyoscyamine (Levsin)

    Scopolamine

    Methscopolamine (Pamine)

Tricyclic antidepressants

    Amitriptyline (Elavil)

    Desipramine (Norpramin)

    Doxepin (Sinequan)

    Imipramine (Tofranil)

    Nortriptyline (Pamelor)

Selective serotonin reuptake inhibitors (SSRIs)

Herbal remedies and alternative therapies

    Peppermint oil

    Ginger

    Aloe

    Acupuncture

Miscellaneous

    Carbamazepine (Tegretol)

    Phenytoin (Dilantin)

    Tramadol (Ultram)

    Gabapentin (Neurontin)

    Pregabalin (Lyrica)

estimated that as much as twenty thousand tons of it is used each year in the United States alone. Aspirin acts to reduce fever and inflammation in the body. A second category of analgesic contains acetaminophen (for example, Tylenol). Acetaminophen was introduced in 1893, although it has only become really popular in the last 50 years. It is used to treat mild to moderate pain of various causes. Like aspirin, it reduces fever, but it has minimal anti-inflammatory effect. The third category is nonsteroidal anti-inflammatory drugs (NSAIDs, such as Motrin, Advil, Ibuprofen, and Aleve). These medications are used for mild to moderate pain; they reduce fever and treat inflammation.

All three types of analgesic are generally effective at treating the everyday aches and pains that we all occasionally suffer, including mild headaches, muscle aches and pains from a cold or flu, muscle pain from doing too much heavy lifting, or joint pain from arthritis. These products are also considered relatively safe if taken at the recommended doses for short periods of time. However, chronic use of either aspirin products or NSAIDs increases the risk of internal bleeding, most commonly from an ulcer in the stomach or small intestine. Chronic use or short-term high-dose use of acetaminophen (especially when combined with alcohol) can injure the liver. Unfortunately, none of these agents seems to provide any significant relief from the recurrent abdominal pain that typifies IBS. Physiologically, this makes sense, because both aspirin and NSAIDs are designed to treat inflammation, and irritable bowel syndrome is not an inflammatory condition.

Smooth-Muscle Antispasmodic Agents

Over the last two decades, the group of prescription medications labeled smooth-muscle antispasmodic agents has evolved into a mainstay of therapy for treating patients who have IBS and abdominal pain. These agents act throughout the GI tract to relax smooth muscle. By relaxing the smooth muscle of the gut, these agents can help relieve the spasms (hence the name antispasmodic) and cramps that are often associated with abdominal pain. Some patients who have IBS and diarrhea find that these medications also help with the sensation of urgency that can accompany diarrhea. Other patients report that antispasmodic agents help with bloating and distention. These medications function primarily by blocking the neurotransmitter vital to muscle contraction, acetylcholine, so, in fact, they are anticholinergic agents (see below).

Ample theoretical grounds exist for prescribing antispasmodic medications, but research studies of them during the last two decades have been few and small scale, although positive. Several small studies in Europe showed that they improved abdominal pain. In addition, a meta-analysis of the data from all of the published research studies found that smooth-muscle antispasmodics improved symptoms of abdominal pain for patients who had IBS. Unfortunately, none of the medications tested in the European studies is currently available in the United States. One study performed in the United States over 25 years ago did show that 40 mg of one of these drugs, dicyclomine hydrochloride (Bentyl), taken 4 times a day improved symptoms of abdominal pain in patients who had IBS. Approximately two-thirds of the patients enrolled in that study suffered side effects, but the dose they were taking is higher than that prescribed by most physicians. In summary, although they are widely used, we have little data on these agents from research studies performed in the United States.

Many patients who have IBS find that their symptoms improve with antispasmodic drugs, particularly if those symptoms are precipitated by meals and sensations of fecal urgency. Despite the limited evidence available to support their use, these medications are commonly prescribed by physicians. This practice may reflect the fact that these drugs provide greater benefits in the clinical setting than have been reported in the research studies or simply that few other options exist.

What recommendations can be given regarding the use of smooth-muscle antispasmodics? For the majority of patients, these medications are best used as needed (p.r.n.) rather than on a regular basis. Some people find that the beneficial effects of antispasmodics wear off over time if they are used on a daily basis. (This raises the issue of whether one develops a tolerance to these medications, a question that has not been studied.) When used for meal-induced symptoms, antispasmodics should be taken 30 to 60 minutes before meals so that peak blood levels of the drug coincide with peak symptoms. Because these medications improve symptoms of abdominal pain for some patients who have IBS, and because they have an extremely low potential for addiction, they can safely be used on an intermittent basis to treat abdominal pain in patients who have IBS. However, they will not cure IBS. Side effects of these agents include dry mouth, dry eyes, difficulty concentrating, urine hesitancy, and fatigue.

Hyoscyamine and Dicyclomine

Hyoscyamine is one of the most commonly prescribed smooth-muscle antispasmodics. It is available in three formulations: a sublingual (under-the-tongue) tablet, a slow-release form, and a liquid. The sublingual tablet (Levsin SL; NuLev) dissolves within minutes and reaches its peak effect in approximately 45 to 60 minutes, although the drug remains in the bloodstream for hours. The liquid (elixir) acts more quickly than the slow-release or sublingual forms. In our experience, the sublingual tablet and liquid can effectively minimize the cramps and urgency that develop after eating a meal. Some patients keep supplies of sublingual tablets at home, in their car, and at work, in order to be prepared at all times. The slow-release, long-acting form (Levsin SR) is taken orally either once or twice a day, depending on symptoms. Dicyclomine (Bentyl) is another commonly prescribed smooth-muscle antispasmodic. It comes in both pill and liquid forms and can be taken from one to four times a day. Its effects are similar to hyoscyamine.

Because both hyoscyamine and dicyclomine work by blocking the neurotransmitter (acetylcholine) that causes smooth muscles to contract throughout the body, these medications have a number of possible side effects. Common side effects are dry mouth or dry eyes, feeling sleepy or fatigued, urinary hesitancy, and difficulty concentrating. At higher doses, some patients note that they feel somewhat groggy throughout the day, become constipated, or have difficulty urinating. As with any medication, side effects can develop in some patients but not others who take the same dose. This can occur because of differences in the individuals' size, age, other medications that are taken, use of alcohol or narcotics, frequency of dosing, and length of time the medication has been used.

Hyoscyamine and dicyclomine are generally safe to take with other medications; however if used with other medicines that have similar side effects (like anticholinergics or TCAs—see below), side effects could be worse. It is important to note that these medications *should not be used if you have glaucoma*, because they can worsen that eye disorder.

Librax and Donnatal

These two smooth-muscle antispasmodics are different from the two described above because they are mixtures of drugs rather than single agents. Librax is a mixture of chlordiazepoxide and clidinium. Chlordiazepoxide is a benzodiazepine, which is a class of drug that helps people to relax and eases anxiety. (Valium is one of the best-known benzodiazepines, although there are many others.) Clidinium is similar to hyoscyamine and dicyclomine. Librax is used to treat symptoms of abdominal pain, cramps, and urgency. It can be especially helpful for people who are also nervous or anxious, because the benzodiazepine component (chlordiazepoxide) helps to relieve anxiety. Librax is prescribed much less frequently than are dicyclomine and hyoscyamine, because many physicians are concerned about patients becoming addicted to the chlordiazepoxide component of the medication. Benzodiazepines, if not monitored carefully and used appropriately, can be addictive.

Donnatal is made up of four agents and is available in pill and liquid forms. Its components are hyoscyamine (an antispasmodic agent), atropine (an anticholinergic agent—see below), scopolamine (an anticholinergic agent), and phenobarbital (classified as an anticonvulsant, usually used to treat seizures). The inclusion of an anticonvulsant seems odd; however, research studies have shown that some medications used to treat seizures also ease nerve pain to a small degree. In addition, phenobarbital can induce mild sedation, which can be helpful for patients whose severe symptoms keep them from sleeping. Donnatal is rarely the first agent prescribed for patients who have IBS; rather, it is generally reserved for patients who have tried other medications but have not had any improvement and for patients who have particularly severe symptoms. Combination agents are sometimes more effective in treating abdominal spasms, cramps, and pain than any single agent.

Some patients and care providers feel that Donnatal causes fewer side effects than some of the other anticholinergic agents. This may be because the amounts of each component medication are much smaller than if the agents were used individually. Like Librax, Donnatal is best used on an as-needed basis for brief periods of time. Typical side effects are similar to those of Librax, although people may feel somewhat more fatigued or groggy on Donnatal, due to the inclusion of phenobarbital. Note that these medications should be used cautiously by people who have IBS and constipation, as opposed to those who have IBS and diarrhea, because they may worsen constipation.

Robinul (Glycopyrrolate)

Although this medication is classified as an anticholinergic agent (described in the next section), it is often used to treat spasms in the GI tract.

Anticholinergic Agents

This category encompasses a large group of prescription medications, some of the most common being atropine, glycopyrrolate, scopolamine, and dicyclomine (dicyclomine is described above). Anticholinergic agents (as described in Chapter 17) block the effects of acetylcholine, a neurotransmitter that plays a critical role in gut motility. It signals the smooth muscle to contract. As we've discussed, this contraction is sometimes too strong in patients who have IBS, and the exaggerated contractions can be quite painful. When the effects of acetylcholine are blocked by anticholinergic agents, the smooth muscle of the GI tract relaxes. This reduces spasms, slows gut motility, and relieves the sense of discomfort or urgency associated with having a bowel movement in people who have IBS.

Robinul (Glycopyrrolate)

As noted in the previous section, Robinul is another medication used to treat spasms and overly strong contractions in the GI tract. However, it is less commonly prescribed than the other antispasmodic agents, because most health care providers think of it as a medication to reduce the production of saliva and bronchial secretions (conveniently in some circumstances, one of the most common side effects of smooth muscle antispasmodics is a dry mouth). No studies have compared Robinul to any of the other antispasmodic medications, so it is not possible to make a valid recommendation about which medication is better. Robinul is generally prescribed in 1-mg doses, taken twice daily.

Unlike the opiates (such as those in Imodium and Lomotil), anticholinergic agents do not have any potential for addiction, even if used for long periods of time. However, like the smooth-muscle antispasmodics, anticholinergic agents act throughout the body, which increases the likelihood that side effects will develop, especially if the dose of the medication is increased or taken more frequently. Potential side effects of anticholinergic agents include dry mouth, dry eyes, change in vision, difficulty urinating, fatigue, sleepiness, and, rarely, constipation.

Tricyclic Antidepressants (TCAs)

Many people who have IBS become skeptical or even offended when they hear the word *antidepressant*. This is not surprising, because a large number of people who have IBS have been told that they are "crazy" or that their intestinal problems are "all in your head." The symptoms of IBS are real; they are not "all in your head." The tricyclic antidepressants (TCAs), although used extensively in the past to treat depression, are actually not very effective for that condition, especially when compared to the newer antidepressant drugs. However, several research studies have demonstrated that these medications, when used in low doses, improve symptoms of nerve pain. Most importantly, research studies have shown that TCAs can be very effective at treating chronic abdominal pain in patients who have IBS. While we continue to refer to these drugs by their original purpose, when used to treat IBS they are not being prescribed because the patient is depressed.

The exact mechanism by which TCAs relieve abdominal pain in patients who have IBS is unknown. They may affect the nerves that lead from the gut to the spinal cord and then the brain, or they may act directly on the brain, influencing how people sense pain in the gut, possibly by altering the thresholds for sensing pain in the central nervous system.

In contrast to both the smooth-muscle antispasmodics and the anticholinergic agents, which are best used as needed rather than taken regularly, tricyclic antidepressants are utilized most effectively with a routine schedule. It is safe to combine TCAs with most of the medications described above, and many patients find significant relief of their symptoms by taking a small dose of a TCA each evening and then using an antispasmodic as needed for intermittent episodes of cramping, spasm, or pain.

Many of the side effects of TCAs are the same as for the antispasmodics and anticholinergic agents: dry mouth, dry eyes, fatigue, and difficulty concentrating. Some patients find that their blood pressure decreases a small amount, while other patients may gain weight on these medications. One of the side effects most likely to occur is mild sedation. For that reason, most clinicians who prescribe TCAs ask patients to take them at night, so that they do not feel tired during the day. Since a large number of people who have IBS have some degree of insomnia, taking a TCA at night can have the advantage of improving that symptom as well.

Generally, TCAs can be used by patients who have IBS with diarrhea, constipation, or alternating bowel habits. At the low doses in which they are usually taken, they don't cause constipation. However, some patients require higher doses for their abdominal pain, and as the dose is increased, constipation is more likely to develop. People who have IBS and constipation may find that TCAs improve their abdominal pain but worsen their constipation.

TCAs do not work immediately. Both patients and physicians need to remember that it may take four to six weeks before any significant benefits are noted. In addition, the dose may need to be slowly increased, extending the trial period to 12 to 16 weeks. Also, TCAs do not work in everyone. Some patients respond very well to these agents, whereas other patients do not respond at all. Some people respond to one TCA but not to another. Therefore, a patient and physician may decide to try a different TCA if the first one prescribed does not lead to any improvement in abdominal pain. Common TCAs include amitriptyline, nortriptyline, and desipramine.

Since TCAs are generally used in low doses to treat abdominal pain, patients with coexisting depression usually do *not* notice any improvement in that condition. However, tricyclic antidepressants are safe to take with other antidepressants, for example, the class of drugs known as SSRIs.

Selective Serotonin Reuptake Inhibitors (SSRIs)

A newer class of drugs for the treatment of depression, selective serotonin reuptake inhibitors (SSRIs) are among the most commonly prescribed drugs worldwide. These medications are also effective in treating some people who have mild anxiety, obsessive-compulsive disorder, somatization disorders, and social phobias. Because many people who have moderate to severe IBS also suffer from depression, anxiety, or a somatization disorder, it seems only natural to evaluate the use of these medications in treating IBS. However, only a few studies have been done, primarily looking at how these medications improve pain and quality of life for patients who have IBS. The data available are limited and to some degree conflicting. One study of 23 patients who had IBS but did not have depression showed that citalopram (Celexa) significantly improved symptoms of IBS compared to a placebo. However, another study of 54 patients who had IBS found that citalopram did not improve IBS symptoms during an eight-week study period. A third study of 72 patients who had IBS found that paroxetine (Paxil) improved quality of life for these patients, although it did not improve their abdominal pain during the 12-week study. A fourth study found that fluoxetine (Prozac) did not improve symptoms of abdominal pain in patients who had IBS. No studies have been conducted using some of the other popular SSRIs, such as sertraline (Zoloft), venlafaxine (Effexor), desvenlafaxine (Pristiq), or escitalopram (Lexapro).

Thus, limited and even conflicting data exist on whether patients will have an improvement in their IBS symptoms when treated with an SSRI. This points out why further research is needed in the field of IBS in general and, in particular, with regard to the treatment of abdominal pain. A large research study involving hundreds or even thousands of patients will be required to sort out this complicated issue. I suspect that, once sufficient data are collected and evaluated, we will find that SSRIs lead to an improvement in patients who have IBS and suffer from coexisting anxiety and depression. When these disorders are under better control, most patients find that they can cope with their abdominal pain much better. Direct effects on abdominal pain may be discovered as well, possibly through the actions of SSRIs in the brain.

If you and your health care provider decide that you should try an SSRI, it is important to be aware that you may not notice *any* improvements in your mood or pain for at least three to six weeks. Your dosage will probably need to be adjusted at routine follow-up visits. Because these medications take a while to work, a reasonable therapeutic trial of any single agent usually requires a minimum of 8 to 12 weeks; by then you will know whether the medication has truly helped. Some patients find that the first SSRI they try does not work but that the second or third agent does. You will need to work closely with your health care provider to find the most appropriate medication and the best dose for you. Although these medications are generally safe, some patients develop side effects, which can include mild diarrhea (which generally goes away within a few days without treatment), headaches, sedation, difficulty sleeping, vivid dreams, and loss of interest in sex.

Herbal Remedies and Alternative Therapies

Peppermint oil, an age-old remedy for many conditions, is recommended and used by many people who have IBS for alleviation of abdominal pain and bloating. A small research study performed nearly 30 years ago found that peppermint oil, when placed on a small strip of smooth muscle, caused the muscle to relax. This finding led to several small clinical trials of the effects of peppermint oil in patients who have IBS. Those studies noted modest improvement in some patients' abdominal pain. Other studies, however, have not shown any improvement. An analysis of all published medical studies of peppermint oil (a meta-analysis) showed no significant improvements in abdominal pain and bloating in people who have IBS. Thus, the data from research studies, when taken as a whole, do not support the theory that peppermint oil significantly improves IBS symptoms in most patients.

Peppermint oil is a safe medication and is reasonably inexpensive. Many patients who have IBS do find that it provides some relief from their symptoms. If you decide to try peppermint oil, make sure that you buy it from a reputable health food store, and get the enteric-coated formulation. The enteric coating delays release in the GI tract. If the oil is released too soon, it is rapidly broken down in the stomach, and is of little or no value for the relief of abdominal pain. The most common side effect of peppermint oil, ironically, is heartburn. Peppermint oil can relax the lower esophageal sphincter (the smooth-muscle valve at the end of your esophagus), thereby increasing the risk that stomach acid will reflux, or regurgitate, into the esophagus.

Very few other alternative medications or treatments have been evaluated in people who have IBS. One well-designed, randomized, placebo-controlled trial found that patients who had IBS and were treated with a standard Chinese herbal formulation (a combination of more than 20 herbs) noted improvement in multiple symptoms of IBS compared to patients who had IBS and were treated with a placebo. An Ayurvedic preparation of two herbs was found to be superior to placebo in the treatment of patients who had IBS and diarrhea in a six-week, double-blind, randomized, controlled trial. Ginger and aloe (liquid) are commonly used by people who have IBS, although there are no controlled trials evaluating their efficacy. Acupuncture has given symptomatic relief to some people who have IBS. A recent placebo-controlled trial testing acupuncture's influence on rectal sensation found no effect.

More and more people are using natural remedies and alternative treatments when conventional medications have failed to provide relief. If you elect to do so, please make sure that you bring any herbal medications (or their labels) to your next doctor's appointment, to ensure that the medication is not dangerous or incompatible with another medication you are taking.

Narcotics

Maria's story, presented at the beginning of this chapter, illustrates how difficult it can be to get relief from chronic abdominal pain. The story also reminds us that narcotics are very effective at relieving nearly every type of bodily pain. If narcotics are so good at combating pain, why not treat the abdominal pain of IBS with them?

There are several good reasons why narcotics should not be used to treat chronic or recurrent abdominal pain. (Note that the treatment of abdominal pain from cancer is a very different matter, not appropriate for discussion here.) First, narcotics are addictive. That means that the body quickly becomes used to the dose of medication initially prescribed and requires an ever-increasing amount to attain the same degree of effect. This phenomenon is called tolerance. Medically, tolerance is defined as a decrease in the effectiveness of a medication with repeated administration. That is, the body begins to "tolerate" a certain amount of the drug rather than being altered by it and thus requires more and more of the medication. This would result only in increasing expense if it were not for the many other disadvantages to taking a narcotic drug.

Narcotics have significant side effects. The most common ones are constipation, fatigue, sedation, delayed reflexes, and inability to think properly. In many cases these side effects themselves can be treated. For example, patients on narcotics may need to take additional medications every day to treat their constipation (stool softeners, milk of magnesia, Miralax, tegaserod). However, other side effects cannot be easily treated—medications are not available to improve memory or concentration or to prevent the fatigue and grogginess commonly found in patients taking narcotics.

Especially important in the case of medications to which the body becomes tolerant is the fact that overdoses of narcotics can be fatal. More disadvantages of ever-increasing doses of narcotics are that the body may become insensitive to warning signs of another medical problem and that the possibility of dangerous drug interactions may arise.

Narcotics can have significant economic side effects that most people could not endure for more than a very short time, let alone recurrently or chronically. Many patients taking narcotics find it impossible to work, because they can't concentrate or think properly or because they cannot safely drive, work in potentially dangerous settings, or operate heavy machinery. In many kinds of jobs, people are not allowed to work if they are being treated with narcotics, because of the known problems with delayed reflexes, difficulty concentrating, and poor memory. In addition, many patients find that narcotics take away their normal motivation and desire to perform their daily tasks and chores. Thus, patients may obtain temporary relief from pain, but they may find themselves unable to live their lives.

For all of these reasons, the vast majority of health care providers believe that narcotics should not be used to treat abdominal pain in patients who have IBS. Although this may seem cruel and cold-hearted, given the severity of some patients' pain, the side effects and potential dangers of these medications greatly outweigh the benefits for people who have IBS.

Other Medications Used to Treat IBS Pain

Because the options for treating abdominal pain are still somewhat limited, health care providers have turned to medications used to treat other conditions, hoping that they might improve symptoms of IBS. All of the medications discussed in this section are available only by prescription. Because they have not been specifically evaluated in patients who have IBS, their use in treating IBS is considered off-label and somewhat experimental.

Tramadol (Ultram) is a non-narcotic analgesic designed to treat acute pain after surgery or the pain of a bone fracture or other orthopedic injury. It is also occasionally used to treat chronic pain. Some patients who have IBS find it useful, but others develop prohibitive side effects of nausea and vomiting. Tramadol cannot be used at the same time as an SSRI due to the potential for a serious, although uncommon, side effect (serotonin syndrome). Theoretical concerns exist that chronic use of tramadol could be addictive, although most addiction specialists do not believe that this is true.

Phenytoin (Dilantin) and carbamazepine (Tegretol) are anticonvulsant agents used to treat people who have seizure disorders. These medications act to "quiet" the nerves involved in the transmission of pain sensation. Some people who had seizure disorders reported that their unrelated chronic pain improved while on these medications. Consequently, they are sometimes prescribed with pain relief as the primary goal. As mentioned above, these medications have not been specifically tested with people who have IBS. Thus, we do not know the likelihood of IBS pain symptoms improving with the use of these medications.

Gabapentin (Neurontin) is a newer anticonvulsant. It is similar to carbamazepine and phenytoin, and like them, it may improve pain by modulating the transmission of pain messages from the GI tract to the spinal cord and brain. Neurontin appears to have a better safety record and fewer side effects than the older anticonvulsants and is being used much more commonly to treat conditions that involve chronic nerve pain. The collective clinical experience of many gastroenterologists is that Neurontin may be a good choice for the treatment of chronic pain, if medications are required and if tricyclic antidepressants and smooth-muscle antispasmodics are not effective.

Lyrica (pregabalin), a newer medication similar to gabapentin, is now being used to treat chronic pain syndromes. It appears to help the chronic abdominal pain associated with IBS in some patients, although large studies designed to evaluate its efficacy and safety in people who have IBS have not been performed.

Duloxetine (Cymbalta) was first approved by the FDA for the treatment of depression. It is in a different class of medications, called SNRIs (serotonin norepinephrine reuptake inhibitors). It has also been shown to improve symptoms of diabetic neuropathy (the painful nerve problems in the feet and hands that many people with Type 1 diabetes have) and fibromyalgia. Some individuals who have IBS note an improvement in their pain symptoms while on duloxetine although, once again, large studies to properly evaluate the efficacy and safety of this medication in patients who have IBS have not been performed.

Medications to Treat Global IBS Symptoms (Including Abdominal Pain)

As mentioned throughout this book, IBS is a complicated disorder characterized by lower abdominal pain and disordered defecation (meaning constipation, diarrhea, or both). People who have IBS often have other gastrointestinal symptoms, including excess gas, bloating, distention, fecal urgency, or straining. Every patient has a different story and a different combination of symptoms that vary in frequency and intensity. Symptoms typically wax and wane in frequency and intensity, and treatment can be complicated. One symptom may require the use of one class of medications, whereas another symptom may require the use of a different class of medications. This type of treatment is not only complicated, but it also increases costs to the patient and the likelihood of medication interactions and side effects. Ideally, all of the symptoms of IBS in an individual patient would be fully treated by one medication.

For many people who have IBS and constipation, lubiprostone is very effective at relieving these "global" IBS symptoms (see Chapter 16). This medication has been on the market since 2005 and was approved for the treatment of IBS with constipation in women in 2006, so it has a long track record of safety. Linaclotide, another medication for IBS with constipation, was shown in several large research studies to improve the global symptoms of patients who have IBS and constipation. Although only recently approved (August 2012) and thus having a shorter "real world" track record, linaclotide also appears to be effective and safe. Finally, for patients who have IBS and diarrhea, alosetron has been very helpful with improving global IBS symptoms and diarrhea in women (see Chapter 17).

Summary

- Abdominal pain or discomfort is the one symptom shared by all people who have IBS and the most common reason for a patient to seek the advice of a health care provider.
- The abdominal pain of IBS may develop due to overly strong muscular contractions in the GI tract, a hypersensitive GI tract, or a heightened awareness of pain in the central nervous system.
- Relieving the abdominal pain of IBS can be challenging. Available agents include smooth-muscle antispasmodics, tricyclic antidepressants, SSRIs, and medications (alosetron, lubiprostone, and linaclotide) that focus on the multiple, global symptoms of IBS.
- Over-the-counter medications (aspirin, acetaminophen, anti-inflammatory agents) are not effective for treating abdominal pain associated with IBS.
- Narcotics should not be used to treat the abdominal pain of IBS.

CHAPTER 19

Treatments for Gas and Bloating

When she was 47 years old, Bonnie was referred to my clinic because of her symptoms of gas, bloating, loose stools, and lower abdominal pain. She said that the symptoms started approximately one year before our appointment and that she was somewhat embarrassed to even talk about them. Because of her excess gas, she was finding it hard to be around others, and she was worried that her symptoms represented something dangerous.

As I continued to ask Bonnie about the reasons for her visit, Bonnie admitted that she had read in a magazine that bloating is a sign of ovarian cancer. She is not usually a nervous or anxious person, but the magazine article made her worry about her symptoms. Bonnie told me that she typically had two to three somewhat urgent, loose stools each day and that these were always preceded by spasms and cramps in her lower abdomen. The stools were never bloody.

When her symptoms began, she had had a severe sinus infection and had taken several courses of antibiotics. Around the same time, she had started a new diet, because she had gained several pounds during the previous few years. None of Bonnie's family members had a history of cancer or celiac disease, although both of her parents were lactose intolerant. On physical examination, I noted that her abdomen was slightly distended and tympanic (when I tapped on it, it sounded like a drum, which indicated that gas was present in her GI tract). Her internist had ordered a complete blood count (CBC) and celiac blood tests, and these were both normal. Bonnie's gynecologist had performed a careful examination and ordered a pelvic ultrasound just to be on the safe side; both were normal.

When I asked Bonnie about her diet, she told me that she drank several glasses of low-fat milk each day (to provide calcium and vitamin D) and that she had a dish of ice cream every night. She had recently decided to become a vegetarian and she consumed large amounts of fresh fruits, fresh vegetables, beans, and whole-grain foods. She didn't like the taste of coffee, so to help stay alert at work she often drank three to four cans of a caffeinated cola drink each day. Bonnie also started off each morning with a large glass of orange juice, and when she went to the gym, she often drank a commercial sports drink afterward to rehydrate.

At the suggestion of a friend, Bonnie had tried digestive enzymes to help with her symptoms, but these did not help. Before work meetings, she would sometimes use an over-the-counter product such as Gas-X or charcoal capsules, but she was not sure that these helped either. She wondered what the cause of her problem was and what could be done to help.

Bonnie's case is not unusual. Although it is ideal to have one simple explanation for the cause of someone's symptoms, I knew that it was likely that Bonnie's symptoms had developed for several reasons. One, she had been treated with several courses of antibiotics just before the onset of her symptoms. Her normal gut flora was probably changed by the antibiotics, which can create problems with gas and bloating. Two, Bonnie was consuming a fairly large quantity of dairy products each day. It was probable that she was lactose intolerant and that the undigested milk sugars were fermenting when they reached the colon, creating excess gas and bloating. Three, Bonnie was consuming a large amount of fructose each day in the form of orange juice, commercial sodas, and sports drinks (the latter two are usually made with high-fructose corn syrup). Many people who have IBS are fructose intolerant. When fructose is not absorbed in the upper GI tract, it breaks down in the colon and causes gas. Four, Bonnie had become a vegetarian one year ago, around the time she started noticing symptoms. She was trying to eat very healthfully by avoiding fats and red meat. However, she had substantially increased her intake of beans, fruits, and vegetables. All of these products contain insoluble fiber, which cannot be digested and ends up being fermented in the colon. In addition, dried and canned beans (red beans, black beans, garbanzo beans, lentils, and kidney beans) contain complex carbohydrates, and most individuals do not have the enzyme needed to break these down completely in the GI tract.

After we discussed her treatment options, Bonnie said that she did not want to try probiotics, antibiotics, or other medications to treat her symptoms. Rather, she wanted to try to identify the cause of her symptoms. We both agreed that it was likely that dietary factors were playing a role. I told Bonnie that she could go on a strict elimination diet (see Chapter 10) to get rid of most of the troublesome substances all at once, or she could try to eliminate the worst offenders. She chose the latter, and shortly afterward, Bonnie stopped her intake of all foods and liquids with dairy, instead substituting Lactaid, rice, soy, or almond milk products. Bonnie also stopped drinking commercial sodas and orange juice (which contain high-fructose corn syrup and natural fructose, respectively) and substituted water or unsweetened green tea. Finally, she eliminated all dried and canned beans, and she limited her fiber intake to no more than 30 gm per day (which is still above the recommended daily dose of 25 gm).

When Bonnie modified her diet in these ways, her symptoms essentially resolved. She still had occasional spasms and cramps with some urgency when she had a bowel movement, but she said that these symptoms were tolerable. She no longer had problems with bloating and gas. In addition, by cutting out the juice and soft drinks, Bonnie lost two pounds every month, until she was back to her previous weight.

Treating the symptoms of gas and bloating can be one of the most difficult tasks for gastroenterologists. Everybody makes gas in the intestinal tract; on average, a person makes approximately 750 to 1,000 ml of gas each day. Not surprisingly, most gas forms after the ingestion of food. Foods that are high in insoluble fiber are more likely to create gas than food products that consist of protein and simple carbohydrates.

Many different gases are present in the GI tract. The five most common are nitrogen, oxygen, hydrogen, carbon dioxide, and methane. Nearly all of the nitrogen and oxygen within the upper GI tract comes from swallowed air. Carbon dioxide in the GI tract comes from swallowed air and from carbonated beverages. It is also a side product of the neutralization of acids and alkalis (bases) and of bacterial fermentation of undigested foodstuffs. Hydrogen gas is also produced as a result of bacterial fermentation, as is methane (although much less common).

Most intestinal gas forms in the colon due to the action of the colonic microflora, which consist of the approximately five hundred to one thousand different species of bacteria that normally reside within the colon. There are more live bacterial cells in the colon than there are live nonbacterial cells in the entire rest of the human body; if collected and weighed, the normal bacteria in the colon would amount to 4 to 5 pounds. These bacteria serve a variety of functions—they help protect the colon and they aid in the immune system of the gut. One of their major roles is to complete the digestion of unabsorbed foodstuffs. When that occurs, gas is produced.

What Is Bloating?

Bloating is defined as a sense of gassiness or a sense of being distended. Distention is when the abdomen is clearly swollen and larger in size than normal, all due to the presence of excess intestinal gas. Some people who have irritable bowel syndrome feel gassy and bloated, but their abdomens are never distended; other people who have IBS may feel gassy and bloated and also develop distention. Individuals who have bloating and distention usually feel better in the morning, because there is little food in the GI tract at the beginning of the day and thus less gas can be formed. Predictably, as the day goes on and people eat and drink, gas forms, leading to sensations of being gassy and bloated and the physical manifestation of distention.

Bloating is one of the most difficult gastrointestinal conditions to treat. Some treatment options for IBS actually worsen bloating (for example, products with excess fiber). Dietary modification, rather than medication, is often the best treatment for people who have bloating (see Chapter 15). Probiotics and antibiotics may improve symptoms of bloating in some individuals. Unfortunately, medications designed specifically to alleviate gassiness and bloating are usually ineffective in most patients. Trial and error may be the only way to find which medication, if any, may improve your symptoms.

Some of the most commonly used medications for bloating are available over the counter. See Table 19.1 for a list of medications used to treat bloating.

Probiotics

Some studies have shown that probiotics, live bacterial supplements, improve the health and balance of native intestinal microflora. Probiotics are found in yogurt or can be taken in capsule form. The theory behind the use of probiotics for bloating is that excess gas may develop from an imbalance of the normal bacteria in the GI tract or from the lack of a specific bacterium and that probiotics may rebalance or replace these bacteria.

Research studies on the use of probiotics to treat bloating have shown mixed results. In two studies of people who had IBS and diarrhea, a probiotic (VSL#3) containing eight different strains of three bacterial species (*Streptococcus, Bifidobacterium,* and *Lactobacilli*) improved symptoms of abdominal bloating. *Lactobacillus plantarum* 299V was found to improve bloating and distention in only one of three studies that were performed. Another study found that *Lactobacillus* GG did not improve symptoms in a group of 24 patients who had IBS. *Bifidobacterium infantis* (sold as the probiotic Align) has shown some ability to improve symptoms of bloating and abdominal discomfort in people who have IBS and diarrhea. Flora-Q is another probiotic being heavily marketed to treat a variety of gastrointestinal disorders, but there are no large prospective studies evaluating its efficacy in individuals who have IBS.

Antibiotics

Some researchers and physicians strongly believe that bloating is due to the presence of too much bacteria in the intestinal tract (see Chapter 11) and that antibiotic therapy should therefore improve symptoms of bloating by destroying the overabundant bacteria. Indeed, some health care

Table 19.1. Medications Used to Treat Bloating

Antiflatulents

   Simethicone (Mylicon, Gas-X, Phazyme)
   Charcoal
   Enzyme replacements

Smooth-muscle antispasmodics

   Hyoscyamine (Levsin)
   Dicyclomine (Bentyl)
   Librax (chlordiazepoxide + clidinium)
   Donnatal (phenobarbital + atropine + hyoscyamine + scopolamine)

5-HT3 antagonists (that is, Alosetron)

Chloride channel activators (for example, lubiprostone)

Guanylate cyclase C activators (for example, linaclotide)

Probiotics

Antibiotics

---

providers routinely use antibiotics to treat symptoms of bloating. But bacterial overgrowth of the GI tract is an uncommon condition, and in most cases it does not cause bloating. I do not recommend antibiotics as a first-line treatment for patients who have bloating because antibiotics can be expensive and entail risks with routine use, such as adverse reactions, medication interactions, the possibility of developing a severe infection of the colon (C. *difficile* colitis), and the potential to develop resistance to the antibiotic. Antibiotic resistance can be very dangerous if a person develops a severe infection and cannot be treated with the necessary antibiotic because he or she no longer responds to it. When I am concerned about bacterial overgrowth in patients who have persistent bloating and have failed to respond to dietary interventions (see Chapter 15) as well as trials of over-the-counter medications and probiotics, I schedule a hydrogen breath test (see Chapter 11). If this test is positive, I treat the patient with antibiotics.

Simethicone

Over-the-counter products like Gas-X and Phazyme contain simethicone, which breaks up large gas bubbles into smaller ones in the stomach. Smaller bubbles are easier to belch or burp up when gas is in the stomach. However, simethicone rarely helps when gas is in the small intestine or colon, and that is the major problem for most people who have IBS.

Charcoal

Activated charcoal is used in many different filtering systems to clean water or air in kitchens and bathrooms. It is also sold in capsule form to be swallowed, because it can absorb some intestinal gas and thus improve its odor. Some patients find that charcoal improves their symptoms of bloating to a small degree. Charcoal capsules generally need to be taken before each meal. They can darken the stool (a worrying side effect for some patients because very dark stool can be a sign of internal bleeding).

Enzyme Replacements

Some people develop bloating because they do not have enough of the right enzymes to break down specific food products properly. For example, people who have lactose intolerance do not have enough of the enzyme lactase so, to avoid GI problems when they eat milk products, they may need to take additional lactase (see Chapter 15 for more information). Lactose intolerance is present in at least 30 percent of people who have IBS.

Fructose intolerance is another enzyme deficiency that is fairly common in people who have IBS (one study reported that up to 50 percent of people who have IBS and diarrhea are fructose intolerant) and that can lead to symptoms of gas and bloating. Unfortunately, there is no medication to treat fructose deficiency (or the other enzyme deficiencies that may contribute to the development of gas and bloating).

The most popular over-the-counter enzyme replacement is Beano. This product contains galactosidase, an enzyme that helps break down complex sugars, including raffinose and stachyose. These two sugars are found in many of the cruciferous vegetables (broccoli, cauliflower, cabbage) and legumes (beans, peas) that often cause intestinal gas. Available in both tablet and liquid forms, Beano is typically taken before any meal that contains food that may cause gas (for example, beans). Beano does not break down fiber, however, which is a major source of gas production in the GI tract.

Other enzyme replacements are available over the counter in health food stores or may be prescribed by a physician. These replacements include pancreatic enzymes, such as lipase, protease, or amylase (Creon, Pancrease, and Viokase). The normal human pancreas makes more than enough of the enzymes needed to break down ingested foods and liquids and to promote the absorption of all necessary nutrients. Enzyme replacements are beneficial for people whose pancreas has been injured and cannot produce enough enzymes (a condition called pancreatic insufficiency). However, there is no evidence that people who have IBS have a higher-than-normal incidence of pancreatic insufficiency.

Overall, I would not recommend enzyme replacements as routine treatment for the bloating experienced with IBS. These medications have never been scientifically evaluated in a group of patients who have IBS.

Smooth-Muscle Antispasmodics

The theory behind the use of antispasmodic medications (described in Chapter 18) to treat gas and bloating is that spasms of the colon or small intestine can trap gas, thereby leading to sensations of bloating. By relaxing the smooth muscle of the GI tract, the spasms are resolved and the gas can be expelled more easily. Some patients taking antispasmodics do report some relief of gas and bloating, but most do not. As a group, smooth-muscle antispasmodics are useful for relieving abdominal pain, but they cannot be recommended specifically for relief of gas and bloating.

Medications to Treat Global Symptoms of IBS (Including Gas and Bloating)

As mentioned throughout this book, many people who have IBS experience a variety of coexisting symptoms. When some patients who have IBS and constipation are treated with lubiprostone (Amitiza) or linaclotide, they also note a significant improvement in their symptoms of gas and bloating. Other people who have IBS and diarrhea report an improvement in bloating and gas symptoms when treated with alosetron (Lotronex). See Chapters 16 and 17 for more information on the use of these prescription medications.

Summary

- Bloating is a common symptom in people who have IBS. In fact, it is the second most common reason individuals who have IBS seek medical attention (abdominal pain is the number one reason).
- Bloating is a sensation of gassiness; distention is the physical manifestation of excess intestinal gas (or gas that is difficult to eliminate).
- Dietary factors often play a role in symptoms of gas and bloating. Lactose intolerance, fructose intolerance, and insoluble fiber are the worst offenders.
- Probiotics have been shown to improve symptoms of gas and bloating for many people who have IBS.
- Antibiotics can be safely used to treat symptoms of gas and bloating; a breath hydrogen test is useful to help guide treatment.
- Although frequently used and quite safe, over-the-counter agents that are advertised to decrease problems with gas and bloating are rarely effective.

CHAPTER 20

Probiotics and Antibiotics: Frequently Asked Questions

Treating irritable bowel syndrome is challenging not only because the symptoms are so varied among patients but because new therapies are constantly being developed. Physicians a decade ago weren't even talking about using probiotics or antibiotics to treat IBS symptoms. Once considered an "alternative" therapy, probiotics are now considered a standard treatment option for IBS by many health care providers. Researchers are actively studying probiotics and antibiotics to answer critical questions about the usefulness of these agents in treating IBS symptoms. Probiotics are sold at nearly all pharmacies and grocery stores, often with somewhat overstated claims about their benefits. Although probiotics and antibiotics have been briefly discussed in earlier chapters (see Chapters 17 and 19), so many patients have questions about these two classes of medications that in this chapter I will answer a list of frequently asked questions.

Probiotics

What is a probiotic?

Probiotics are live organisms that, when ingested in adequate amounts, can affect the health of a person who has IBS. In other words, probiotics are supplements of living bacteria taken to alter, and presumably improve, the balance of native intestinal microflora (see below for a definition of microflora and gut flora). Although they are bacteria, they are classified as nonpathogenic (that is, not pathogens), meaning that they are not considered dangerous and will not cause an infection.

My doctor keeps mentioning the "gut flora." What is that?

The gut flora (also called the gut microflora) are most accurately referred to as the gut microbiota. The gut microbiota is a large group of bacteria that normally resides within the gastrointestinal tract (primarily the large intestine). Estimates vary as to the precise number of different bacterial species within the gastrointestinal tract, but most authorities agree that there are approximately five hundred to one thousand different species of bacteria in the colon. Collectively, the number of live bacteria in the human colon is larger than the number of all other live cells combined throughout the rest of the body. The total number of bacteria that reside within the colon is staggering—over 10^{13} to 10^{14} cells—and weighs more than 4 pounds.

What is the role of the gut microbiota?

The gut microbiota have many different functions. These bacteria play a vital role in maintaining the health of the cells that line the colon. In addition, gut microbiota support the immune system of the gastrointestinal tract and aid in the processes of digestion and absorption of key nutrients.

How do probiotics work?

Unfortunately, this is a question that remains unanswered. Different probiotics probably work differently, and although various people who have IBS may have similar symptoms, every person's gut microflora are probably different from every other person's. Many different theories have been proposed about why probiotics may improve symptoms in some people who have IBS. Researchers theorize that probiotics may

- add a previously deficient bacterial species
- restore the balance of "good" and "bad" bacteria
- improve gut immune function
- make the lining of the colon (referred to as the "barrier") stronger and healthier
- improve the health of the cells that line the colon (the colonic epithelial cells)

Is there evidence that probiotics work?

In two separate randomized, placebo-controlled trials, the probiotic *Lactobacillus plantarum* 299V improved bowel habits and symptoms of abdominal pain in patients who had IBS in one of the studies but not the other. Two small studies of patients who had IBS and diarrhea showed that the probiotic VSL#3 appeared to improve symptoms of abdominal bloating and abdominal gas. By far the best studied probiotic for treatment of IBS symptoms is *Bifidobacterium infantis*. Two large, randomized, placebo-controlled studies in patients who had IBS (either with diarrhea predominance or alternating diarrhea and constipation) have shown that *Bifidobacterium infantis* 35624 improves symptoms of bloating, gas, and abdominal pain when compared to a placebo. *Bifidobacterium infantis* 35624 is currently sold under the trade name Align. More recently, the probiotic *Bifidobacterium lactis* DN-173-010A was tested in patients who have constipation-predominant IBS; it showed significant benefits for symptoms of bloating and constipation. More trials are needed to support this preliminary evidence for *Bifidobacterium lactis* with individuals who have IBS.

What is the best probiotic for treating IBS symptoms?

I generally recommend *Bifidobacterium infantis* (sold as Align) to my patients who have IBS and diarrhea symptoms and to those who have IBS and alternating symptoms of constipation and diarrhea. I tell people who have IBS and constipation that Align may help some symptoms of gas and bloating but that it probably won't help their constipation symptoms (although *Bifidobacterium lactis* may). VSL#3 remains another option, although it is generally more expensive than Align, and there are fewer data to support its use at this time. Finally, because of the negative studies published to date, I do not recommend *Lactobacillus* to my patients.

How much probiotic should I take?

Each new research study on the role of probiotics in the treatment of IBS raises more questions than answers. Just as no two people or medications are identical, no two probiotics are the same. Even for probiotics that seem very similar (because they are the same species of bacteria—*Bifidobacteria*), the different strains (the subtypes of bacteria within each major category) may have vastly different and even contrasting effects (for example, as noted above, *Bifidobacteria infantis* appears to act differently from *Bifidobacteria lactis*). Because all of the products are different from each other, it is impossible to make a sweeping statement that all probiotics must be used on a specific schedule for a certain time period. Rather, each probiotic must be evaluated individually. For example, some probiotics need to be used daily for 90 days to assess effectiveness, whereas others may need to be used twice daily for only 45 days.

For how long should I take a probiotic?

The length of treatment will vary from probiotic to probiotic. Most research studies involving probiotics have lasted only 4 to 12 weeks. No studies have evaluated long-term safety and effectiveness (after 6 to 12 months of continuous use). Because options are limited, I generally recommend a 90-day trial of any probiotic to determine whether or not it is effective. If after 90 days no benefits are noted, then the probiotic should be stopped and a trial with another probiotic started. If a patient notices an improvement (whether an improvement in gas, bloating, or diarrhea) in IBS symptoms using a probiotic, then I generally recommend that the person continue the probiotic for at least six months. At that point, if symptoms are under control, then the probiotic can be stopped. However, many people note a slow return of symptoms after stopping the probiotic (regardless of type), and then they may begin taking them again.

Can I use probiotics with my other medications?

Yes. No significant interactions with other medications have been identified.

Are probiotics safe?

Probiotics of many different forms (such as yogurt with live cultures) have been used for more than one hundred years by millions of individuals without any apparent side effects. Thus, on face value, probiotics appear quite safe. However, the probiotics contained in a capsule are somewhat different from probiotics that are in a natural food like yogurt. Only a few published research studies have addressed the safety of probiotics, and these only looked at a small number of probiotics.

Some concern about probiotics arose recently when patients who had severe acute pancreatitis may have become sicker or even died due to administration of probiotics. These patients were extremely ill to begin with, though, and they were administered large doses of probiotics through a tube directly into the small intestine. The apparent cause of death in some of these patients was decreased blood flow to the gastrointestinal tract (intestinal ischemia), *not* infection by a bacteria. There was no control group in this study, no patients were given a placebo, and only one dose was given. So, we don't really know if these patients became sicker or died from the probiotic, because the study had only a small number of patients (which makes accurate statistical analysis difficult), because there was no control group, and because a larger dose than usual of probiotic was used. In addition, patients who have severe acute pancreatitis are completely different from patients who have IBS, so it is not helpful to apply the data from the pancreatitis group to a population who has IBS. Future trials will need to assess long-term safety of probiotics, but at present, they seem quite safe for nearly all populations (see below).

Are there any groups of patients who should not take probiotics?

Due to concern about giving an immunosuppressed patient a live bacteria, I do not recommend using probiotics for patients who have a known immune deficiency, patients who have cancer or are undergoing treatment for cancer, patients who have a short gastrointestinal tract (this is called short gut syndrome), and newborn infants. Although I may be overly cautious, the theoretical risks of probiotics to these people, even if very low, outweigh the potential benefits of probiotics.

Can I buy probiotics from a grocery store, a pharmacy, and over the Internet?

Yes. Probiotics are readily available from a multitude of sources. A word of caution: a probiotic is defined as a live organism that, when ingested, promotes improved health. Many probiotics now available on the market fail to meet that definition because they do not contain live organisms. Because probiotics are not regulated like food or medications, there is no guarantee that they will be shipped or stored under the appropriate conditions to guarantee that they remain healthy or even alive until you ingest them. One small study found that nearly 50 percent of probiotics purchased off the shelf were already dead. In addition, some probiotics have been found to be contaminated with other bacteria. Thus, you have the potential to ingest a bacteria that could make you sick or not help you at all.

As mentioned above, few probiotics have been tested in humans using scientific protocol. Some probiotics that were tested yielded negative results (meaning that they did not improve symptoms). But since probiotics are not under strict control like medications, they can still be sold even if they are not effective. Only one probiotic has been conclusively shown to survive passage through the gastrointestinal tract to reach the colon: *Bifidobacterium infantis* (sold as Align). So, it's possible that a probiotic, even if alive and used in adequate amounts, might not survive passage into the large intestine and thus may not provide any benefits. As you contemplate using a probiotic, read the label carefully to determine what quality control measures are in place to guarantee safe arrival of the bacteria, and discuss your choice with your health care provider.

How are probiotics regulated?

The Food and Drug Administration (FDA) is responsible for ensuring the safety of over-the-counter and prescription medications. Although regulation is a daunting task, the rules and regulations enforced by the FDA are part of the reason why medications available in the United States are generally safe. However, probiotics are not considered medications, and as such, they are not regulated by the FDA. Probiotics are considered foods (like yogurt and kefir) or dietary supplements. They do not have to undergo the rigorous testing involving thousands of patients that is required for traditional medications used to treat IBS symptoms (such as lubiprostone, alosetron, or linaclotide). In addition, unlike over-the-counter and prescription medications, which are advertised and sold only for certain conditions based on clinical studies and scientific evidence, manufacturers of probiotics can make any claim they want because they are not regulated. For these reasons, I recommend only a select few probiotics, those that have been researched using clinical studies involving people who have IBS.

What is a prebiotic?

A prebiotic is a substance that provides nutrients to a probiotic. Prebiotics are typically foods such as whole grains, complex carbohydrates, or fiber. Many patients and physicians believe that probiotics work better if a prebiotic is consumed just before taking the probiotic, but scientific evidence to support this is lacking.

Could I get a stool transplant to improve my IBS symptoms?

Many individuals who have IBS are asking their doctors whether a stool transplant might help with their symptoms. As discussed earlier, the natural bacteria in the large intestine play a role in generating symptoms for many people who have IBS. However, these bacteria also ferment foods. When fermentation occurs, gas is produced, and this can cause the colon to stretch (distend), leading to intestinal cramps, spasms, bloating, pain, and urgent diarrhea. Since fecal flora seem to play such a critical role in symptom development, it is reasonable to wonder whether they could all be replaced with a different type of bacteria or with healthier bacteria.

The technical name for a stool transplant is fecal microbiota transplantation (FMT), and it is considered a probiotic technique. First described in 1958, it has recently received a lot of attention in the lay press. To perform a stool transplant, a fresh stool sample is taken from a healthy donor (a healthy first-degree relative is best), mixed with saline, processed and filtered and then infused into the patient during a colonoscopy. The theory is that "transplanting" or replacing a sick person's normal microbiota with healthy bacteria will improve the patient's intestinal symptoms. Casting aside the "yuck" factor, this therapy has been used to successfully treat severe *Clostridium difficile* (*C. diff*) infections that were resistant to standard antibiotic therapy. More than 90 percent of patients who had a severe *C. diff* infection (one that had failed antibiotic therapy) and who were treated with FMT stated that they would undergo an FMT again if necessary. Although FMT in people with severe ulcerative colitis or Crohn's disease has been much less well studied, very limited data show that FMT may improve symptoms for them, as well.

No studies have yet evaluated FMT for people who have IBS. Although this will probably be an area of research in the future, physician researchers are approaching this topic cautiously, for many reasons. One, stool transplantation has some small risks associated with the procedure (undergoing a colonoscopy). Two, we still have much to learn about the gut microbiota; it is possible that, in an attempt to improve the health of patients, we may expose them to other disorders. Since FMT involves transferring five hundred to one thousand different types of bacteria from one person to another, the theoretical risks involved are huge. Three, at present we can only culture 10 to 20 percent of stool bacteria. Thus we cannot currently effectively "screen" a healthy donor to see if they have a disease that could be transmitted to the patient. For example, some practitioners are concerned that an autoimmune disorder such as rheumatoid arthritis could be transmitted from a seemingly healthy donor to a patient. For these reasons, stool transplantation is not yet a viable option for people who have IBS, but it may be in the future.

Antibiotics

How do antibiotics work to treat IBS?

As with probiotics, no one really knows how antibiotics work to improve IBS symptoms. Currently, three main theories exist. One, some patients who have IBS have small intestinal bacterial overgrowth (SIBO; see Chapter 11). If a person has symptoms of gas, bloating, or diarrhea due to SIBO, then eliminating or reducing the offending bacteria from the small intestine with a course of prescription antibiotics makes sense. Two, some individuals may develop IBS symptoms because of an overabundance of bacteria in the large intestine. An antibiotic may be able to temporarily reduce (or suppress) the large number of bacteria, and this will normally improve symptoms of gas and bloating. Three, some people who have IBS may have an imbalance of certain bacteria in their colon (more "bad" bacteria than "good" bacteria), and an antibiotic could reduce or eliminate the problematic bacteria.

What is the best antibiotic for IBS symptoms?

It is difficult to decide which antibiotic is best, because people who have IBS, even those with similar symptoms, have different intestinal microflora and will therefore respond to antibiotics differently. Current technology does not allow us to accurately measure or grow all of the different bacterial species in the colon. In fact, we can only accurately grow or culture 10 to 15 percent of the 500 to 1,000 species that reside within the human colon. Ideally, we could analyze a stool sample from a patient who has IBS and then recommend a specific antibiotic based on that analysis. Although that scenario may be possible in the future, currently it is not. Given these research deficiencies, I generally recommend one of two antibiotics for individuals who have IBS. Both of these antibiotics are considered nonabsorbable, meaning that very little of the medication (less than 1 percent) is absorbed from the gastrointestinal tract. Nonabsorbable antibiotics stay in the GI tract and generally do not cause any side effects outside the GI tract. The two antibiotics I currently recommend are rifaximin (also called Xifaxan) and neomycin. Keep in mind that, at the time this book was written, neither of these antibiotics, nor any other type of antibiotic, had been approved by the FDA for the treatment of IBS.

What is the best dose of an antibiotic for my IBS symptoms?

If you and your health care provider decide to use an antibiotic to try to improve your IBS symptoms, then I suggest trying either neomycin or rifaximin. Neomycin has been around for decades and is considered safe. In addition, since it is available as a generic prescription medication, it is usually fairly inexpensive. I generally recommend using 500 mg of neomycin 3 times daily for 10 days. Some physicians prescribe a higher dose (1,000 mg) for a longer period (up to 14 days), although there are no scientific studies comparing one regimen or time course to the other. One potential concern with neomycin is that patients may develop resistance to the medication, meaning that they may respond well to it initially but then not respond as well when it is prescribed again. For this reason, health care providers who choose to use an antibiotic use rifaximin first.

Used in Europe for more than 30 years, prescription rifaximin is currently approved by the FDA for the treatment of "traveler's diarrhea" (for that disorder, it is considered safe and effective). Rifaximin has been tested in five large studies of people who have IBS. Two of the randomized, placebo-controlled studies involved a total of 1,258 patients. The results of these studies showed that rifaximin was much better than a placebo at treating IBS symptoms of gas, bloating, pain, and diarrhea. Although patients in these studies only took rifaximin for 14 days, many of them noted an improvement in their symptoms for 8 to 10 weeks after finishing the 2-week course of medication. As mentioned above, although not currently approved for the treatment of IBS, rifaximin can be taken 3 times daily at 550 mg for 14 days.

How long should I take an antibiotic?

If you and your health care provider decide to use neomycin, I generally recommend just one course of this prescription antibiotic (500 mg taken 3 times daily for 10 days). Many patients do not respond to a second course of neomycin, even if their original symptoms initially improved. Rifaximin appears to be different, however. Many patients originally treated with rifaximin (550 mg 3 times daily for 14 days) note a recurrence of their symptoms 8 to 12 weeks after finishing the original course of antibiotics. A second course of rifaximin at that point may once again improve IBS symptoms in most patients (more than 50 percent). A few patients have been treated three or even four times with an antibiotic such as rifaximin to improve their symptoms of gas, bloating, and distention. Results vary; some patients report improvement after each course of the antibiotic, while others note that their level of response is less with each course of antibiotics. At the time of this book's publication, a large research study was under way to evaluate the safety and efficacy of repeated courses of rifaximin in people with non-constipation IBS.

Are all antibiotics the same for the treatment of IBS?

No. Antibiotics have risks (see below) and should not be used interchangeably for the treatment of IBS. In addition, other than those involving neomycin or rifaximin, no good scientific studies have evaluated the safety or efficacy of antibiotics for the treatment of IBS. So, unless there is definitive proof of small intestinal bacterial overgrowth (SIBO) in a patient who has IBS, I don't recommend the use of any other antibiotic for the treatment of IBS symptoms.

Can I take antibiotics with my other medications?

Both neomycin and rifaximin are safe to use with nearly all other medications. However, other antibiotics have potential drug or diet interactions. For example, taking metronidazole (Flagyl) with alcohol can cause flushing, nausea, and vomiting, and some antibiotics can interfere with oral contraceptive agents. Many antibiotics cause vaginal yeast infections in women because they change the normal balance of "good" bacteria in the vagina. Review these potential interactions carefully with your health care provider.

Are there any groups of patients who should not take antibiotics for their IBS symptoms?

Patients who have a prior history of *C. difficile* colitis, those whose immune systems are suppressed, and those on multiple medications should be cautious about using any type of antibiotic, even the nonabsorbable antibiotics (neomycin and rifaximin) described above. Note that although physicians and patients are concerned about the use of antibiotics and the potential complication of *C. difficile* colitis (see below), no case of *C. difficile* colitis has occurred in any of the rifaximin IBS studies.

Are there any risks associated with taking antibiotics?

Absolutely. There are several reasons why antibiotics should not be taken unnecessarily. One, inappropriate antibiotic use may lead to the development of antibiotic resistance, which means that the next time you need a specific antibiotic, you may not respond to that antibiotic (this could be a life-threatening concern). Two, antibiotics can change the composition of intestinal microflora, therefore altering digestion, changing the absorption of nutrients, and creating symptoms of gas and bloating. Three, inappropriate use of antibiotics can cause antibiotic-associated diarrhea. This type of diarrhea is a temporary condition that develops due to a change in intestinal microflora. It usually resolves on its own without any treatment. Four, antibiotics can cause *Clostridium difficile* colitis (also called *C. difficile* colitis, or *C. diff*, for short). *Clostridium difficile* colitis develops when the virulent bacterium *C. difficile*, which is normally found in the colon but is suppressed by "good" bacteria, grows unrestrained. The growth of this bacterium causes severe diarrhea that is potentially life threatening and requires treatment with antibiotics. For these reasons and more, antibiotics should not be used indiscriminately or liberally dispensed for the treatment of IBS symptoms.

CHAPTER 21

Complementary and Alternative Medicine

If you watch the evening news, read a daily newspaper, scan the Internet, or use an iPhone or tablet, you are likely to hear or read a report discussing the merits of complementary and alternative medicine. The phrase "complementary and alternative medicine," abbreviated CAM, has come into use to describe a broad range of therapeutic interventions, among them herbal remedies, acupuncture, naturopathic medications, and homeopathy. In contrast, the kind of medicine practiced by M.D.s is called allopathic medicine.

CAM is spoken of pejoratively by some people in both the lay and medical communities. The term *alternative* has been understood by some to mean "untested, unproven, unorthodox, or dangerous." These charges are not necessarily so, and we should look at alternative medicines as just that, alternatives to the allopathic therapies. We should, however, judge alternative therapies by the same standards we judge conventional treatments with regard to safety and effectiveness. The term *complementary* brings to some minds thoughts of quackery or crazy ideas. However, complementary medicine should also be taken as just that, a complement to more conventional therapies. An example of complementary medicine would be the use of relaxation techniques to lower blood pressure, coupled with modern Western medications used to treat elevated blood pressure. The combination has been shown to be quite effective, often more so than medication alone.

The last two decades have witnessed an explosion in the use of complementary and alternative medicine in the United States. In the last 10 years alone, the number of people who use some form of CAM therapy has increased from 10 percent of the U.S. population to 35 percent of the population. Some questionnaire studies have reported that as many as 50 percent of patients who have functional gastrointestinal disorders, such as irritable bowel syndrome, have used some type of CAM. This groundswell of support for CAM has occurred for a variety of reasons. Many patients are interested in using medications that they consider to be more "natural" and less dangerous than modern pharmaceuticals. Many are frustrated by the failure of Western medications to cure their health problems. Some people have a general distrust of medical technology and the medical profession. Also, in some circumstances, CAM therapies can be less expensive; they do not require a prescription from a doctor, and many people use them without consulting any health care provider. This also allows the patient to be completely in charge of her or his own health care, which has both advantages and disadvantages, of course.

Some legitimate concerns exist about the use of CAM therapies. Because CAM therapies are usually not covered by insurance, for some patients CAM therapies may be more expensive than traditional medications. Although widely available, most CAM medications are not tested, certified, or regulated by the Food and Drug Administration (FDA). Thus, their safety over both the short term and the long term is unknown. Few CAM therapies are subjected to the rigorous testing or controlled experiments that prescription medications are required to undergo. Since CAM therapies have generally not been compared, in formal studies, to placebos or to other medications on the market, it is hard to determine whether they are as effective, or possibly even more effective, than the prescription medications currently available.

Because CAM encompasses so many different therapies, it is impossible to generalize about whether they are good or bad, safe or unsafe. And because they are so numerous and varied, it is not possible to review them all here. However, in the following sections, some of the most popular therapies are described, with a note about whether any research supports their use in the treatment of IBS. We will consider acupuncture, aromatherapy, biofeedback, herbal remedies, homeopathy, hypnosis, manipulation therapy, and naturopathy. Although probiotics used to be considered an alternative therapy, given their popularity and the fact that some probiotics have been subjected to rigorous scientific study, I now consider probiotics another sensible therapeutic choice (like other allopathic medications), and I discuss them in Chapters 17 and 20.

Acupuncture

This technique originated in Asia thousands of years ago. During this procedure, extremely thin needles are inserted into the skin and subcutaneous tissue (the connective tissue underneath the skin) at various specific points on the body. These points may be on the ears, the abdomen, or the legs, for example. The points are thought to be locations of energy (this energy is called qi and pronounced "chee"). The theory behind acupuncture is that energy vital to the body is distributed to various points in the body, and illness occurs when these points are blocked or disturbed. Insertion of a needle is thought to liberate the blocked energy, restoring the flow of energy and thus bringing the body back into balance.

Acupuncture is occasionally coupled with pressure (acupressure), with electrical stimulation through the needle (electroacupuncture), or with heat, which is produced by burning herbs over the acupuncture site (moxibustion). Among its uses are the treatment of addictions (narcotics, alcohol, and tobacco), headaches, hypertension, stress, nausea, and vomiting. Studies have shown that acupuncture helps combat and relieve nausea and vomiting after surgery and during pregnancy.

To my knowledge, only six studies have evaluated the efficacy of acupuncture for treating IBS symptoms. Two of these studies were from China and included more than 200 patients; one found that acupuncture was better than a traditional Chinese herbal medication (TXYF) used to treat IBS symptoms, and the other study reported that acupuncture plus psychotherapy was better than psychotherapy alone at treating IBS symptoms. Other acupuncture studies found that real acupuncture was better for treating symptoms of IBS than "sham" acupuncture (a placebo form of acupuncture in which patients are treated either with a needle that does not break the skin or with a real acupuncture needle, inserted at a site thought to be irrelevant to the GI system). One study performed in the United States demonstrated that acupuncture was equivalent to sham acupuncture at improving IBS symptoms but was only slightly better at improving IBS symptoms than simply observing the patient (meaning following the patient on an outpatient basis but not providing any specific treatment). A meta-analysis of all of the data on acupuncture and IBS has showed that acupuncture does not appear to be any better than a placebo (sham acupuncture) for relieving the symptoms of IBS. Nonetheless, there are some patients who report significant improvements in their IBS symptoms after acupuncture.

No acupuncture study has compared acupuncture to an oral medication, nor has any study lasted as long as the research trials now required by the FDA to gain approval for a new medication. I tell my patients that, if all traditional treatments have failed, or if they don't want to use any medication (but are open to traditional Chinese medicine), then acupuncture may be of benefit. However, I also tell them that I can't provide any good data to support its use.

If you decide to seek the assistance of an acupuncturist, you should receive treatment *only* from a reputable person who uses sterile, single-use-only needles (the acupuncturist should never reuse the acupuncture needles). You should feel free to ask the person about his or her needles, training, certification, and results.

Aromatherapy

In aromatherapy, naturally distilled essences of plants are used to promote healing and positive changes in physical, emotional, and mental health. These essential oils can be applied to the skin or be inhaled. There are no studies available in the medical literature evaluating the benefits of aromatherapy for people who have IBS.

The best-studied oil involved in the treatment of IBS is peppermint oil, but traditionally peppermint oil has been taken orally, not inhaled or applied to the skin. (If you wish to try ingesting peppermint oil, you should take an enteric-coated form; otherwise the oil may be destroyed by stomach acid.) Some studies have shown that peppermint oil, when ingested, can improve symptoms of pain and bloating in some patients who have IBS; others have shown no benefit.

Biofeedback

Biofeedback includes any therapy in which sensors measure functions of the body (such as heart rate, respiration rate, and blood pressure) while the patient, through mental concentration, tries to change the parameter being measured. For example, patients who have hypertension often practice relaxation techniques while connected to a blood pressure monitor. Biofeedback has been shown to be successful at treating hypertension in some people. It also has helped people learn to control symptoms of anxiety. Biofeedback may improve IBS symptoms in some people, most likely by promoting relaxation and reducing stress and anxiety. There are no well-controlled trials comparing this form of treatment to standard medications for the treatment of IBS. Several studies have shown that biofeedback can help relieve constipation in individuals who have pelvic floor dysfunction, which often coexists in women who have IBS and constipation.

Herbal Remedies

Herbal remedies are used worldwide. Many modern pharmaceuticals are based on traditional herbal medicines. Historical studies have documented that herbal preparations were routinely used in ancient Egypt, Rome, and Greece, and it is quite likely that many herbal agents were used long before then. Thousands of herbs have been put to medicinal uses. The most important fact to know if you are contemplating using any herbal product, even if sold under a familiar brand name, is that herbal medicines are not required to undergo safety testing or rigorous scientific testing to determine efficacy prior to being marketed to the public. Before using any herbal preparation, you should read about it in more than one reputable information source. There may be side effects you should know about or potential serious interactions with foods or other medications. Remember, if the substance is strong enough to have a positive effect on your body, it is strong enough to have a negative one. For example, although herbs such as kava, chapparal, and yohimbe were recommended in the past to treat a variety of illnesses, all three of these herbs were found to cause liver damage, which in some cases was severe enough that it led to liver failure and death. Although herbs are natural, they can be dangerous and even deadly (just as allopathic medications can).

Common herbs and a few of their uses include saw palmetto to treat prostate enlargement, ginger for nausea, aloe for constipation, garlic for its antibiotic properties, gingko to increase memory, peppermint oil for abdominal pain, and St. John's wort for depression. Although these herbs are widely used, most clinical studies do not demonstrate any significant benefits from any of them. One large American double-blind, placebo-controlled trial showed no significant benefit of St. John's wort when compared to a placebo. A list of herbs that should be *avoided* or used *only* with great caution and under the direct supervision of a physician can be found in Table 21.1.

Homeopathy

Homeopathic medicine is rather counterintuitive. It uses a tiny amount of a specific substance that would normally cause the symptom that is being treated. An extremely dilute (that is, watered-down) solution of the substance is ingested, and it is thought to promote healing by the body itself. There is very little scientific evidence to support this type of therapy. No medical journal in the United States that is peer reviewed (meaning that the articles have been read, reviewed, and approved by scientists or physicians who are considered experts in the field) has accepted an article on homeopathy for publication. One point at issue is that the substances are so dilute that critics suspect there is no active ingredient left in the solution. At present, there are no known trials on homeopathy and IBS.

Hypnotherapy

Hypnosis has been used to treat many medical problems over the centuries. It is generally considered safe. Positive effects on IBS symptoms have been reported and may relate to a calming effect and a reduction in stress and anxiety. Use of hypnosis in treating IBS is described more completely in Chapter 22.

Table 21.1. Herbal Remedies That Require Extreme Caution and Supervision

Almond (*Prunus dulcis*)	Ma huang (*Ephedra sinica*)
American hellebore (*Veratum viride*)	Mandrake (*Mandragora officinarum*)
Belladonna (*Atropa belladonna*)	Mayapple (*Podophyllum peltatum*)
Birthwort (*Aristolochia clematitis*)	Monkshood (*Aconitum napellus*)
Boxwood (*Buxus sempervirens*)	Nutmeg (*Myristica fragrans*)
Chaparral (*Larrea tridentata*)	Poke (*Phytolacca americana*)
Digitalis (*Digitalis purpurea*)	Scopolia (*Scopolia carniolica*)
Germander (*Teucrium chamaedrys*)	Scotch broom (*Cytisus scoparius*)
Indian hemp (*Apocynum cannabinum*)	Tonka beans (*Dipteryx odorata*)
Jaborandi (*Pilocarpus microphyllus*)	Wahoo (*Euonymus atropurpurea*)
Kava (*Piper methysticum*)	Yohimbe bark (*Pausinystalia
Lily of the valley (*Convallaria majalis*)	yohimbe*)

Manipulation Therapies

This category includes a wide range of therapies, most of which are essentially massage therapy. The general theory is that manipulation of muscles, tendons, and subcutaneous tissue promotes healing by releasing blocked energy and toxins. Various forms include reflexology, Rolfing, shiatsu (a combination of acupressure and massage), Swedish massage, and trigger point therapy. Manipulation therapy has generally been shown to be safe and effective in relieving muscular stress, pain, and fatigue. It nearly always has a calming effect on the patient and so could be beneficial if anxiety is a factor contributing to a person's IBS symptoms. At present, there are no well-controlled trials on manipulation therapy and the treatment of IBS.

Naturopathy

Naturopathy is not a single therapy but rather a philosophy that emphasizes nutrition, the use of herbal remedies, manipulation, and relaxation techniques to release the body's inner vitality. No controlled trials exist comparing naturopathic approaches to the treatment of IBS to conventional medical therapies. Because naturopathy represents a combination of several different types of therapies, objectively assessing its benefits in comparison to any other single therapy will be difficult. However, it seems to be common sense that eating a healthier diet, performing relaxation techniques, and massaging sore and tired muscles will normally improve one's overall health and outlook on life.

Summary

- Complementary and alternative medicine (CAM) therapies are now routinely used by at least 35 percent of the adult population of the United States.
- Some CAM therapies may be safe and effective for certain IBS symptoms, but most have not been subjected to the same rigorous testing by which conventional treatments have been evaluated.
- Although data supporting its use is limited, acupuncture may help some people who have IBS. Additional studies to assess its safety and efficacy are needed before clear-cut recommendations can be made.
- Herbal supplements should be used with caution. Some herbal supplements have the potential to cause severe liver injury or even death.

CHAPTER 22

Psychological, Hypnotherapeutic, and Psychiatric Therapies

Many medical conditions are simple in nature. They can be handled with a single kind of treatment, and the symptoms go away. A good example is the common and annoying condition called athlete's foot. This is a simple fungal infection, often picked up in locker rooms or gyms. Once symptoms develop (itching and burning in the areas between the toes) and the characteristic red, flaky rash is seen, the diagnosis is made (usually by the patient) and treatment is started. A topical antifungal agent, purchased without a prescription, is applied to the affected area once or twice a day, and within days to weeks the infection is cleared up. The infection is limited to the skin; other organ systems are not involved and additional therapies need not be employed.

Irritable bowel syndrome is entirely different from that scenario. As we have learned, irritable bowel syndrome affects multiple parts of the GI tract, often all at the same time. Multiple types of symptoms occur and can differ dramatically from one person to the next. The symptoms can be accompanied by significant psychological effects that can in turn dramatically affect the course of the disease. IBS is frequently underdiagnosed (symptoms are ignored by the health care provider or attributed to another disease process); in addition, it is often misdiagnosed and thus treated inappropriately. Even when the condition is correctly diagnosed, the symptoms can be difficult to control in some people.

We all wish that a single therapy could be used to treat all of the symptoms of IBS and that all patients could be cured, but we are painfully aware that this is not the case, at least not yet. Although several available medications can significantly improve some of the symptoms of IBS, they are not effective in all patients, nor are they effective to the same degree in all of those who do respond to them. For that reason, researchers, clinicians, and patients have looked to alternative and complementary therapies for help in the treatment of IBS. Some of these therapies are reviewed in Chapter 21. This chapter will focus on therapies to improve the mental and physical health of individuals who have IBS. Maggie's case illustrates some of these treatment options.

Maggie, who is now a 24-year-old law student, started having problems with abdominal discomfort, bloating, diarrhea, and urgency as a high school student. Sometimes her symptoms were so severe she could barely finish a meal before having to run to the bathroom with diarrhea. Separate one-month trials of a wheat-free diet and then a lactose-free diet did not improve her symptoms. She saw her family doctor, who reviewed her history (nothing worrisome came to light), performed a thorough physical examination (which was normal), performed some simple blood tests (all of which turned out normal) and then made the diagnosis of IBS. He recommended a regimen of small, frequent meals in conjunction with as-needed doses of an antidiarrheal medicine (Imodium) and a smooth-muscle antispasmodic (dicyclomine). Maggie's symptoms improved dramatically during the next several years.

In college, however, Maggie's symptoms worsened. She noticed that they flared before an exam or before a major paper was due. On a bad day, she might have 10 loose, watery bowel movements with significant abdominal cramping and urgency. These episodes left her feeling drained and wiped out. Maggie went to the college health clinic and was referred to the university health center, where she saw a gastroenterologist. As it had been several years since any blood work had been done, Dr. Marzetta ordered a complete blood count, thyroid tests, a sedimentation rate (ESR), and an antibody test for celiac disease. Fortunately, all of the test results were completely normal. Dr. Marzetta also ordered some simple stool cultures (fecal leukocytes and ova and parasites) and scheduled a colonoscopy, to make sure that Maggie did not have inflammatory bowel disease. The stool studies all yielded normal results, and the colonoscopy, including biopsies at intervals throughout the colon, showed no abnormalities. This reassured Maggie, and she and Dr. Marzetta decided to use a combination of a different antidiarrheal agent, Lomotil, and sublingual hyoscyamine to treat the abdominal discomfort. They also discussed the fact that Maggie's symptoms seemed to get worse during times of stress. Maggie admitted that she got anxious at times; in fact, her brothers and sisters had nicknamed her "Nervous Nellie" and her parents said that she had always had a "sensitive stomach."

Maggie tried these new medications for a while, but she continued to experience symptoms. By this time, Maggie was starting to become a little depressed; she worried that she would suffer from these symptoms all of her life. Back at college, she saw a counselor. They decided to try treating the mild anxiety and depressive symptoms with a low dose of sertraline (Zoloft). This medication made Maggie a little groggy, so paroxetine (Paxil) was tried next, which dramatically improved Maggie's mood. Over the next year, the combination of small and frequent meals, Paxil, Lomotil, and hyoscyamine worked well for Maggie, and she graduated with honors.

After moving to a new city and starting law school, however, all of her symptoms worsened again. She tried increasing the doses of Lomotil and hyoscyamine, but the higher doses made her feel sleepy and gave her a dry mouth. She saw a local gastroenterologist, who started her on amitriptyline (Elavil), one of the tricyclic antidepressants that often eases diarrhea; however, even a very low dose made her feel groggy the next day, and she had to stop taking the medication.

Maggie came in to see me during her winter break. She accurately reported her history, including that several of the medicines she had used had improved her IBS symptoms but caused side effects that made it difficult for her to function. She also admitted that her symptoms worsened during stressful situations. Maggie was beginning to realize that, for her, IBS was likely to be a longstanding problem. She stated that her goals were to minimize her symptoms, improve her overall health and sense of well-being, and minimize medication use. We talked about a wide range of therapies and the risks and benefits of each. Maggie decided that she would focus on a regimen of routine exercise (something new for her), diet (low-fat, low-fiber, no caffeine, small frequent meals), and cognitive behavioral therapy, in addition to continuing a low dose of Paxil and using Imodium as needed.

Over the next several months, Maggie attended weekly and then every other week counseling sessions, and she noted a significant improvement in her symptoms. Her mood lightened, she felt more confident, and when she did have GI symptoms she was less anxious that they would escalate out of control. She took Imodium before a major examination or a mock trial, and it kept her symptoms manageable. Her abdominal discomfort was nearly gone. Even though she had an occasional flare of her IBS, the episodes were much less severe than in the past and, significantly, were not distressing to her. Using a combination of diet, exercise, medications, and behavioral therapy, Maggie had broken the vicious cycle in which gut problems made her anxious and the anxiety aggravated her gut (this is a good example of the brain-gut connection described in Chapter 2).

Effective treatment of people who have IBS must address both the physical symptoms of abdominal pain, bloating, diarrhea, and constipation and the emotional and mental aspects that often accompany this chronic disorder. The symptoms of IBS are ones that can be emotionally upsetting in themselves, and they can seriously disrupt daily life and work routines, causing additional distress. The tendency of the disorder to recur episodically and the frustrating process of trial and error to find an effective treatment that many patients go through can be sources of anxiety and stress. And, as Maggie's case illustrates, the emotional stress of the disorder fuels the symptoms.

The following sections describe psychological, hypnotherapeutic, and psychiatric treatments that may improve symptoms for people who have IBS symptoms.

Psychological Elements of IBS

Many people who have chronic IBS symptoms that are considered moderate to severe have coexisting anxiety or depression or suffer from panic attacks or a somatization disorder. Somatization disorders are character-ized by patients inappropriately focusing on minor symptoms, feeling that everything is going wrong in their body, and thinking that no part of their body is healthy. Anxiety disorders are the most prevalent psychiatric problem in the United States after substance abuse disorders. General-ized anxiety disorders occur in about 5 percent (about 1 in 20) of the U.S. adult population. Up to two-thirds of people who suffer from anxiety also suffer from depression.

For many people who have IBS, their physical symptoms become in-extricably interwoven with their mood problems. Symptoms of IBS can create feelings of anxiety: How bad will the episode be? When will the at-tack occur? How long will it last? People become nervous about how they will deal with the attack, and their anxiety increases as they think about how the attack will affect their other activities. Then the IBS symptoms flare and the patient's level of anxiety worsens. All of a sudden, a vicious cycle develops, in which IBS symptoms cause anxiety and heightened anxiety aggravates the GI symptoms. A similar pattern occurs in people with depression and IBS; they find that their IBS symptoms worsen when they are more depressed.

Medications designed to treat IBS symptoms do not directly treat the anxiety and depression suffered by many patients who have IBS, and the IBS symptoms may resist treatment unless the accompanying emotional problems are treated. Psychological management of IBS begins with the recognition that coexisting depression, anxiety, panic disorder, or soma-tization disorder may contribute to the frequency and severity of IBS symptoms.

The brain-gut connection (see Chapters 2 and 3) is always present in IBS, and we believe that visceral hypersensitivity contributes to the disorder, but not everyone who has IBS also has an anxiety disorder or depression or any other emotional problem. So, not every person who has IBS needs psychological or psychiatric therapy. Rather, psychological evaluation is recommended when it appears that anxiety, depression, or somatization is playing a role in the generation or expression of a person's IBS symptoms. Psychological therapy may be very helpful for anyone who answers yes to any of the following questions: Are you frequently anxious? Have you ever been treated for anxiety? Are your gut problems aggravated by stress? Do they get worse when you are anxious? Do you frequently feel depressed? Are your IBS symptoms worse when you are depressed? Do you find that you think about and worry about your health a lot? Are you pretty sure there is something seriously wrong with you, even though your doctor says there isn't? Another type of patient who can be helped by psychological therapy is one who is having trouble accepting the reality of having IBS or who is convinced that somewhere there is a single medicine that is going to make all the symptoms go away forever. Many people who have IBS benefit from a multidisciplinary approach to treating their IBS, involving cognitive behavioral therapy, stress management, and medications to treat both IBS symptoms and any emotional difficulties. These treatments are described below.

Cognitive Behavioral Therapy

Using cognitive behavioral therapy, people who have chronic medical problems can be taught skills and methods for dealing with their symptoms in a positive, rather than a negative, manner. Cognitive behavioral therapy (CBT) aims to help people change behaviors and thought processes that produce and maintain emotional distress. It can improve physical symptoms and eliminate feelings of hopelessness or helplessness and inappropriate fears and actions. In addition, CBT teaches patients how to control many of the negative thoughts that automatically appear when a certain physical symptom develops. Cognitive behavioral therapy is based on two key assumptions: first, that some symptoms can be learned, and that these symptoms represent specific deficits in cognitive and behavioral functioning; and second, that individuals can be taught to modify behaviors and thought patterns that can precipitate or worsen these symptoms, therefore improving the symptoms with a proper course of therapy. For example, some patients who have intestinal urgency and diarrhea start to assume that any episode of diarrhea will lead to severe pain, extreme diarrhea, and fecal incontinence. This automatic, negative thinking dramatically and adversely influences their physical and emotional health. Cognitive behavioral therapy teaches these people effective ways to deal with their symptoms in a positive manner and skills and mechanisms to improve their symptoms. In the end, this means that a small flare of their IBS symptoms does not lead to a downward spiral in their overall health.

People receiving CBT generally attend regularly scheduled group or individual sessions. Each session is run by a behavioral psychologist. Psychologists are trained completely differently from psychiatrists; they are not medical doctors, they emphasize counseling and discussion, and they are not authorized to prescribe medications. Patients are asked to identify their symptoms, are provided with education about their condition, and are taught various strategies for dealing with their symptoms. The message of such a program is that symptoms can be identified and managed in a positive manner. Many CBT programs include techniques to promote relaxation and manage stress. Relaxation therapy teaches patients to incorporate calm into their daily activities, to induce a sense of mental and emotional relaxation whenever they need it. The focus is positive and forward thinking. One goal of CBT is to deal with things proactively, not reactively. Another goal is to reduce avoidance behavior (like the extremely limited diet of Jean, whose story is in Chapter 10). When used as part of treatment for a chronic medical problem, the message of CBT is that patients have the skills and abilities to understand and manage their symptoms on a daily basis. By teaching appropriate management strategies to people who have IBS, CBT can provide them with the tools to prevent small IBS flares from snowballing into major crises.

Hypnotherapy

The use of hypnosis to treat chronic medical problems is relatively new. Most of us are familiar with the concept of hypnosis, but many people have an outdated and incorrect understanding of the practice. The old-fashioned view is of a "parlor trick" in which the hypnotist puts someone in a trance by having him or her focus on a swinging pocket watch and then "planting" suggestions into the person's head. On awakening, the person who was hypnotized is made to perform the suggestion when a specific signal is provided. This process was acted out in countless movies and television shows. This stereotypical view of hypnosis is outdated and factually incorrect, as people who are hypnotized are not really put into a trance, nor can they be made to do something against their will.

Hypnosis is slowly gaining acceptance in the medical community as a reasonable and viable treatment option for a variety of chronic medical problems. It has been used successfully in clinical and research settings to treat high blood pressure, tobacco abuse, alcohol abuse, chronic pain, and other disease states. In these settings, hypnosis is performed by someone who has been specifically trained in the therapeutic use of this technique. Multiple sessions are usually required, typically 1 session a week for 8 to 12 weeks. During each session, the patient is placed into a hypnotic state. This usually takes place in a warm, quiet room without distractions. The patient is first asked to concentrate on an image while the hypnotist relaxes the patient with soothing words. The patient then closes her or his eyes, and the hypnotist verbally guides the patient through slowly relaxing all of the muscles. This process is called "induction." As the session progresses, the hypnotist uses various techniques to place the patient into a deeper state of relaxation. Depending on the patient's personality, susceptibility to hypnosis, and goals, the state of hypnosis will be deeper or lighter. When the patient is very calm and relaxed and not distracted by internal thoughts or external noises, the hypnotist will provide thoughts, suggestions, and guided imagery for the patient to use to improve his or her symptoms. Patients can then use these suggestions to help themselves. Some patients even learn to induce a state of hypnosis on their own.

The exact mechanism by which hypnosis works is not known. Research studies using PET (positron emission tomography) scans have demonstrated that hypnotized people undergo changes in the metabolic activity of certain parts of their brain that are concerned with pain. In 1996, after reviewing the data on hypnotherapy for cancer pain, the National Institutes of Health judged that hypnosis was an effective intervention for alleviating pain from cancer. Over a dozen studies have now been published on the efficacy of hypnotherapy in the management of IBS. However, these studies were all performed in Europe, most in the United Kingdom. The studies consistently showed that hypnosis leads to an improvement in many of the symptoms of IBS, although the results of some studies are limited by design flaws and small numbers of participants.

Recently, researcher Peter Whorwell and colleagues from Manchester, England, published a long-term follow-up study of 273 patients who had IBS and completed a course of gut-directed hypnotherapy. Seventy-one percent of those who responded reported that they had good initial responses to hypnotherapy, and 81 percent of these stated that they had long-term improvement in their IBS symptoms. Despite the fact that the exact mechanism by which hypnosis improves symptoms of IBS remains unknown, these results are quite exciting, and they support the idea that hypnosis should be considered a viable treatment alternative or complement for patients who have IBS. It is especially encouraging that patients receiving hypnotherapy used medications less frequently for their symptoms and sought out consultation with their doctor less often. Although the results of this large study are positive, they do warrant confirmation by a large, multicenter trial.

Theoretically, then, it is a good idea to treat patients who have chronic IBS symptoms with hypnotherapy. Here in the United States, however, this can be quite difficult. It can be difficult to find someone who is well trained in hypnosis. At present, an extremely limited supply of suitably trained and experienced practitioners live in the United States. In addition, it is important to find a hypnotherapist who is interested in using hypnosis to treat IBS, as opposed to helping someone stop smoking. Although the technique may be similar, the actual therapy is quite different for these two very different disorders.

Hypnosis works well for some people but not for all. Some people seem to be more susceptible to the influences of hypnosis than others, just as people differ in their responses to medications. Also, most insurance companies don't pay for hypnosis sessions. In fact, many insurance companies actively discourage practitioners from referring patients for this type of therapy, since it usually requires an out-of-network referral.

Psychiatric Therapy for IBS

Some people who have severe IBS have significant problems with anxiety and depression. Although most primary care physicians feel comfortable treating patients who have mild depression or anxiety, psychiatrists are usually better equipped to treat patients who have severe mental and emotional problems. Psychiatrists begin their training by going to medical school; they are then required to spend an additional year of training in internal medicine, to become familiar with medical disorders. They then spend an additional three to five years focusing on psychiatry. In contrast to psychologists, who are not medical doctors and cannot prescribe medications, psychiatrists are likely to incorporate medications into their treatment plan. Patients who have severe anxiety or depression may require multiple medications or medications that can be accompanied by uncommon side effects. Some may need a period of inpatient care.

People who have severe IBS symptoms and significant anxiety or depression are more likely to note an improvement in their IBS symptoms when they are treated by both their primary care physician or gastroenterologist and also a psychiatrist. An interactive team approach treats the whole person, although the psychiatrist focuses on the complicated mental and emotional issues while the internist or gastroenterologist concentrates on the physical symptoms. Consistently, when anxiety and depression are under control, the patient feels better able to address the symptoms of IBS. This dual treatment approach is more likely to lead to an improvement in both aspects of the person's health.

Summary

- Patients who have severe or difficult-to-control IBS symptoms frequently also suffer from anxiety, depression, or a somatization disorder.
- Effective treatment for these patients must include therapy directed at the emotional and psychological components of this chronic disorder.
- Cognitive behavioral therapy, hypnotherapy, and therapy with a psychiatrist or psychologist are all worthwhile treatment options that may lead to an improvement in IBS symptoms and quality of life.

CHAPTER 23

The Ingredients of an Effective Doctor's Appointment

Most office visits are very different today than they were just 10 years ago. Why is this? Our health care system is overwhelmed by rules and regulations, there are more patients to be seen—and many of them have more severe problems—and diagnostic tests and treatments are more complicated than in the past, requiring more time for scheduling and explanations. All of this leads to a more hectic schedule for both patients and physicians, which translates into visits that seem more harried and less user-friendly than in the past. Long gone are the days of a leisurely office visit with your primary care provider, in which you would first carefully review your health concerns and then undergo a thorough and thoughtful physical examination, followed by a discussion to design a treatment plan and additional time to ask any remaining questions. Instead of a one-hour new patient appointment with your internist, some managed care organizations now require that physicians schedule new patients every 10 to 15 minutes. Due to these time and scheduling restrictions, some health care providers now limit the number of items discussed during an appointment to just two or three; other providers ask patients to come in for one visit where they review allergies, medications, and symptoms and then schedule another visit on another day for a physical examination. At the end of the second visit, a treatment plan is decided on (sometimes with little input from the patient) and, if any time remains, questions are briefly, and sometimes brusquely, answered. It is little wonder that so many people are disenchanted with our health care system.

Physicians will probably not be able to return to the more relaxed and leisurely office visits of the past. Unfortunately, this means that some of the burden for efficient care is shifted onto the patient. More than ever before, as a patient you must be your own best advocate, which means being as prepared as possible for each office visit. Follow the thirteen suggestions listed below to make your visits to your primary care provider or to specialists as useful as possible for you and for your health care provider. Most patients will not need all of the items on the list at each visit; others may find that this list is best suited for the first visit to a new primary care physician or to a new specialist. By following the suggestions below, you can dramatically improve the efficiency of your doctor appointments. Doing so will give you more time to coordinate a treatment plan together with your doctor and get all of your questions answered.

1. Make a list of your symptoms in advance and bring this list with you.
2. Set priorities.
3. Make a list of questions that you want answered.
4. If appropriate, bring a list of recently performed tests and their results.
5. Think about your goals.
6. Bring a list of allergies and any reactions to medications.
7. Bring a list of the medications you are currently taking.
8. Make a list of active medical problems that you are currently being treated for.
9. Arrive at your doctor's office 20 minutes early.
10. Bring a list of any fears or concerns that you have.
11. Try to schedule your appointment so you are the first or second appointment in the morning or the first or second afternoon appointment.
12. Do a little research in advance.
13. Make sure you understand your treatment plan.

Each item is discussed in detail below.

1. Make a list of your symptoms in advance and bring this list with you.

Although this suggestion seems obvious, it's a good one—for two reasons. First, it's fairly common for a doctor who asks a patient "What's bothering you today?" to hear, "Nothing, I'm doing fine." Admittedly, this type of conversation is becoming rarer in today's health care environment, since most doctor visits are prompted now by a specific concern or symptom rather than by a routine annual physical examination (routine annual exams in otherwise healthy adults are rapidly falling out of favor). Second, and more significantly, many people are a little nervous or anxious about going to the doctor, so when they arrive for the appointment they "freeze up" and forget many or all of their symptoms and concerns. If a patient forgets symptoms and concerns, the doctor can't help the patient. People find it frustrating to arrive home only to remember the two or three urgent items he or she meant to talk about with the doctor.

2. Set priorities.

Arrange the list of symptoms or issues that you want to discuss from most important to least important. Don't use valuable office time discussing that small wart on your foot that only bothers you during sandal season, when the more important issue is urgent diarrhea or painful gas and bloating that occurs on a daily basis. If you bring a list of 15 to 20 issues, it is unlikely that your doctor will be able to address all of them. Address the top two or three most important issues, and then bring an updated list of symptoms and issues to your next office visit.

3. Make a list of questions that you want answered.

As you prepare for your visit and think about your symptoms, you probably also think about questions that you want answered. Some patients feel embarrassed about asking questions because they are not sure if they are using the right words or if they are pronouncing the words correctly. Remember that most doctors love to teach! Like artists, scientists, carpenters, chefs, and others, doctors like to talk about their work. They enjoy educating patients—this is what they are trained to do. So, don't feel embarrassed about asking a question, and don't worry about possibly mispronouncing a word. Bring a (reasonably sized) list of specific questions and make sure you get answers to them.

4. If appropriate, bring a list of recently performed tests and their results.

This may not be necessary if you are seeing your long-standing internist for a routine office visit or if you are going to a routine follow-up appointment with your gastroenterologist. However, if you are seeing a specialist for the first time (such as a gastroenterologist) or if you are seeing a physician for a second opinion, it will make your visit much more efficient if you bring a list of all tests performed for your symptoms (for example, colonoscopies, abdominal ultrasounds, CT scans, and/or blood tests), where and when they were performed, and the test results.

5. Think about your goals.

Goals are completely separate from the questions you want answered or from your fears and concerns (see below). Maybe your goal is to improve or eliminate episodes of urgent diarrhea. Or maybe your goal is to minimize bloating. Try to be as specific as possible, because knowing your goal will help your doctor coordinate an individualized treatment plan.

6. Bring a list of allergies and any reactions to medications.

This list is usually reviewed at the first visit and updated at subsequent visits. For most patients, it will only take a few seconds to make such a list; however, some people who have irritable bowel syndrome are very sensitive to medications. It is more efficient to bring a list of allergies and adverse drug reactions that can be quickly reviewed in 30 seconds than to spend 5 to 10 minutes trying to remember which medication caused which side effect.

7. Bring a list of the medications you are currently taking.

If in doubt, or if you don't have enough time, bring the pill bottles. Similar to the suggestion of bringing a list of allergies and adverse drug reactions, your doctor's visit will be much more efficient if you bring a typed list of the medications you are currently taking. Ideally, this list will include the dose of the medication (for example, 81 mg of aspirin or 25 mg of phenergan) in addition to a notation of how and when the drug is taken (such as 30 minutes before breakfast or 1 tablet with each meal). The more specific the information, the better. For example, it is much more helpful to bring a list that says "20 mg of omeprazole taken each day 30 minutes before dinner" than to tell the doctor "I take a pink pill some time during the afternoon."

8. Make a list of active medical problems that you are currently being treated for.

Also bring a list of any surgeries you have had, along with the dates of surgery (this list of surgeries is especially important if you are seeing a gastroenterologist or if your major symptom is abdominal pain). Patients who have had multiple surgeries over time, especially if those surgeries were performed at different institutions, can easily get the type of surgery and the date confused. The first 5 to 10 minutes of an office visit is then spent just reviewing the surgical history, instead of focusing on more pressing symptoms. The more prepared you are, and the less time you spend reviewing your past medical and surgical history with your doctor, the more time you'll have to discuss your current symptoms.

9. Arrive at your doctor's office 20 minutes early.

Every office needs to gather demographic information (age, date of birth, gender, ethnic background, occupation, etc.), and even if you have been to that office before, they will need to check to see if the information they have is up to date. In addition, all offices have to gather insurance information, and this process is becoming increasingly more complicated and more time consuming with each passing year. Although frustrating, this process has to be repeated for each health care provider you see. Arrive early. Let the office staff gather all of your information and update it if necessary. That way you'll be finished with the paperwork when your doctor is ready to see you.

10. Bring a list of any fears or concerns that you have.

This list may be different from your list of questions. Your list of questions may include why you have specific symptoms or why you developed IBS. But many people who have IBS are worried and concerned that having IBS increases their risk for cancer (it doesn't) or that IBS will change into IBD (inflammatory bowel disease—it doesn't do this, either). Write these concerns down and discuss them with your doctor to relieve any unnecessary stress you may be feeling.

11. Try to schedule your appointment so you are the first or second appointment in the morning or the first or second afternoon appointment.

If your provider has a busy schedule, it is probable that as the morning wears on, she or he may fall behind schedule. This can happen because patients arrive late, patients come in with unexpected problems that require more time, or because the doctor must address an urgent or emergent problem. You can minimize your chance of being inconvenienced by scheduling your appointment for first thing in the morning or first thing in the afternoon, after lunch. If your doctor is running late from the morning, he or she will usually be able to catch up during the lunch break (a time most doctors use to finish dictations and notes, make phone calls, and fill out forms). In addition, it is likely that your doctor will be more alert and attentive first thing in the morning or after lunch than late morning or at the end of the day.

12. If you have time, do a little research in advance.

This seems obvious, but if you have had painful heartburn for 3 years, and this is the first time you're going to see a doctor to discuss your symptoms, it is worthwhile to spend 10 or 15 minutes reading about that topic either at the library or online. Sometimes this research time is best spent just learning the language and specific terms that are used to describe that disorder. If you know something about the subject and are familiar with some of the key words and terms, you and your doctor will find it easier to communicate. A brief list of consumer-oriented medical websites is presented at the end of this book.

13. Finally, as you finish your visit, make sure you understand your treatment plan.

Do tests need to be scheduled? If so, when and where? How will you get the results? If a prescription is provided, how should it be taken? Once a day, twice daily, or more often? Should you take it every day or only if you have a symptom? What are the side effects? Can it be used safely with other medications? And, given the cost of medications these days, is there a less expensive option? If you need to return for a visit, when? If you have a question, who should you call?

I provide each of my patients with a written plan at the end of the visit. Office visits can be confusing—new information is provided and questions are answered, and if a patient does not feel well, it may be difficult to concentrate and remember everything that is said. A written plan helps both the health care provider and the patient understand the plan of action, and it also serves as a nice reference for the patient later, if questions come up.

PART IV

Other Issues

CHAPTER 24

IBS and Children

It's not unusual for a parent or teacher to hear a child say, "My tummy hurts." Most of the time, abdominal pain in children represents a brief problem that resolves on its own without any treatment. However, many children suffer from recurrent abdominal pain. It is the most common reason children are referred by their primary care provider to a pediatric gastroenterologist. In the past, the dominant view was that chronic or recurrent abdominal pain in children was a separate and distinct clinical entity from the irritable bowel syndrome found in teenagers and adults. It was believed that children were simply too young to develop IBS. However, as our understanding of the disorder has expanded, our views about IBS and children have also changed. In this chapter, I explain available data about abdominal pain in children and try to answer the question of whether recurrent abdominal pain in children is the forerunner of IBS in adulthood. In addition, I discuss the current diagnostic criteria for IBS in adolescents.

In the late 1950s Dr. Apley, a British pediatrician, observed that a large number of school-age children suffered from recurrent episodes of abdominal pain. He defined recurrent abdominal pain as repeated episodes of pain during a period of three months or more, each of which went away without treatment. He noted that in children who had recurrent abdominal pain, symptoms were likely to first occur at approximately age 5, and in girls there appeared to be a rise in occurrences during puberty. He found that the region around the umbilicus (belly button) was the most common site of pain, although it could develop anywhere in the abdomen. As in adults, the pain could be sharp or dull or aching and could be either continuous during an episode or intermittent. He carefully evaluated these children, but in only 10 percent was he able to identify a specific disease or disorder as the cause of the pain. In this small group (10 percent of all children studied), the most common causes of the pain were inflammatory bowel disease, celiac disease, and lactose intolerance.

For the vast majority of children Dr. Apley examined, however, a distinct cause of the pain could not be identified, so the abdominal pain was assumed to be functional in nature (meaning that no organic cause for it could be identified). He did note that abdominal pain seemed to be more frequent in children who were anxious or high-strung, and that overall, children who had chronic abdominal pain were more likely to have psychological problems than children who did not have abdominal pain.

For many of the children in this informal study, their abdominal pain went away as they grew older; however, a significant proportion had persistent symptoms that lasted into adulthood. Dr. Apley labeled this condition "recurrent abdominal pain of childhood," or RAP, and this description is still used. The current most commonly accepted definition of RAP is at least three distinct episodes of abdominal pain during the course of three months, and the child's activities must be affected by these episodes. For many years health care practitioners debated whether or not RAP was exactly the same as IBS. Recurrent abdominal pain of childhood does represent IBS in some cases; however, RAP is a broader category than IBS and includes three major subcategories: organic diseases (such as inflammatory bowel disease), functional disorders (like IBS and dyspepsia), and idiopathic disorders (conditions of unknown origin).

Another research study that addressed the issue of recurrent abdominal pain in children was conducted in the 1990s, nearly 40 years after Apley made his preliminary observations. This study was performed in part to take advantage of technology that was not available earlier. These technological advances make it easier to recognize medical conditions that were present decades ago but could not be easily or accurately diagnosed. Two such conditions are *Helicobacter pylori* infection (a cause of ulcers) and acid reflux disease. This study, which was done in Europe, evaluated 103 children with recurrent abdominal pain (all of whom were older than 3 years, with an average age of 10 years). The children underwent extensive testing, including blood work to look for celiac disease, blood tests to evaluate liver and pancreatic function, a complete blood count, tests to measure kidney function, sedimentation rate, urinalysis, stool studies (cultures, ova and parasites, fecal leukocytes, occult blood), tests for sickle cell disease (if appropriate), and an ultrasound of the abdomen. In addition, many children underwent invasive testing, including upper endoscopy, colonoscopy, and pH testing (to look for acid reflux disease); these tests were performed on an individualized basis and depended on the presence of certain symptoms and warning signs.

After this extensive battery of tests, an organic problem could be identified in less than a third of the children. In many cases, this organic problem was considered fairly minor (for instance, mild gastritis) or uncommon in children (inflammatory bowel disease, celiac disease). Sometimes the organic problem was one that is also present in approximately the same percentage of all children in the general population, which means that it was unlikely to be the cause of the child's pain. One interesting observation was that pain at night and pain localized to a specific area usually had an organic cause, like inflammation, as opposed to a functional one.

Of the majority of patients whose pain was due to nonorganic causes, over half fulfilled the criteria for IBS. Health care workers determined that 36 percent of the children who entered the study had IBS. These results have been confirmed by two published American studies, which found that 26 to 51 percent of children who meet the criteria for RAP also fit the criteria for IBS. It appears that IBS in children is not uncommon. A 1996 study by the Connecticut Children's Medical Center found that 17 percent of high school students and 8 percent of middle school students reported symptoms consistent with IBS. Other studies have confirmed these data. Overall, it is estimated that 10 to 20 percent of school-age children in the United States have symptoms of IBS.

Irritable bowel syndrome in children is a significant medical condition that warrants thoughtful evaluation and treatment because it can dramatically affect how children behave socially, adversely influence learning and school grades, and increase school absenteeism. In fact, IBS is one of the leading causes of school absenteeism across the country. In addition, IBS in children may necessitate frequent and costly physician visits and can disrupt family and social life.

Many children who have RAP do develop IBS later in life. In fact, one large research study found that approximately one-third of children who had RAP as a child had symptoms of IBS as an adult. This highlights the fact that better treatment options are needed for children in an attempt to minimize or even prevent this progression.

Comparison of IBS in Children and Adults

Irritable bowel syndrome in children is currently defined in much the same way as it is in adults (see Chapter 2), although no studies have verified or validated the Rome criteria for children. One major difference is that children need to have symptoms only once per week for at least two months before diagnosis (in adults, symptoms should be present for at least six months and active for the last three months before diagnosis). In children, IBS generally falls into one of three main types: pain predominant, constipation predominant, and diarrhea predominant. The pattern of alternating constipation and diarrhea found in nearly one-third of adults who have IBS is much less common in children. However, the bowel habits of young children differ from those of adults. The average baby has four to six stools per day during the first year of life. This decreases to an average of one to three stools per day after the age of one, and by age five, most children settle into nearly an adult pattern of bowel habits, meaning that they range from three bowel movements per day to three per week.

Symptoms of IBS are generally the same in children as they are in adults, with the following exceptions: bloating and distention appear to be less common in children than in adults; a pattern of alternating constipation and diarrhea is uncommon in children; and children are more likely to complain of nausea, especially after eating. Nausea after eating is most consistent with the diagnosis of dyspepsia (upper GI complaints), which occurs in 40 percent of adults who have IBS. While the passage of mucus with a bowel movement, occasionally noted in children who have symptoms of IBS, occurs in adults as well, it often generates more concern in children. Adults become aware that passing a small amount of mucus with a bowel movement is not unusual or uncommon; the mucus represents normal secretion from the cells that line the colon, and it coats the stool and facilitates evacuation.

The pathophysiology of IBS in children is thought to be similar to that in adults, although far fewer studies have been performed with children to verify the presence of the abnormalities in gastrointestinal motility and visceral sensitivity seen in adults. One of the reasons that few studies of children who have IBS exist is that researchers are reluctant to employ in children the invasive tests used in many of these diagnostic studies. These tests often require sedation, and they usually require the place-ment of a tube or catheter into the colon or small intestine. Most parents and pediatricians feel that the risks of these tests, although quite small, outweigh any possible benefits for the individual children. Thus, there is much less information available on children than on adults. However, some information is available that is worth discussing.

Like adults, children who have symptoms of IBS and diarrhea experi-ence rapid transit of food through the GI tract, while those children who have symptoms of constipation have slower transit than normal. Children may have disordered motility in both the small intestine and the colon, including either more frequent contractions than normal or the presence of very strong contractions in the small intestine and colon. Strong contractions may cause abdominal cramps, spasms, and pain. The central nervous system is likely to play a major role in the manifestation of IBS symptoms in children as well, and certainly, as in adults, environ-mental influences that produce feelings of fear, anxiety, or stress can in-fluence both gut motility and gut sensation. Two separate studies showed that feelings of fear and depression can delay the normal emptying of the stomach in children, while another study demonstrated that feelings of aggression can stimulate gut motility. Finally, studies have confirmed that visceral hypersensitivity probably plays a critical role in the manifestation of IBS symptoms in children, as it does in adults. In summary, the patho-physiology (abnormal physiology) of IBS symptoms in children appears to be quite similar to that in adults.

Possible Causes and Triggers

The etiology of IBS for children is probably the same as it is for adults. The fact that young children can develop IBS strongly suggests that there is at least a partial genetic basis for the development of IBS. A second important reason for the development of IBS in children is a preceding infectious illness. One study showed that children who have IBS were more likely than their healthy counterparts to have received antibiotics. The antibiotic use probably indicates treatment of an infection. External stressors and internal emotions like anxiety, fear, and depression seem to influence the frequency and severity of IBS symptoms, although, just as in adults, these factors are not the cause of IBS in children.

What external factors might precipitate the onset of symptoms? Very few studies have prospectively evaluated risk factors for IBS in children. A recently published Australian study reported on a group of people who were followed from age 3 to age 26 with routine examinations and questionnaires. Study participants in the highest socioeconomic group were much more likely to develop IBS than those in lower socioeconomic groups. Unfortunately, the study did not isolate which factors about a more privileged upbringing were associated with the development of IBS. More important, it seems that children who have not developed adequate coping skills are more likely to experience symptoms of IBS.

Several good research studies performed in the United States have focused on the relationships between parents who have IBS and their children. These studies were trying to determine whether a child who has a parent with IBS is at increased risk for developing IBS later in life. The answer seems to be an unqualified yes. Although having a parent who has IBS is not a guarantee that a child will develop IBS, it definitely makes it much more likely. There are several reasons why this may be so, beyond an inherited predisposition to the disorder. Children carefully observe their parents and notice their IBS symptoms and the way the parents handle the symptoms. The children may later mimic those same symptoms and responses. Sometimes children are in effect rewarded for being sick, by being given a special toy or treat. During a time when parents are busy, the extra attention a parent gives an ill child may unintentionally encourage the child to feel sick more often. For many children, school can be quite stressful. For some, stress develops at school because of learning difficulties; for others, stress occurs because they are being bullied. In an effort to avoid this stress, some children, consciously or unconsciously, take on illness behaviors. If they are then rewarded as well, the strategy is reinforced.

Diagnosis

The initial steps in diagnosing IBS in children are the same as in adults (see Chapter 7). The health care provider needs to take a thorough history of the child's symptoms and perform a complete physical examination. Most pediatricians believe that a careful evaluation of social and psychological factors is important as well. Children obviously have a shorter medical history to record than adults do, but there are as many, or more, topics to address. They include

- nature of the child's birth (any complications)
- history of the child's growth (normal, slow, periods of weight gain or loss)
- history of infections and how treated
- dates and place of any travel outside the United States
- usual source of drinking water; any episodes of contamination
- history of medication use, especially antibiotics
- history of diet and any dietary changes
- health of other family members (especially a history of parents who have IBS symptoms)
- history of IBS symptoms (first occurrence, frequency, severity, type)
- other physical problems (rashes, joint pain, fevers, vomiting, mouth ulcers)
- nature of nighttime behavior (sleep, GI problems)

Warning signs, or "red flags," that might alert a pediatrician to an organic cause of a child's symptoms, include the following (finding an organic cause means that symptoms are a result of a structural change in an organ):

- dysphagia (difficulty swallowing)
- persistent vomiting
- anemia (low blood count)
- pain that awakens the child from sleep
- nocturnal (nighttime) diarrhea
- ulcers in the mouth
- inflamed or swollen joints
- new rashes
- involuntary weight loss
- a slowing down of the normal growth curve
- unexplained fevers
- delay in attaining puberty

These symptoms, either alone or in combination, may prompt specialized tests and/or a referral to a specialist.

With regard to psychosocial factors, the health care provider will try to determine if symptoms are correlated with times of stress. Have symptoms occurred around the time of stressful events, such as tests at school, problems with friends, being bullied by another child, and/or difficulties at home (financial problems, parents fighting, parents going through a divorce, hospitalization or death of a parent, parent changing jobs, moving of the household)?

Currently, no guidelines specify the tests to be ordered for an evaluation of a child suspected of having IBS. In general, pediatricians take a more conservative approach than do health care providers who treat only adults. This is in part because in children, symptoms often represent a benign or transitory process that resolves on its own without any medical intervention. This approach, which is appropriate for children, is called "watchful waiting." In contrast, physicians who treat adults often work on the assumption that there is an organic problem at the root of the patient's symptoms and that this problem needs to be diagnosed. Thus, diagnostic testing is much more prevalent in adults. This approach is called "test and treat."

For children who have recurrent or chronic abdominal pain and disordered bowel habits, many health care providers initiate the evaluation by performing blood tests, including a complete blood count (CBC) and a sedimentation rate (ESR). In addition, many pediatricians routinely order a urinalysis. For children who have persistent diarrhea, stool samples may be collected to look for evidence of an infection, and additional blood work may be requested to determine whether the child has celiac disease (a wheat allergy).

If abdominal pain persists, an abdominal x-ray may be taken. This can show whether a kidney stone is present, whether the child is severely constipated (e.g., stool is present throughout the entire colon), and whether there is evidence of a mechanical obstruction of the intestinal tract, among other findings. If the persistent symptoms are in the upper abdomen, the pediatrician may order an x-ray study of the upper GI tract (an upper gastrointestinal series). During this procedure, children are asked to swallow approximately a cup of barium solution, and then x-rays are taken as the barium coats the esophagus, stomach, and upper small intestine. This test can be used to look for evidence of an ulcer or other problem that could cause recurrent abdominal pain.

If all of the testing described above has yielded normal results and symptoms persist or if new symptoms develop, the child will usually be referred to a pediatric gastroenterologist, a physician who specializes in treating gastrointestinal disorders in children. At this point, the child may be scheduled for an upper endoscopy (EGD) if upper abdominal symptoms predominate or a colonoscopy if symptoms of lower abdominal discomfort, persistent diarrhea, or constipation predominate. In children, these tests are usually performed under general anesthesia rather than with conscious sedation. During general anesthesia, the patient is completely unconscious, and his or her breathing is assisted with the use of a ventilator. The patient is carefully monitored by an anesthesiologist, a nurse, and the physician performing the test. Colonoscopy would be especially important in evaluation of patients who have persistent diarrhea, because of the concern that the child could have inflammatory bowel disease (IBD).

Organic abnormalities are rarely found in children. In one study, only 4 percent of children who had recurrent abdominal pain and underwent colonoscopy and upper endoscopy were found to have an abnormality. Thus, if a careful history and physical examination are performed and warning signs of other disease are absent, and if a child meets the Rome criteria for IBS, then IBS is the likely diagnosis. This diagnostic approach has proven to be reliable for children as well as adults. The results of an Italian study support this approach. The study followed children who had been diagnosed with functional GI disorders and found that only rarely did an organic problem turn out to be the cause of their symptoms instead of IBS. A study from the Mayo Clinic reported similar findings. These data further support the practice of watchful waiting employed by most pediatricians.

Other Disorders

Hirschsprung's Disease

Children who have severe constipation (significant straining at stool, very infrequent bowel movements) of long standing should be evaluated for Hirschsprung's disease. This is an uncommon but well recognized condition that results from a lack of normal nerve supply in the anal and rectal area. Hirschsprung's disease develops before birth, when nerve cells fail to migrate into the anorectal area. The missing cells are those that normally help the internal anal sphincter to relax, thus assisting evacuation. After birth, the smooth muscles in the anorectum cannot relax properly, and children become severely constipated. Hirschsprung's disease can be diagnosed with anorectal manometry (see Chapter 8). In many cases, flexible sigmoidoscopy is performed as well, to make sure there is no evidence of obstruction. In the case of Hirschsprung's disease, taking biopsies requires a surgeon, because the biopsies have to go through the entire thickness of the rectum. Definitive treatment for Hirschsprung's disease involves surgery.

Encopresis

Encopresis is an uncommon problem in which there is repetitive passage of stool at inappropriate times. This evacuation of stool can be either voluntary or involuntary. The condition affects 1 to 3 percent of children over the age of 4. Encopresis is very different from fecal incontinence, which typically occurs in adults due to injury or trauma to the nerves or muscles in the anorectal area. People who have fecal incontinence usually leak small amounts of liquid stool. With encopresis, young children either repeatedly soil their underwear (which parents usually assume are recurrent episodes of diarrhea) or pass a formed bowel movement during the night.

Encopresis is unrelated to IBS and does not indicate any known neuromuscular disorder of the pelvic floor or anorectal area. It usually results from the withholding of stool in the rectum. The retained stool is then released while the child is asleep or at some other inappropriate time. Stool withholding may be voluntary (for any of a variety of reasons) or may represent an inability of the child to sense that there is stool in the rectum, which may represent a nerve disorder. In many cases, children who have encopresis have an underlying psychological problem, such as anxiety, depression, or severe stress or tension. Treatment of encopresis is generally directed at the underlying psychological problem (if present) and combined with bowel training.

Treatment

The treatment for children who have IBS is similar in many ways to that for adults. Both the similarities and differences relate to the use of medications. It is not widely known that most medications used to treat disorders in children have never been tested on children. In fact, less than 25 percent of the medications currently available to the public have been tested directly in children, and even those have not been studied in the trials involving thousands of patients that are now required for approval of a medication for adults. At best, hundreds of children were included in the studies.

Why aren't all medications tested in children before being released? There are four main reasons. One, health care workers are concerned with the safety of testing unproven medications on children. Two, most parents will not give consent for their children to participate in drug trials. Three, the cost of safety trials in children specifically, added to the already high cost of testing in adults, could further increase the cost of the medication. Four, pharmaceutical companies are worried that an even greater danger exists of their being sued when children are involved in drug studies than when the participants are adults. For example, let's say that a company includes children in a medication study that determines that the medication is both safe and effective. However, 15 years later, after tens of millions of doses have been prescribed, new data comes to light showing that the medication can have serious long-term side effects. In the current legal climate, it is virtually guaranteed that a host of lawyers will sue the pharmaceutical company, saying that the medication caused harm to these children during the drug studies (whether it did or not). For all of these reasons, drug trials in children are few and far between. Because of that, most pediatricians are forced to rely on information from adult studies, which they then try to translate into useful information that they can apply to the pediatric population.

Faced with this shortage of information, most pediatricians try other treatment approaches before prescribing medications. After they identify the predominant symptom, whether it is pain, constipation, or diarrhea, the first step is typically some form of dietary intervention focused on eliminating foods thought to be triggering the symptoms. Depending on symptoms, dietary interventions may include a lactose-free diet, a fructose-free diet, a wheat-free diet, a diet free of eggs, or a diet without any caffeine (this includes avoiding soft drinks, cocoa, coffee, and tea). Many physicians also emphasize decreasing the amount of junk food and snack foods. For children who have constipation, bowel training and use of fiber supplements is recommended (and see Chapter 15).

Although no medication is approved by the FDA for the treatment of IBS with constipation in children, many health care providers recommend using a polyethylene glycol product (i.e., Miralax or glycolax) to help with the symptoms of constipation. However, as discussed in Chapter 16, the polyethylene glycol product won't relieve the child's abdominal pain. Other pediatricians recommend the use of lubiprostone, which is FDA approved for the treatment of women who have IBS and constipation and has been shown to be safe and effective. Trials are currently being performed with children, and data should be available in the near future.

Children who have problems with recurrent diarrhea are usually treated with small doses of Pepto-Bismol or Imodium (see Chapter 17) and helped to change their diet. Two recent studies reported that a low-dose tricyclic antidepressant (amitriptyline) improved quality of life and symptoms of anxiety for children who had IBS. However, amitriptyline did not significantly improve symptoms of abdominal pain in either study. A small clinical trial involving children who had IBS found that peppermint oil improved symptoms of abdominal pain, although the study results are weakened by the fact that the study lasted only two weeks.

Most pediatricians want to minimize medication use. They are concerned about overmedication and possible adverse events, such as fatigue, drowsiness, mood changes, and inability to function normally at school and during social activities. However, if initial treatment efforts fail, most will resort to the medications reviewed in the previous chapters, according to the predominant symptom. Because few of these medications have been subjected to rigorous testing in children, specific dosing guidelines for children are not provided in most standard pharmacology texts; the dosing guidelines are based on studies performed in adults. Generally, pediatricians calculate a quarter, third, or half of the lowest recommended adult dose, depending on the age and size of the patient. This is used as the starting dose, and when the patient is seen in follow-up, adjustments up or down can be made, if necessary. Safe, careful medication of children, like that of adults, focuses on starting with a low dose, increasing it slowly if necessary, maintaining regular follow-up with the patient, and watching for side effects and drug interactions. Fortunately, many children who have IBS respond well to simple dietary interventions and reassurance and do not require the use of any medications.

Summary

- Abdominal pain is a frequent but very nonspecific symptom in children. In the vast majority of cases, the pain goes away on its own without any treatment.
- Recurrent abdominal pain (RAP) of childhood represents a broad collection of disorders, including IBS.
- Ten to twenty percent of school-age children are estimated to have symptoms consistent with the diagnosis of IBS.
- Symptoms of IBS in children are similar to those in adults, with a

few exceptions. Bloating and abdominal distention and IBS with alternating constipation and diarrhea are less common in children, and nausea is more common in children.

- Children who have IBS are often evaluated and treated more con-servatively than adults who have IBS symptoms. A "watch and wait" approach prevents unnecessary diagnostic testing of children.

CHAPTER 25

What Does the Future Hold?

The practice of medicine is both a science and an art. The science of medicine is built on numbers, which are easily measured and derived from laboratory research, clinical trials, diagnostic tests, and clinical experience. The art of medicine, which has an intuitive aspect, is formed from the practitioner's myriad emotional, social, educational, and professional experiences. The elements of the art of medicine are much harder to quantify and are obviously more subjective.

To practice the art of medicine, one must have the time to be a careful listener. The astute physician is a good detective, searching out seemingly insignificant details that could later play a major role in the diagnosis and treatment of a patient. To be a good practitioner, one must be able to convey caring and compassion, so that the patient is comfortable communicating honestly. In addition, the provider must be able to provide an opportunity for each patient to tell her or his own story. These things are difficult to accomplish in the current health care climate, in which insurance companies and managed care organizations view the practice of medicine as a business and time spent with patients as something to be strictly rationed.

The field of medicine is also characterized by change, in both its scientific underpinnings and our understanding of people. The evaluation and treatment of people who have irritable bowel syndrome are prime examples of this. During the last two decades, we have witnessed dramatic changes in our approach to conducting research in this area, and we have made great strides in treating this chronic disorder that is frustrating and discouraging for so many people. We now have a better understanding of why IBS develops and how symptoms reflect disordered physiology. We're more comfortable with the concept of the brain-gut axis and how emotions and moods can influence gut activity. That IBS is commonly associated with other disorders, such as fibromyalgia, migraine headaches, and interstitial cystitis, has come to light in recent years, and our understanding of these relationships has increased our diagnostic capabilities. We are beginning to understand why some people seem to be at a greater risk of developing IBS than other people. And, we are getting better at diagnosing IBS without subjecting patients to unnecessary tests.

All of these changes have improved our ability to treat individuals who have IBS. Meanwhile, changes in the philosophy of medical care have made doctors better at understanding and treating the whole patient, rather than viewing the patient only as a symptom, such as constipation or abdominal pain or bloating. Given these remarkable changes during the last two decades, further advances can be expected in the next decade. I believe that significant progress will be made on multiple fronts in both the basic science and the patient care arenas of IBS. A driving force behind efforts in these directions is the realization by patients and physicians that the current treatments for IBS remain unsatisfactory for many people.

Public Awareness

For years, IBS was considered by some patients and physicians to be a catch-all or "wastebasket" diagnosis. Some patients believed that because their doctor could not find a cause, their symptoms were given the label "IBS" for want of a more definitive diagnosis. In addition, because so few treatments were available ("take fiber" and "take more fiber"), there appeared to be little interest in obtaining a better understanding of the disease. "Why bother, since there's no treatment anyway" was not an uncommon response of physicians and scientists.

The understanding and treatment of IBS have already benefited from one of the greatest advances in the field of medicine in the last two decades, the wider distribution of health care information. Educational efforts have greatly raised the public's awareness of common medical conditions such as high blood pressure, heart disease, colon cancer, breast cancer, and acid reflux disease. Increasing public awareness of common medical problems has many benefits. It lets patients know that they are not the only ones dealing with this problem. Suffering with symptoms and believing that you are the only one with the condition can be discouraging and frightening. Knowing that your collection of symptoms has a name is empowering, because it enables you to locate vital information that allows you to actively participate in your care.

Increasing public awareness generates interest in research. Unfortunately, funding for scientific research is scarcer than in years past. The amount of funding available for research in a specific area is often based on how common a specific disorder is and how severely the problem affects people's lives. Demonstrating the high prevalence of IBS, how it affects patients economically, and how it interferes with their daily activities may translate into more funding for research. Also, learning what symptoms are part of which disorder allows people to recognize when their symptoms may be warning signs of serious diseases and increases the likelihood that they will seek medical help earlier than they would have if they had not been properly informed.

All of these points support the broadening of education about IBS. Educational programs are now being conducted by the American College of Gastroenterology and the American Gastroenterological Association (see the Patient Resources section for further details). The International Foundation for Functional Gastrointestinal Disorders (IFFGD), along with other IBS support groups, has also initiated educational programs for the public. Although pharmaceutical companies are often faulted for neglecting some of the health care problems that the United States now faces, many companies provide funding and other resources to educate patients.

Physician Education

Physicians are now considerably more comfortable evaluating and treating people who have IBS than they were 15 years ago. Nearly all doctors were taught years ago that IBS was a diagnosis of exclusion, which meant that all patients who had IBS had to be put through a lengthy battery of tests to exclude all other diseases that could cause the common symptoms of pain, bloating, and either constipation or diarrhea, and only when *all* other possible causes had been excluded could a patient be diagnosed as having IBS. This inevitably led to a delay in treating patients' symptoms and was unnecessarily expensive, as many patients underwent tests that were not necessary—and didn't change either the diagnosis or the treatment. Also, since some diagnostic tests have risks, when people undergo repeated diagnostic procedures, serious side effects can occur.

Over the last several years, increased education about IBS has also been directed at physicians and other health care professionals. Professional education is important, because many health care providers are not as informed as they could be about this disorder. A research study from our laboratory showed that physicians in various specialties differ in their ability to recognize IBS and that they evaluate, test, and treat people who have IBS quite differently. This indicates that physicians have still not achieved consensus on how to safely and effectively diagnose and treat patients who have IBS. Continued educational efforts will improve the ability of all health care providers to diagnose IBS without extensive testing and thus to begin treatment sooner. Education will also improve the quality of treatment received by patients who have IBS, by making health care providers aware of the range of treatments that are available. It will also let them know that this chronic condition can be difficult to treat medically but should never be treated surgically. This last point is important to make, because several studies have demonstrated that people who have IBS are more likely to undergo unnecessary and risky surgery than patients of the same age and sex who do not have IBS.

Research

A great deal of what is known about any medical problem was learned in research labs. Basic science research investigating IBS has been limited, in part because IBS seems not to exist in animals other than humans. However, research studies during the last several years have investigated elements of IBS—the mechanisms of abdominal pain and heightened visceral sensitivity—in both humans and other animals. Ongoing research is examining how the GI tract responds to certain medications, how the brain responds to stimulation within the GI tract, and why people with certain blood types seem to respond better to one type of medication than another. In addition, studies are under way to determine how stress and hormones influence gut function.

With increased public and professional awareness of IBS, clinical research studies will probably also continue to evolve, depending on research funds, of course. A number of key questions remain to be answered: What is the genetic basis for IBS? Is there a genetic explanation for why some people respond to one type of IBS medication while others, with seemingly similar symptoms, do not? Could blood tests be developed to determine whether an individual has the potential to develop IBS? Could a blood test determine whether a person will respond to a type of medication? Could a blood test be developed to detect IBS? This last question is especially important for patients who have abdominal pain and diarrhea, because one of the most important clinical concerns is whether the patient has inflammatory bowel disease rather than IBS. A similar question is whether a stool sample could provide enough information to determine whether somebody has IBS or IBD. Are there ways to prevent IBS from developing after a viral or bacterial gastroenteritis? Can other risk factors be identified and treated, thereby preventing IBS from developing?

In regard to the pathophysiology of IBS, physician-scientists are performing interesting studies to determine how people who have IBS sense pain in their gut and what happens in their brain. Previous studies have shown that the central nervous systems of people who have IBS sense pain differently from those of other people. Continued research in this area is likely to shed more light on the physiology of IBS and eventually lead to better treatments for pain. Several studies are underway looking into why patients who have IBS often have the associated conditions of fibromyalgia, interstitial cystitis, chronic pelvic pain, or migraine headaches. Understanding how these painful conditions are related may help minimize testing, prevent unnecessary surgery, and improve treatment. In addition, clinical research is exploring kinds of treatments that previously were considered alternative—cognitive behavioral therapy, hypnosis, and acupuncture are all areas currently under investigation.

New Treatments

Behavioral Therapies

Everyone knows that stress can affect their GI tract. Some people develop abdominal pain during times of stress, others develop diarrhea, and nearly everyone has experienced the sensation of "butterflies" in their stomach when they were excited or anxious. Exactly why this occurs is not known. However, we do know that stress can alter levels of various hormones and neurotransmitters in the body, one of which is corticotropin-releasing factor (CRF, also known as corticotropin-releasing hormone, or CRH). CRF is important to the body's response to stress and can affect gut motility. Preliminary data from several small research studies have shown that CRF levels in the blood were different in the participants who had IBS than in the healthy volunteers. Theoretically, if CRF levels can be lowered, the probability of diarrhea might be lowered too. Relaxation therapy and stress reduction therapy might prove to be valuable ways to decrease stress, CRF levels, and gut motility.

Looking at cognitive behavioral therapy (CBT), a large multicenter research trial recently found that CBT is effective in treating the chronic abdominal pain that affects people who have IBS. Other studies have shown that CBT can improve other symptoms in patients who have IBS. A large multicenter trial funded by the National Institutes of Health is now under way to evaluate the effectiveness of different types of CBT for people who have IBS. The results of this study may dramatically change physicians' practices when it comes to recommending CBT and may also change how CBT is performed.

Diet

Once forsaken as a "dead" area of research in IBS, diet is now the focus of several studies. The exciting results obtained from the low-FODMAP diet have stimulated new research efforts into the role of diet in IBS. The close relationship between ingesting food and experiencing symptoms for many people who have IBS raises many questions. Can foods cause IBS? Are some foods more likely to produce symptoms in patients who have IBS than in healthy volunteers? If a specific food is the culprit, could an individual be desensitized to that food? For example, some people who have IBS notice the onset of symptoms or the worsening of symptoms after eating certain foods. Such patients are often referred to an allergist or immunologist to determine whether or not they are truly allergic to these foods. While the diagnostic tests currently available can indicate if someone is allergic to a food, these tests are not capable of determining whether the person has a sensitivity to the food. Thus at present, we can rely only on symptoms to tell us whether a person is sensitive or intolerant to a specific food. Although many scientists and physicians are interested in studying the question of food sensitivity in patients who have IBS, funding for research in this area is severely limited. Future research may promote the development of a blood test that could detect these food sensitivities.

Medications

During the development of a new drug, the initial goals are safety and effectiveness. As a drug continues through the various phases of development, additional goals must be met, including that the drug acts as specifically as possible with minimal side effects. The connection between genetic inheritance and IBS is now being explored, and researchers are asking whether a drug could be designed specific to a person's genetic makeup. This would mean that some people who have IBS and constipation would receive "drug A," because they have a certain genetic makeup (verified by a blood test), while others who have IBS and constipation would receive "drug B," because they have a different genetic makeup. The emerging area of science that involves both pharmacology (the study of medications) and genetics is called pharmacogenomics. This field will become significantly more important in the next decade and may yield some discoveries that can be applied to the treatment of IBS.

Below are descriptions of some medications now being studied that may prove helpful in treating IBS.

Medications for constipation. Plecanitide is a new medication that stimulates guanylate cyclase receptors. Preliminary data show that this medication improves symptoms of constipation and abdominal pain. Large multicenter prospective trials need to be conducted to determine whether or not this medication is safe and effective.

Prucalopride is a serotonin agonist (more specifically, a 5-HT4 agonist) that was approved for use in Europe in October 2009 for the treatment of chronic constipation. Three large studies have shown that it is safe and effective in both women and men. It is not yet available in the United States, and studies with patients who have IBS and constipation still need to be performed.

Velusetrag is another serotonin agonist that, in preliminary studies, has been shown to be effective at treating symptoms of constipation. Large prospective studies with patients who have IBS are needed before this medication will become available on the market.

Medications for diarrhea. JNJ-27018966 is a new compound being developed for the treatment of IBS and diarrhea. In preliminary research studies, people who have IBS noted a significant improvement in diarrhea, urgency, and abdominal pain. A large multicenter prospective study is currently under way, and results will probably be available in late 2013.

Dextofisopam is a medication that acts on benzodiazepine receptors in the brain. Results from a study in patients who had IBS and diarrhea or IBS and mixed symptoms were encouraging, because the medication was much better than a placebo at improving symptoms of diarrhea and abdominal pain. Additional study of dextofisopam is needed.

Medications for pain. Abdominal pain is often the most distressing symptom for patients who have IBS. The GI tract is densely populated with opioid (narcotic) receptors, which is one reason narcotics are so effective at treating postoperative pain (such as after an appendectomy or hysterectomy). However, narcotics are quickly addictive, and patients can develop a tolerance for narcotics, requiring ever-higher doses to relieve their pain (see Chapter 18). Researchers are actively investigating other medications that act on these opioid receptors to reduce pain, hoping to find some without the side effects and complications associated with chronic narcotic use.

Alvimopan (a mu-opioid receptor antagonist) is a medication that acts on opioid receptors and, in this case, blocks the mu-receptors. Alvimopan has been shown to ease pain in some patients who have IBS, and in a recent (small) research trial, it also improved symptoms of chronic constipation.

Alternative Therapies

A desire to improve symptoms without the use of oral medications has led patients who have chronic IBS symptoms to search for alternative therapies. Many patients and physicians strongly believe that symptoms of IBS are caused by an overgrowth, or imbalance, of bacteria in the GI tract (see Chapter 11). Several researchers have made very convincing arguments for the role of bacterial overgrowth in the pathogenesis of IBS, although other researchers have not been able to duplicate their study results, and many clinicians remain unconvinced. Antibiotics that act specifically on the gut, with few extra-intestinal side effects, are currently being tested in populations who have IBS. As mentioned above, rifaximin has been shown to improve symptoms of gas, bloating, distention, pain, and diarrhea in many patients who have IBS-D or IBS-M (IBS with mixed symptoms of constipation and diarrhea). A large multicenter trial is currently under way to assess the safety and efficacy of rifaximin for long-term use.

Over one-third of all people in the United States now use some form of alternative medication for their health care needs. Many of these individuals use herbal remedies. The advantages, disadvantages, and dangers of herbal remedies are discussed in Chapter 21. As people who have IBS explore options for treating their symptoms, herbal medications will be used more often. The cautionary note I would make is that these substances should be purchased from a reputable source, and users should research them in authoritative sources before taking them.

Probiotics is the final type of therapy that warrants mention. This is an area in which, I believe, we will witness exceptional growth in the next few years. Although probiotics are commonly used by patients and practitioners, many critical questions need to be answered regarding their role in treating the symptoms of IBS (see Chapter 20). That being said, well-designed studies demonstrating the effectiveness and safety of the probiotic *Bifidobacterium infantis* are encouraging. Future trials will need to determine which probiotic is best for which patient, in addition to identifying the optimal dose and duration of treatment.

Research into the development and treatment of IBS is active and will probably become even more so over the next decade. New therapies are on the horizon. The fact that pharmaceutical companies are actively looking for new agents to treat symptoms of IBS is encouraging. Patients and practitioners can be optimistic that new treatments will be developed to relieve symptoms and improve quality of life for people who have IBS. We have begun to, and in the future we will be increasingly able to, make sense of IBS.

Summary

- Educational efforts and research (both clinical and basic science) have contributed to an increasing public awareness of IBS.
- Treatment for IBS is no longer limited to medications.
- Advances in our understanding of how different foods can influence IBS symptoms now make it possible for many people who have IBS to better control their symptoms on their own.
- Both probiotics and antibiotics can influence the gut microbiota (the bacteria that reside in the large intestine), which in turn can dramatically affect IBS symptoms.
- New medications for the treatment of the different subtypes of IBS will probably be approved in the next five years.

Appendix:
About Clinical Trials and
Scientific Research

Most of us take modern medicine for granted. For example, antibiotics, vaccines, and CT scans are all now recognized as key components of clinical medicine. However, penicillin, the first widely recognized antibiotic, was not clinically available until 1940, and the polio vaccine was not introduced until 1954. It surprises many people to learn that the first CT scans were not clinically available until 1974. These three vital aspects of present-day clinical medicine have contributed to exciting health care advances. Each is also the direct result of research in both the basic sciences and the clinical arena.

The term *research* appears throughout this book with regard to diagnosing IBS, treating patients, and seeking new therapies. This appendix gives a very brief overview of research, describing basic science and clinical research, explaining how research studies are conducted, and defining some terms commonly used in research.

Studies that explore the basic workings and physiology of the human body constitute *basic science* research. These research projects may investigate the structure of red blood cells, how nerves regenerate, or how medications are absorbed into the body. Basic science research studies are immensely important in understanding how our bodies and our individual organ systems function. In addition, these studies are critical to understanding why our bodies do not always function normally and why diseases occur. However, the information obtained from basic science research studies may not directly translate into a change in the practice of clinical medicine. Thus, a research study may determine that a unique combination of 13 different chemicals is vital to the development of nerve cells in a tissue culture plate in the laboratory but may not have any practical significance for how patients are treated by their physicians.

In contrast, *clinical research* is designed to answer questions that are directly relevant to patient care, and it often leads to improvements in care.

Clinical research studies generally have four distinct phases. The first phase is to ask a simple question that is clinically relevant, that is, a question whose answer may lead to a change in the practice of clinical medicine. In the field of IBS, this could be as simple as, "What percentage of patients who have IBS also have fructose intolerance?" If it is found that a large percentage of patients who have IBS are fructose intolerant (and patients who have IBS and diarrhea do often suffer from fructose intolerance), then physicians may start counseling their patients who have IBS to avoid fructose, in the hope of ameliorating their symptoms.

The second phase is developing a research protocol, a road map for the research study. It states who can and cannot enter the study, how the study subjects will be evaluated, what specific questions will be asked, what the intervention will be (*intervention* is defined below), and how the results will be measured. The design of the protocol is critical, as a poorly designed study will inevitably lead to poor results, in the form of data that are either not interpretable or not usable.

The third phase in the research project is to recruit appropriate participants and enter them into the study. This sounds easy, but it can be very difficult. Let's say that you want to study whether a new medicine improves symptoms in patients who have IBS and diarrhea. You may decide to place an advertisement in the local paper asking for people who have IBS and diarrhea to call your office. During the initial part of the screening process, you would exclude patients who have IBS and constipation or IBS and alternating symptoms, because they might develop side effects from the new medication, fail to respond to it, or develop an adverse effect. You would also need to make sure that the patients truly have IBS, not an infectious diarrhea and not inflammatory bowel disease (patients frequently get IBS and IBD mixed up). Participants would need to meet other inclusion and exclusion criteria as well. Finally, potential participants need to be informed about the risks and benefits of entering a research study, and they must agree to show up for all of the visits. In some research studies, at least 5 to 10 people need to be screened to identify one patient who is appropriate to enter the study.

In the fourth phase, the data from the study are collected, analyzed, and recorded in a written report. Only then can it be made available to clinicians and other researchers. It can take years from the time a study first begins until the data are analyzed and written up. As you can tell from this description, clinical research often moves very slowly.

Many patients who have IBS express interest in becoming involved in a research study. People enter research studies for a variety of reasons. Some are seeking a personal benefit; some are motivated by a desire to help others. Here are the most common reasons people enroll in a research study.

Some people enter a research study to learn more about the specific disease being studied. During the study, participants interact with professionals who are very interested in the disorder under investigation. They are often able to provide information about the condition that is not easily accessible elsewhere.

People sometimes join a research study to get better health care than would otherwise be available to them. Participants in a research trial usually undergo a comprehensive history and physical examination and simple laboratory tests or diagnostic studies. This process occasionally uncovers medical problems that the patient was not previously aware of.

Often, patients enroll in a research study in hopes of receiving the new medication being tested. It is important to know that nearly all clinical research studies involve a randomization process (described below); this means that some volunteers will receive a placebo (defined below) rather than the active medication. However, many research studies are now constructed so that patients who were randomized to placebo during the trial have the opportunity to get the active medication at the end of the study.

If a research study is looking for volunteers to undergo testing for a particular condition and a person is concerned that he or she might have that condition, because a relative did, that person may decide to enroll in the study so that he or she can have a specialized test that would likely not be ordered by a primary care provider or paid for by insurance companies.

Fortunately, many people enroll in research studies because they know that by doing so they are helping advance the field of medicine and contribute to human knowledge. They realize that they may not receive any direct benefits, but the knowledge that they have directly contributed to an advance in science is very rewarding.

Lastly, some people enter research trials because they are paid to participate. Being paid may serve as an added incentive and a compensation for people who have other reasons, too, or it may be the principal motivation. For many college students, participating in research studies can be an easy source of extra income.

After reading all of the reasons that people enter research studies, you may feel motivated enough to call your local medical center and sign up for one of the research studies being conducted there. However, it is important to realize that there are potential disadvantages to participating in a research study. First of all, some studies require multiple visits and multiple tests, and these can consume a large amount of time. Second, because most studies place people in groups randomly, you may be put into the placebo group, so if you are entering a study in the hopes of receiving a new medication for your medical problem, you may be disappointed. Most importantly, although safeguards are in place to protect research subjects, there is always the very small possibility that you will have a severe side effect or suffer a complication from entering a research study. Such risks are always carefully explained to research subjects, and complications are very uncommon, but they do happen. I am a strong believer in conducting research and have been a subject in a few research studies myself (as a medical student), but it is important that you understand both sides of the issue.

Most academic medical centers, university hospitals, and large private practice medical groups have ongoing research projects. A research coordinator is usually employed to help manage these projects, and that person can provide you with a list of active research projects at that institution.

If you are interested in research or in joining a research study, you will encounter certain terms with very specific meanings. Below are definitions of some commonly used terms.

Hypothesis. In scientific studies, the hypothesis is a modified version of the question being asked in the study. However, a hypothesis is much more specific and involves some type of a test or experiment with measurements of the outcome. The hypothesis in a research project is often stated so that one condition is compared to another with reference to statistical significance. For example, the original study question may have been, "Will drug X improve symptoms in patients who have IBS?" The study hypothesis, however, might be: "Can drug X improve symptoms of constipation at least 25 percent better than a placebo?"

Observational study. An observational research study simply observes and records behavior; there is no intervention during the study. Thus, an observational research study could involve recording the use of alternative medications over time. Observational studies can be useful for recording the behaviors of large groups of people, but they don't attempt to provide insight into the actual behavior.

Experimental study. An experimental study always involves an intervention or action. First, symptoms, behaviors, or patterns are observed and recorded, and then an intervention or experiment, such as a medication, a diagnostic test, a change in diet, or the introduction of a new exercise routine, is imposed. Then, the participants are monitored for a specified time period, to see if the intervention had an effect.

Variables. In research studies, a variable is a trait or characteristic that can be altered. Ideally, in each experiment, only one variable is changed at a time, while others are held constant (intentionally not changed). This provides the most precise measurement of how the changed variable has affected the outcome. For instance, if you wanted to refine your favorite cake recipe, you would not alter the amount of several ingredients at once. Rather, you might first change the amount of salt you add and then see whether you like that change. The next time, you might alter the amount of baking powder, and again note the effect on the result.

Longitudinal study. In longitudinal studies, measurement over a period of time is critical to the design of the study (compare to *cross-sectional study*). Longitudinal studies continue for days, weeks, months, or even years.

Cross-sectional study. Cross-sectional studies involve measurement at a specific point in time. A cross-sectional study might study a single type of behavior in multiple populations, but only on a single day.

Retrospective study. Retrospective research studies ask a research question but try to asnwer it with data that have already been collected. Retrospective studies do not involve collecting new data, recruiting or enrolling new subjects, or studying new medications. They are often used to answer broad-based research questions that involve large populations of people. For example, one could ask what the prevalence of IBS was in the Medicare population during the 1970s and 1980s. Researchers can easily obtain data from government sources regarding patients who were covered by Medicare during these two decades, and then can identify those patients who were diagnosed with IBS. Note that this type of study is not very good at answering questions like why certain patients develop a disorder.

Prospective study. Prospective studies are designed to collect new information over a specific period of time and, in clinical research, generally involve following patients who have a specific medical condition. Prospective studies may track blood pressure, cholesterol levels, or body weight or measure the influence of a new medication. Clinical research studies investigating new medications are always prospective in nature. The best clinical research employs prospective methods.

Subjects. Participants in a research study are called subjects. They may have no health problems, or they may have a particular type of medical problem.

Inclusion criteria. The inclusion criteria are the characteristics that potential participants must have to be eligible to be included in the research study.

Exclusion criteria. Exclusion criteria are the characteristics—symptoms, signs, diagnoses, or test results—that will exclude a person from being eligible to enter the research study.

Bias. In research studies, bias is defined as "systematic error." The goal of all research studies is to design the study as carefully as possible, so that errors (bias) will not be unintentionally introduced. Bias can occur at any level of a research study, which is why so much time and effort is needed to design a good clinical research study. Let's consider a simple research study that involves measuring the incidence of IBS symptoms among patients at a specialized research center in the Midwest. This center sees only patients referred by gastroenterologists. The center publishes a study stating that 100 percent of their patients have severe daily abdominal pain that cannot be treated in any way. Are the results applicable to all patients who have IBS? The answer is no. The results of this study are flawed because there is significant bias (systematic error) in the study. There are many biases, and some are easy to recognize. One, it is a specialized research center and its patients are likely not representative of all patients who have IBS. Two, the center is in the Midwest, and its patients may differ in some relevant ways from patients who have IBS in, say, the South or the Southwest. Three, these patients were referred by gastroenterologists for specialized attention, which means they had probably already not improved with over-the-counter medications, therapy provided by their primary care provider, and medical therapy by their gastroenterologist. Thus, there was a "selection bias" that guaranteed a study population who had more persistent symptoms than the population of all people who have IBS.

Intervention. In research studies, an intervention is an action that is imposed on the research participants; the consequences are then measured. An intervention can take many forms. It might be watching a videotape on the benefits of wearing seat belts, to see if it would change the viewers' behavior. In IBS studies, interventions often include using medications, and then measuring the change in the patients' symptoms.

Randomized. In a randomized trial, study participants are selected at random to enter one of the treatment groups, either the active medication group or the placebo group (see below). This means that participants are not selected based on race, sex, age, weight, or any other characteristic. Random selection occurs purely by chance. Most research studies now use computer-generated tables to randomly assign study participants to the different treatment groups. Randomization prevents bias, which can either falsely exaggerate or minimize study results.

Placebo. A placebo is essentially a sugar pill. It looks exactly like the study medication (same color, size, shape, texture). The placebo does not have any active ingredients in it, only inactive ones. A good research study always compares the intervention (for example, a medication) to a placebo.

Placebo effect. This is a fascinating topic that was not well understood for many years. In the distant past, when patients were enrolled in a research study, they were all given the study medication and then evaluated for their response. Many research studies were published showing that the medication had remarkably good benefits. However, when the medicine became available to the public, the impressive results from the research studies were not duplicated. This caused a great deal of confusion until scientists and physicians realized that there is a phenomenon called the "placebo effect." When patients are given a study medication, they often feel better just because they are involved in a research trial: they are having more frequent doctor visits, being seen by more experienced clinicians, often being provided with additional advice and counseling, or may just be convinced that the medication is going to work. If we are told that a medication is going to make us feel better, we are more likely to feel better, regardless of whether we receive the actual medication or a sugar pill. This is the placebo effect. The placebo effect can be as high as 50 percent in some studies; that is, 50 percent of patients who received the placebo feel better. This shows the importance of designing the study so as to compare the intervention, whether it is surgery or a medication, to a placebo, as a control against inflating the benefits of the intervention.

Placebo controlled. Studies that are placebo controlled have a placebo included in the study design. Many studies compare a single intervention (Drug A) to a placebo; others compare several types of intervention (Drug A at ¼ dose, Drug A at ½ dose, Drug A at full dose) to a placebo. Placebo-controlled studies are the best type of clinical research study, because placebos help adjust the results for the "placebo effect" (see above).

Blind and **double blind.** Blinding in a study means that participants are unaware of whether an active medication (the study drug) or a placebo (a sugar pill) is being administered. In some studies, only the subjects are "blinded," whereas in other studies only the practitioners dispensing the substance and evaluating the patients are "blinded." In a *double-blind* study, both subjects and practitioners are unaware of who is receiving the active drug and who is getting the placebo. Blinding is important because it helps the true effects of the medication to be properly judged. If the study subjects are blinded, they will not know whether they are receiving active medication or a placebo. All of the pills will look identical in color, size, and shape and will be taken in the same number and at the same time each day. If the physicians dispensing the substances don't know whether their patients are taking the active medication or the placebo, the physicians can't unintentionally influence their patients with subtle signals about whether the medication is going to work or not. Such subliminal messages can inflate the real effects of the medication. Double blinding thus minimizes bias from both patients and providers.

Patient Resources

Many groups and organizations are now available to provide information, to answer questions, and to give support to people who have IBS. The list below is divided into four sections. All of the websites are free; they do not require a subscription of any kind. The fourth section provides a source or two on each of the medical conditions commonly associated with IBS. These lists are obviously not all-inclusive. At the time this book was written, these sources were accurate and up to date.

A general note about websites: like all other sources of information (books, magazines) there are reputable websites and not-so-reliable ones. It can be difficult to know which sites you can trust to provide honest, unbiased, up-to-date information. Some reasonable guidelines are as follows:

- Websites produced by medical institutions (for instance, the Mayo Clinic), government agencies (like NIH), and nonprofit organizations are generally very reliable. Keep in mind, however, that it is difficult to keep all areas of a website current at all times, so look to see when the website you are consulting was last updated.
- Websites should include references and reports of scientific studies that are current. Ideally, there will also be some interpretation of these studies on the website, so that you don't have to review and interpret a complicated article by yourself.
- Avoid websites that advertise specific products or sell medications or supplements. The information on these sites is typically biased and is designed to persuade you to purchase their product.
- Be cautious when viewing websites with multiple links to other websites. Often, these sites are designed to steer you to webpages that sell their products.

General Health Information

1. *The Merck Manual of Medical Information*, Second Home Edition, is a very comprehensive source of medical information for laypeople. It is available in both book form and on the website *www.merck.com*. After you have accessed the website, click on "Merck Manuals" and then search the specific topic that you're interested in.

2. The National Women's Health Information Center website, *www.womens health.gov*, covers a large number of topics. It is informative and up to date, although some of the subjects are covered rather superficially. In addition, when searching for some topics, you may end up with an overwhelming number of links. That being said, this is a good place to start for answers to general women's health questions.

3. The U.S. Preventive Services Task Force has a website that provides information on whether certain tests and diagnostic studies are recommended under specific conditions. So, if you are interested in whether you should have a colonoscopy, Pap smear, or prostate biopsy, go to *www.uspreventiveser vicestaskforce.org/*. The site also provides current recommendations regarding vaccinations.

4. The Drug Information Database at the American Academy of Family Physicians (*www.familydoctor.org*) is an excellent place to get information about how to safely take medications. Information is available for both prescription and over-the-counter medications.

5. For questions on herbs, dietary supplements, and alternative medications, check the Memorial Sloan Kettering Cancer Center website, *www.mskcc .org/cancer-care/integrative-medicine/about-herbs-botanicals-other-products*. This center has compiled a large database of information on the benefits and potential side effects of herbs and alternative medications.

6. A great source of general information for all medical conditions is *www .mayoclinic.com*.

7. Another general medical website that provides up-to-date information on a variety of medical problems, including IBS, is *www.webmd.com/medical*.

8. If you need information about the nutritional content of a specific food, search the U.S. Department of Agriculture's Food and Nutrition Information Center website, *www.fnic.nal.usda.gov*.

9. For consumer health information from the faculty at Harvard Medical School, see *www.intelihealth.com*.

10. The Cleveland Clinic produces *www.clevelandclinicmeded.com*, which provides information on many medical conditions and has a good tutorial on IBS.

IBS Information on the Internet

1. The national IBS support group site provides information on IBS and offers chat rooms where people can discuss their symptoms with other people who have IBS. The address is *www.ibsgroup.org*.

2. Another website that carries general information on IBS is *www.aboutibs .org*.

3. At *www.healingwell.com*, you can find answers to frequently asked questions about IBS. Once you have accessed the site, enter "IBS" into their "search site" box.

4. The website at *http://emedicine.medscape.com/article/180389-overview* is routinely updated to provide new information on the treatment of IBS.

5. The American Gastroenterology Association is an organization consisting of researchers, scientists, physicians, and allied health personnel involved in diagnosing and treating people who have diseases of the GI tract. It is the largest such organization in the United States. Many of its members have an interest in functional GI disorders. The organization has created a website that is available to the public (*www.gastro.org*).

6. The National Library of Medicine has an online tutorial to help answer questions about IBS. It is an interactive site with easy-to-understand illustrations. The website can be found at *www.nlm.nih.gov/medlineplus/tutorial .html*.

8. At *www.centerwatch.com/clinical-trials/listings/condition/90/irritable-bowel -syndrome-ibs* you can find a listing of active research studies in the field of IBS.

9. The National Institutes of Health has dedicated a website to children who have IBS. Go to *www.digestive.niddk.nih.gov/ddiseases/pubs/ibschildren/*.

10. The American College of Gastroenterology, the largest clinical gastroenterological organization in the United States, has a website that provides a nice introduction to IBS and answers common questions. Its address is *http:// patients.gi.org/topics/irritable-bowel-syndrome/*.

11. The site at *www.iffgd.org* is run by the International Foundation for Functional Gastrointestinal Disorders. This site offers up-to-date information for both patients and physicians on IBS and other functional GI disorders (dyspepsia, noncardiac chest pain, etc.). The foundation also has a toll-free phone number, 1-888-964-2001, which you may call to request information.

12. The website *www.fmsfonline.org/hypnosis* provides a wealth of information about hypnosis. It does not focus on IBS.

Books on Diet and IBS

1. *Eating for IBS: 175 Delicious, Nutritious, Low-Fat, Low-Residue Recipes to Stabilize the Touchiest Tummy*, by Heather Van Vorous, was published in 2000. Many patients find this book's dietary suggestions helpful, and the consensus is that the recipes are good.

2. *Tell Me What to Eat If I Have Irritable Bowel Syndrome: Nutrition You Can Live With*, by Elaine Magee, was published in 2000. Some patients greatly enjoyed this book, while others felt it did not provide as much useful information as they had hoped. It offers some common-sense advice regarding diet.

Information about Medical Conditions Associated with IBS

1. Fibromyalgia: The Arthritis Association has a website (*www.arthritis.org*) with information on fibromyalgia. Their toll-free telephone number is 1-800-282-7800.

2. Interstitial cystitis: *www.cobfoundation.org/* is an English website. It is easy to use and up to date. The National Institutes of Health offers information at *http://kidney.niddk.nih.gov/kudiseases/pubs/interstitialcystitis/*.

3. Chronic pelvic pain: At *www.womenshealthmatters.ca/*, if you click on the "site map," it will direct you to the area that focuses on chronic pelvic pain. This site also contains information about interstitial cystitis and incontinence.

4. TMJ syndrome: *www.tmj.org* is maintained by a support group that provides medical information about this chronic problem.

5. Migraine headaches: *www.webmd.com* (click on the box labeled "condition centers") and *www.migrainepage.com* are up-to-date sites providing information on migraines and other types of headaches.

6. Celiac disease: *www.celiac.org* and *www.naspgn.org* both provide current information on celiac disease. In addition, you can contact the Celiac Sprue Association directly, at 402-558-0600 or P.O. Box 31700, Omaha, Nebraska 68131-0700.

Glossary

abdomen The area between the chest and the hips that contains the stomach, small intestine, large intestine, liver, gallbladder, pancreas, and spleen.

acid reflux The movement of caustic gastric acid from the stomach into the esophagus.

acupuncture The insertion of needles into various parts of the body, at very specific sites, to cause healing or a change in sensation in other parts of the body.

acute A term used to describe a disorder, disease, or process that is sudden in onset and often severe but lasts only a short time.

aerophagia The abnormal swallowing or gulping of air.

allodynia The misinterpretation of normal sensation as being painful.

allopathic medicine A therapeutic type of medicine in which a specific disease or disorder is treated by producing a second condition that is antagonistic or incompatible with the first condition. Common examples include giving antibiotics to treat a bacterial infection or treating high blood pressure with a medicine designed to reduce blood pressure. Essentially all Western-trained physicians are allopathic physicians.

amylase A digestive enzyme that breaks down starch.

anemia A low blood count as measured by hemoglobin or hematocrit.

anismus Dyscoordination of the muscles in the pelvic floor. Also called pelvic floor dyssynergia. The term *anismus* is rarely used now; pelvic floor dyssynergia is the preferred term.

anorectal manometry (ARM) A test to evaluate neuromuscular function of the anorectum and the pelvic floor muscles.

antibiotic A type of medication that acts to kill bacteria in the body.

anticholinergic agents Medications that block the effects of acetylcholine, one of the major neurotransmitters in the GI tract.

antispasmodic agents A class of medications that help relax the smooth muscle of the GI tract and thus help prevent spasms in the GI tract.

anxiety A prevalent condition in the U.S., affecting up to 5 percent of the population. Characterized by excessive worry, restlessness, inability to concentrate, poor sleep, irritability, and feeling "keyed up" or "on edge."

aromatherapy A form of alternative medicine that uses a variety of herbs, oils, and fragrances to promote healing, relaxation, and stress reduction.

arthralgia Pain or discomfort in a joint. This is different from arthritis, which is an inflammatory condition of a joint.

autoimmune disease Any number of processes or conditions where the body's immune system mistakenly believes that a normal part of the body is "foreign" and starts to attack it, creating inflammation.

autonomic nervous system (ANS) The portion of the nervous system that allows various parts of the body, for example, your heart rate and blood pressure, to function on their own without conscious thought. The ANS can be divided into the sympathetic nervous system and the parasympathetic nervous system.

bacterial overgrowth (also called small intestine bacterial overgrowth, or SIBO). A condition in which an inappropriately large number of bacteria reside in the small intestine. This condition can lead to bloating and diarrhea and may lead to nutritional deficiencies in mild cases or malnutrition in severe cases.

barium A radio-opaque substance used to coat the inside of a hollow organ, such as the esophagus or stomach, so that it can be visualized on an x-ray. A radio-opaque substance is one that x-rays do not penetrate well, so it shows up on an x-ray as a white area.

barium enema An x-ray test in which barium (see above) is inserted into the rectum and then coats the colon so that abnormalities in the colon can be identified.

biofeedback A training technique that teaches patients how to gain control over autonomic (that is, self-regulating) functions of the body. In gastroenterology, biofeedback is often used to treat patients who have pelvic floor dysfunction.

biopsy The technique whereby a small piece of tissue is removed from an organ or structure so that it can be examined with a microscope. During a colonoscopy, a biopsy of your colon or rectum may be taken.

bloating The sensation of gassiness.

borborygmi Rumbling or gurgling noises from the GI tract produced by peristalsis and movement of fluid and gas.

brain-gut axis The bidirectional nerve pathway that connects the brain to the gut.

breath test (also called a breath hydrogen test). A test that measures the excretion (elimination) of hydrogen from the GI tract. Used to diagnose patients who have lactose intolerance, fructose intolerance, or bacterial overgrowth.

celiac disease A wheat allergy. Patients may have mild symptoms of bloating or more severe symptoms of unintentional weight loss, iron deficiency anemia, diarrhea, and/or osteoporosis. Celiac disease is treated by eliminating all wheat products from the diet.

central nervous system (CNS) Consists of the brain and the spinal cord.

chromosome One of the threadlike structures in the cell nucleus that transmits genetic information. Each chromosome consists of a double strand of DNA (see DNA entry) along with proteins called histones. The nucleus of each human cell usually contains 46 chromosomes.

chronic A term used to identify a disorder, disease, or process that continues for a long time or recurs frequently.

chronic fatigue syndrome (CFS) A condition characterized by severe fatigue, lack of energy, and decreased exercise endurance that is not relieved by rest. The cause of CFS is unknown.

chyme The semifluid mass of partly digested food that passes from the stomach into the small intestine.

coccyx The last three to five vertebrae in the vertebral column. These are rudimentary (vestigial) in nature. Commonly referred to as the tailbone.

cognitive behavioral therapy (CBT) A type of psychological therapy where patients learn to address their problem in a proactive, positive manner. Stress reduction and relaxation techniques are often taught as well.

colitis A nonspecific term that indicates the presence of inflammation in the colon. This is not an appropriate term for patients who have IBS, since the colon is not inflamed. This word is best reserved for patients who have true inflammatory bowel disease, that is, Crohn's disease or ulcerative colitis.

colonoscopy The technique of using a flexible lighted tube to visualize the colon.

complementary and alternative medicine (CAM) A diverse group of treatments and therapies that complement or provide alternatives to traditional Western medicine. This includes hypnotherapy, acupuncture, herbal medicine, etc.

conscious sedation The technique of using intravenous medications to make a patient feel comfortable and relaxed during a procedure, such as a colonoscopy, but not to induce sleep.

constipation A common condition affecting 15 percent of adult Americans. Defined in a number of different ways, including infrequent bowel movements (fewer than three per week), excessive straining at stool, feelings of incomplete evacuation, or pain with defecation.

Crohn's disease A type of inflammatory bowel disease. In contrast to people who have IBS, patients who have Crohn's disease have an inflammatory process in their GI tract. This may occur anywhere from the mouth to the anus.

CT scan CT is an abbreviation for computed tomography, a special type of x-ray test that can visualize the internal organs.

cystoscopy A procedure where the interior of the bladder is visualized using a special lighted instrument (a cystoscope).

defecation The act of having a bowel movement.

depression A mental state characterized by feeling sad or blue, often accompanied by feelings of despair, loneliness, or worthlessness. Approximately 5 percent of U.S. adults meet clinical criteria for depression.

diaphragm The muscle between the chest and the abdomen. It is the major muscle that the body uses for breathing.

diarrhea Defined in a number of different ways, but typically characterized by frequent stools (more than three per day) that are loose and watery.

digestion The process the body uses to break down food into simple substances that can be absorbed into the body and used for energy, growth, and cell repair.

digestive system The organs in the body that break down and absorb food. Organs that make up the digestive tract (gastrointestinal tract) are the mouth, esophagus, stomach, small intestine, large intestine, rectum, and anus. Organs that help with digestion but are not part of the digestive tract are the tongue, salivary glands, pancreas, liver, and gallbladder.

distention The physical state of being stretched or swollen.

dizygotic twins (*di* means "two") Twins derived from two separate fertilized embryos, in contrast to twins that develop from a single fertilized egg that divides into identical parts (monozygotic twins).

DNA (deoxyribonucleic acid) The material found in the nuclei of cells that makes up the chromosomes and contains the genetic material.

duodenum The first part of the small intestine. It is connected to the stomach by a circular muscle called the pylorus.

dyspareunia Pain with intercourse.

dyspepsia A condition that affects up to 20 percent of adults at some point in their lifetime. Characterized by meal-associated upper abdominal discomfort or pain; may be associated with nausea and a feeling of fullness or being "overstuffed." This condition frequently overlaps with IBS.

dysphagia   Difficulty swallowing. This may occur because of severe heartburn, the presence of a stricture (narrowing) of the esophagus, or even cancer of the esophagus.

efficacy   The extent to which an intervention (that is, medication, a procedure, a device, or surgery) produces a beneficial result.

elimination diet   A diet used by some health care providers to determine whether a patient has food allergies or food sensitivities. The diet begins with eating only simple foods that rarely cause symptoms in anyone (for example, water, broth, white rice, and boiled chicken), and then different foods are slowly added back to the diet as the patient monitors symptoms.

empiric therapy   The practice of using a combination of symptoms and signs to make a diagnosis and then initiating treatment for the presumed problem, without any objective tests being performed.

endoscope   A flexible, lighted tube with a lens on the end. It is designed to look into your stomach and esophagus (upper endoscopy) or your colon (colonoscopy).

endoscopy   A procedure that uses an endoscope to diagnose or treat a condition within the intestinal tract.

enteric nervous system (ENS)   The part of the nervous system within the GI tract that controls gut function.

eructation   The medical term for belching or burping.

esophagogastroduodenoscopy (EGD)   A procedure that uses an endoscope to look into the esophagus, stomach, and upper small intestine (duodenum). Also called upper endoscopy.

esophagus   The muscular tube that connects the mouth to the stomach. Approximately 10 inches long.

etiology   The cause of a disease or disorder.

fecal incontinence   The unintentional leakage of stool.

fecal urgency   The sudden and intense urge to have a bowel movement. Common in patients who have IBS and diarrhea.

fibroymyalgia   A syndrome of fatigue and pain in the muscles and fibrous connective tissues. The cause is unknown.

flatulence   The presence of an excessive amount of gas in the lower gastrointestinal tract.

flatus The passage of gas from the lower intestinal tract.

flexible sigmoidoscopy A flexible lighted tube designed to visualize the lower colon (descending and sigmoid colon) and rectum.

fructose A simple (single) sugar (a monosaccharide) found in many fruits.

fructose intolerance The clinical condition in which a person cannot adequately digest fructose. This may lead to gas, bloating, and diarrhea.

functional bowel disorders A group of common, chronic conditions (IBS, dyspepsia, aerophagia) that affect the gastrointestinal tract. These disorders cannot be explained by an organic lesion (that is, an ulcer), by a blood disorder (for example, anemia), or by an x-ray test such as a CT scan. The name is appropriate, since patients develop symptoms because their intestinal tract does not function normally.

fundus The uppermost part of the stomach.

gas In clinical practice and for the lay public, gas usually refers to either the feeling of being bloated or distended ("gassiness") or to the passage of gas from the intestinal tract.

gastric Related to the stomach.

gastrocolic reflex The reflex between the stomach and the colon. Normally, ingesting food or liquid stimulates the stomach, which then initiates a reflex in the colon, leading to contractions and peristalsis. In many patients, this is commonly interpreted as an urge to have a bowel movement. Patients who have IBS often have a heightened or exaggerated gastrocolic reflex, which explains the sense of urgency they develop after eating a meal.

gastroenterologist A doctor who specializes in diagnosing and treating diseases of the digestive system.

gastroenterology The study of the digestive tract and its associated organs, including the liver, pancreas, and gallbladder.

gastroesophageal reflux disease (GERD) The movement of caustic gastric juices from the stomach back up into the esophagus. This movement may occur because of transient relaxation of the lower esophageal sphincter, the presence of a weak lower esophageal sphincter, or poor motility in the body of the esophagus. Prolonged episodes of reflux may cause esophagitis, esophageal ulcers or erosions, strictures, Barrett's esophagus, or even cancer of the esophagus. GERD is also called esophageal reflux or heartburn.

gastrointestinal tract (GI tract) The large, muscular tube that extends from the mouth to the anus. It includes the mouth, esophagus, stomach, small intestine, large intestine, rectum, and anus. Also called the alimentary tract or digestive tract.

heartburn A burning sensation caused by stomach acid after it moves into the lower esophagus and irritates the lining of the esophagus. It is usually felt in the upper abdomen, in the lower chest, or behind the breastbone (the sternum).

Helicobacter pylori (H. pylori) Bacteria commonly found in the stomach that can cause ulcers and are associated with an increased risk of developing stomach cancer; not related to IBS symptoms.

herbal medicine The practice of using herbs to treat various medical conditions and diseases.

homeopathy A system of therapy which is based on the belief that a substance that can provoke certain symptoms or induce an illness in a patient may be effective at treating different illnesses that have similar symptoms.

hypnosis An artificially induced trance or a period of deep concentration in which certain states of awareness are temporarily suspended. Used by some practitioners to treat patients who have functional bowel disorders by providing them with advice and suggestions during a period of increased susceptibility.

hypnotherapy The practice of using hypnosis to treat a variety of medical conditions.

ileum The third portion of the small intestine; follows the duodenum (the first part) and the jejunum (the second part).

incidence The number of new cases or events that occur during a specified time period.

incomplete evacuation The sensation some people have after a bowel movement, in contrast to the feeling some people have after a complete or "full" evacuation.

incontinence The accidental leakage of material from the bladder (urinary incontinence) or rectum (fecal incontinence).

inflammatory bowel disease One of two separate conditions, either Crohn's disease or ulcerative colitis. Both of these disorders typically cause diarrhea and abdominal pain. However, both of these conditions are characterized by inflammation in the GI tract and thus are completely distinct disorders from IBS.

inflammatory colitis An outdated term used many years ago to describe IBS. However, since the intestinal tract is not inflamed, inflammatory colitis is an inaccurate term that should not be used to describe people who have IBS.

interstitial cystitis A condition of the bladder characterized by pain, urinary urgency, and urinary frequency. Often seen with people who have IBS.

ischemic colitis An inflammatory condition of the colon that develops due to inadequate blood flow (ischemia).

jejunum The second portion of the small intestine (after the duodenum).

lactose A disaccharide, made up of the simple sugars glucose and galactose. Lactose is found in dairy products such as milk and cheese.

lactose intolerance The clinical condition in which a patient is unable to break down the sugar commonly found in milk products. This may lead to gas, bloating, and diarrhea.

lower esophageal sphincter (LES) A circular muscle, approximately 1½ inches in length, located at the junction of the esophagus and the stomach. When contracted, it prevents stomach acid from refluxing up into the esophagus. If it relaxes too frequently, or for prolonged periods of time, then gastric acid can easily rush up into the esophagus and cause heartburn.

manipulation therapy The process of using massage to promote healing and release of blocked energy. Examples include Rolfing, shiatsu, and reflexology.

Manning criteria A set of criteria used to diagnose IBS. No longer used in research studies or clinical practice since the advent of the Rome criteria.

microflora or **microbiota** The normal population of bacteria that resides in the intestinal tract (primarily the large intestine).

migraine headache A type of headache characterized by pain in the head (usually only on one side), nausea, vomiting, and light sensitivity. Some patients also notice "flashing" lights and peculiar smells (burnt rubber, eggs).

monozygotic twins Also called identical twins. Twins that develop from a single fertilized egg, which then divides into identical parts that develop into individuals with the same sex and the same genetic components.

motility The normal process, coordinated by nerves and smooth muscle, that results in coordinated contractions in the digestive tract. Motility results in the normal movement of food and liquids through the upper GI tract and liquid and solid waste through the lower GI tract.

mucus A clear liquid made by cells that line the intestinal tract. Mucus coats and protects tissues in the gastrointestinal tract.

mucus colitis An outdated term for IBS. Used in the past because some patients note that they pass mucus during or after a bowel movement. This term is inaccurate and should be discarded.

myalgia Muscle ache or discomfort.

natural history The normal and natural course of a disease or disorder over time if treatment is not provided.

naturopathy The practice of healing using only natural agents (that is, no drugs).

nervous colitis An outdated term for IBS that should be discarded.

panic disorder A disorder characterized by extreme anxiety, agitation, fear, and often feelings of dread. Patients may also experience sweating, difficulty breathing, and an increased heart rate.

parasympathetic nervous system One of the two major divisions of the autonomic nervous system (the other being the sympathetic nervous system). In general, the parasympathetic nervous system leads to a quieting of body functions (for example, decreased heart rate), although it plays a major role in stimulating peristalsis in the GI tract.

pathophysiology The alteration or abnormality of function seen with a medical disease or condition.

pelvic floor The group of muscles (puborectalis, pubococcygeus, and iliococcygeus) that support the internal organs in the pelvis (bladder, urethra, rectum, vagina, cervix, uterus, prostate gland, and anal canal).

pelvic floor dyssynergia A condition that may cause constipation. Characterized by inappropriate contraction of the external anal sphincter muscle during attempted defecation or inability to relax the internal anal sphincter.

pelvis The cup-shaped ring of bone formed by the hip bones (pubic bone, ischium, and ilium) on both sides and in front and the sacrum and coccyx behind.

perforation A hole that develops in a hollow organ such as the colon, stomach, or esophagus. A perforation may develop due to an ulcer in the stomach or may result from a foreign object in the GI tract or trauma to the GI tract (a sharp object, accidentally swallowing a sharp bone, endoscopy).

peripheral nervous system This consists of the autonomic nervous system (ANS) and the somatic nervous system.

peristalsis The muscular contractions of the gastrointestinal tract that move materials from the esophagus to the rectum.

pharynx The space behind the mouth. It serves as a passageway for food from the mouth to the esophagus and for air from the nose and mouth to the larynx and then into the lungs.

physiology A general term that refers to the normal functioning and vital processes of an entire organism (for example, a person) or a specific organ (for instance, the liver).

placebo A mostly inert substance (a pill with no intentionally active ingredients) that can be given as a medicine due to its suggestive effects. Commonly used in research trials to allow a better understanding of the true effects of the medicine being tested.

positron emission tomography (PET) scan A special type of radiologic test that can detect changes in the activity or metabolism of a cell. This test requires the injection of a radioactive material called a tracer. It is most frequently used to help detect cancer.

postprandial The period of time after eating a meal.

prevalence The number of cases of a disease (or disorder) that exist in a population at a specific time.

probiotic A live microbial organism (bacteria) introduced to promote health in the GI tract.

prognosis The long-term outcomes of a disease, either with or without treatment.

prokinetic agents A class of medications that act on the gastrointestinal tract to increase contractions and peristalsis in the GI tract. These agents may help to empty the stomach or to increase peristalsis in the small or large intestine.

prolapse When an organ sinks down out of the normal position. Most commonly refers to prolapse of the uterus (when it moves lower in the pelvic cavity), the bladder, or the rectum. Excessive prolapse of any of these organs usually requires surgery.

pylorus The circular muscle at the junction of the stomach and the duodenum. When contracted (closed), it prevents gastric contents from leaving the stomach and entering the duodenum.

quality of life A global term used to measure satisfaction and happiness with our daily lives and all of the daily activities we try to perform. An important concept in IBS research studies, because it allows patients to describe how a specific illness or disorder affects them.

Rome criteria The most recent and accurate set of diagnostic characteristics for irritable bowel syndrome, including symptoms, duration, and frequency.

scybala Hard, rocky, pellet-like stools (singular scybalum).

serotonin One of the most important neurotransmitters in the GI tract. Serotonin (also called 5-hydroxytryptamine) plays a critical role in both normal and abnormal gut function.

sign What a physician finds on physical examination (in contrast to a symptom—see below).

sitz marker study An x-ray study that measures transit of materials through the colon. Patients swallow a gelatin capsule that contains radio-opaque markers. X-rays of the abdomen are then performed at specific times to measure the movement of the markers through the colon. Typically performed in patients with constipation who have not responded to standard therapies.

smooth muscle One of the three types of muscle in the body, the others being cardiac (heart) muscle and skeletal muscle. Smooth muscle lines the entire GI tract, from the upper esophagus to the anorectum.

SNRIs (serotonin norepinephrine reuptake inhibitors) A class of medications used to treat depression.

somatic Refers to the muscles, bones, and joints in the body.

somatic nervous system (also called the voluntary nervous system). This system is responsible for transmitting information from the brain to skeletal muscle.

somatization disorder An uncommon disorder in which psychological or psychiatric problems (for example, anxiety or depression) are translated into physical problems. Patients who have a somatization disorder suffer from multiple, recurrent physical complaints and symptoms without an underlying organic cause. Many patients who have somatization disorders believe that all of their body is sick and dysfunctional.

sorbitol A sugar that is poorly broken down in the upper GI tract in some people. If large amounts are ingested, then bloating, gas, cramps, and diarrhea may ensue.

spastic colitis An old, outdated term for IBS. Factually incorrect, because the colon is not inflamed in IBS.

SSRIs (selective serotonin reuptake inhibitors) The class of medications most commonly used to treat depression.

stomach The J-shaped muscular organ designed to hold food, mix and grind food, and then empty the ground-up food into the small intestine. The stomach also produces a variety of chemicals, the most important of which is hydrochloric acid. This is the acid responsible for causing heartburn when it refluxes into the lower esophagus.

sympathetic nervous system One of the two major subdivisions of the autonomic nervous system (the other being the parasympathetic nervous system). In general, stimulation of the sympathetic nervous system leads to a state of arousal and heightened sensations throughout the body (for instance, increased heart rate and increased awareness) except in the GI tract, where sympathetic stimulation leads to decreased activity.

symptom A feeling or sensation that a patient may report to a health care provider.

syndrome A collection of symptoms and signs that occur together.

TCAs (tricyclic antidepressants) This class of medications was used to treat depression in the past. However, they were generally not very effective at treating depression. These agents can, however, be very helpful with treating chronic pain, especially the chronic abdominal pain of IBS and dyspepsia.

TMJ syndrome (temporomandibular joint syndrome) A painful condition of the jaw that is often associated with difficulty opening the mouth.

trigger points Also called tender points. These are specific points on the body which, when pressed, cause significant pain or discomfort in patients with fibromyalgia.

ulcer A sore on the lining of the esophagus, stomach, or intestine. Often caused by excess acid, medications, poor blood flow, or the bacterium *Helicobacter pylori*.

ulcerative colitis A form of inflammatory bowel disease (the other major one being Crohn's disease). This condition is very different from IBS, because with ulcerative colitis, the colon is inflamed. This can cause chronic bleeding from the colon.

unstable colitis / unstable colon These are older terms used to describe IBS. They should be discarded, since they are factually incorrect (patients who have IBS do not have colitis, which is an inflammatory condition of the colon).

upper endoscopy See **esophagogastroduodenoscopy**

upper esophageal sphincter The circular band of muscle at the top of the esophagus. It is usually contracted and helps to prevent acid from moving from the esophagus into the lungs and mouth.

upper GI series (upper gastrointestinal series) An x-ray study that usually employs barium as the contrast agent. A patient swallows the barium, which coats the esophagus, stomach, and upper small intestine. X-rays are then taken to look for abnormalities, such as ulcers, erosions, strictures, or cancer, in the lining of these organs.

urgency The sudden feeling of needing to use the bathroom immediately, often for fear of having an accident.

video defecography An x-ray test designed to measure function of the anorectum and the pelvic floor. Thick barium paste is inserted into the rectum, and then x-rays are taken as the patient attempts to expel the material.

viscera Refers to the internal organs (colon, small intestine, stomach, etc.). Viscus is the singular form.

visceral hypersensitivity This refers to the finding that patients who have IBS have a lower threshold for sensing pain in their GI tract.

zygote A fertilized egg. The cell that develops from the union of an egg with a sperm.

References

Chapter 2. What Is IBS?

Brandt LJ, Bjorkman D, Fennerty MB, et al. Systematic review on the management of irritable bowel syndrome in North America. *Am J Gastroenterol* 2002;97:11(suppl):S7-S26.

Drossman DA. Review article: an integrated approach to the irritable bowel syndrome. *Aliment Pharmacol Ther* 1999;13(suppl 12):3-14.

Drossman DA, Camilleri M, Mayer EA, Whitehead WE. AGA technical review on irritable bowel syndrome. *Gastroenterology* 2002;123:2108-2131.

Longstreth GF, Burchette RJ. Family practitioners' attitudes and knowledge about irritable bowel syndrome. *Fam Prac* 2003;20:670-674.

Longstreth GF, Yao JF. Irritable bowel syndrome and surgery: a multivariable analysis. *Gastroenterology* 2004;126:1665-1673.

O'Sullivan MA, Mahmud N, Kelleher DP, Lovett E, O'Morain CA. Patient knowledge and educational needs in irritable bowel syndrome. *Eur J Gastroenterol Hepatol* 2000;12:39-43.

Schuster MM. Defining and diagnosing irritable bowel syndrome. *Am J Manag Care* 2001;7:S246-S251.

Chapter 3. Why Do I Have IBS?

Ali A, Richardson D, Toner B. Feminine gender role and illness behaviour in irritable bowel syndrome. *J Gender Culture Health* 1998;3:59-65.

Almy TP, Mullin M. Alterations in man under stress. Experimental production of changes stimulating the "irritable colon." *Gastroenterology* 1947;8:616-626.

Camilleri M, Atanasova E, Carlson PJ, et al. Serotonin-transporter polymorphism pharmacogenetics in diarrhea-predominant irritable bowel syndrome. *Gastroenterology* 2002;123:425-432.

Chang L, Heitkemper MM. Gender differences in irritable bowel syndrome. *Gastroenterology* 2002;123:1686-1701.

Coates MD, Mahoney CR, Linden DR, et al. Molecular defects in mucosal serotonin content and decreased serotonin reuptake transporter in ulcerative colitis and irritable bowel syndrome. *Gastroenterology* 2004;126:1657-1664.

Crane C, Martin M. Illness-related parenting in mothers with functional gastrointestinal symptoms. *Am J Gastroenterol* 2004;99:694-702.

Drossman DA, Leserman J, Nachman G, et al. Sexual and physical abuse in women with functional or organic gastrointestinal disorders. *Ann Int Med* 1990;113:828-833.

Drossman DA, Talley NJ, Leserman J, et al. Sexual and physical abuse and gastrointestinal illness. *Ann Int Med* 1995;123:782-794.

Gwee KA, Graham JC, McKendrick MW, et al. Psychometric scores and the persistence of irritable bowel after infectious diarrhoea. *Lancet* 1996; 347:150-153.

Gwee KA, Leong YL, Graham C, et al. The role of psychological and biological factors in postinfective gut dysfunction. *Gut* 1999;44:400-406.

Heitkemper MM, Cain KC, Jarrett ME, et al. Symptoms across the menstrual cycle in women with irritable bowel syndrome. *Am J Gastroenterol* 2003;98:420-430.

Houghton LA, Jackson NA, Whorwell PJ, et al. Do male sex hormones protect from irritable bowel syndrome? *Am J Gastroenterol* 2000;95:2296-2300.

Kanazawa M, Endo Y, Whitehead WE, et al. Patients and nonconsulters with irritable bowel syndrome reporting a parental history of bowel problems have more impaired psychological distress. *Dig Dis Sci* 2004;49:1046-1053.

Lackner JM, Gudleski GD, Blanchard EB. Beyond abuse: the association among parenting style, abdominal pain, and somatization in IBS patients. *Behav Res Ther* 2004;42:41-56.

Lembo T, Zaman MS, Chavez NF, et al. Concordance of IBS among monozygotic and dizygotic twins. *Gastroenterology* 2001;120:A636.

Levy RL, Jones KR, Whitehead WE, et al. Irritable bowel syndrome in twins: heredity and social learning both contribute to etiology. *Gastroenterology* 2001;121:799-804.

Levy RL, Whitehead WE, Von Korff MR, Feld AD. Intergenerational transmission of gastrointestinal illness behavior. *Am J Gastroenterol* 2000;95:451-456.

Locke GR, Zinsmeister AR, Talley NJ, et al. Familial association in adults with functional gastrointestinal disorders. *Mayo Clin Proc* 2000;75:907-912.

Miller V, Whitaker K, Morris JA, Whorwell PJ. Gender and irritable bowel syndrome: the male connection. *J Clin Gastroenterol* 2004;38:558–560.

Morris-Yates A, Talley NJ, Boyce PM, et al. Evidence of a genetic contribution to functional bowel disorder. *Am J Gastroenterol* 1998;93:1311–1317.

Neal R, Barker L, Spiller RC. Prognosis in post-infective irritable bowel syndrome: a six-year follow-up study. *Gut* 2002;51:410–413.

Pata C, Erdal E, Yazici K, et al. Association of the 1438 G/A and 102 T/C polymorphism of the 5-HT2A receptor gene with irritable bowel syndrome. *J Clin Gastroenterol* 2004;38:561–566.

Rodriguez LA, Ruigomez A. Increased risk of irritable bowel syndrome after bacterial gastroenteritis. *BMJ* 1999;318:565–566.

Ruigomez A, Rodriguez LA, Johansson S, Wallander MA. Is hormone replacement therapy associated with an increased risk of irritable bowel syndrome? *Maturitas* 2003;44:133–140.

Spiller RC, Jenkins D, Thornley JP, et al. Increased rectal mucosal enteroendocrine cells, T-lymphocytes, and increased gut permeability following acute *Campylobacter* enteritis and in post-dysenteric irritable bowel syndrome. *Gut* 2000;47:804–811.

Tornblom H, Lindberg G, Nyberg B, Veress B. Full-thickness biopsy of the jejunum reveals inflammation and enteric neuropathy in irritable bowel syndrome. *Gastroenterology* 2002;123:1972–1979.

Whitehead WE, Bosmajian L, Zonderman AB, et al. Symptoms of psychologic distress associated with irritable bowel syndrome. Comparison of community and medical clinic samples. *Gastroenterology* 1988;95:709–714.

Chapter 4. How Common Is IBS?

Drossman DA, Li Z, Andruzzi E, et al. U.S. householder survey of functional gastrointestinal disorders. Prevalence, sociodemography, and health impact. *Dig Dis Sci* 1993;38:1569–1580.

Mitchell CM, Drossman DA. Survey of the AGA membership relating to patients with functional gastrointestinal disorders. *Gastroenterology* 1987;92:1282–1284.

National Ambulatory Medical Care Survey. National Center for Health Statistics: NAMCS description. Available at www.cdc.gov/nchs/about/major/ahcd/namcsdes.htm.

Saito YA, Locke GR, Talley NJ, et al. A comparison of the Rome and Manning criteria for case identification in epidemiological investigations of irritable bowel syndrome. *Am J Gastroenterol* 2000;95:2816–2824.

Talley NJ, Zinsmeister AR, Van Dyke C, Melton LJ. Epidemiology of colonic symptoms and the irritable bowel syndrome. *Gastroenterology* 1992;101:927–934.

Chapter 5. What Is My Prognosis?

American Gastroenterological Association. *The Burden of Gastrointestinal Diseases.* Bethesda, Md. 2001.

Bertram S, Kurland M, Lydick E, et al. The patient's perspective of irritable bowel syndrome. *J Fam Prac* 2001;50:521–525.

Brandt LJ, Bjorkman D, Fennerty MB, et al. Systematic review on the management of irritable bowel syndrome in North America. *Am J Gastroenterol* 2002;97:11(suppl):S7–S26.

Creed F, Ratcliffe J, Fernandez L, et al. Health-related quality of life and health care costs in severe, refractory irritable bowel syndrome. *Ann Intern Med* 2001;134:860–868.

Frank L, Kleinman L, Rentz A, et al. Health-related quality of life associated with irritable bowel syndrome: comparison with other chronic diseases. *Clin Ther* 2002;24:675–689.

Gralnek IM, Hays RD, Kilbourne A, et al. The impact of irritable bowel syndrome on health-related quality of life. *Gastroenterology* 2000;119:654–660.

Harvey RF, Mauad EC, Brown AM. Prognosis in the irritable bowel syndrome: a five-year prospective study. *Lancet* 1987;1:963–965.

Lacy BE, Rosemore, J, Robertson, D, et al. Physicians' attitudes and practices in the evaluation and treatment of irritable bowel syndrome. *Scand J Gastroenterol* 2006;41:892–902.

Owens DM, Nelson DK, Talley NJ. The irritable bowel syndrome: long-term prognosis and the patient-physician interaction. *Ann Intern Med* 1995; 122:107–112.

Sandler RS, Everhart JE, Donowitz M, et al. The burden of selected digestive diseases in the United States. *Gastroenterology* 2002;122:1500–1511.

Talley NJ, Gabriel SE, Harmsen WS, Zinsmeister AR, Evans RW. Medical costs in community subjects with irritable bowel syndrome. *Gastroenterology* 1995;109:1736–1741.

Chapter 6. The Anatomy of Digestion

Chey WY, Jin HO, Lee MH, et al. Colonic motility abnormality in patients with irritable bowel syndrome exhibiting abdominal pain and diarrhea. *Am J Gastroenterol* 2001;96:1499–1506.

Kellow JE, Phillips SF. Altered small bowel motility in irritable bowel syndrome is correlated with symptoms. *Gastroenterology* 1987;92:1885–1893.

Kellow JE, Phillips SF, Miller LJ, et al. Dysmotility of the small intestine in irritable bowel syndrome. *Gut* 1988;29:1236–1243.

Mertz H, Morgan V, Tanner G, et al. Regional cerebral activation in irritable bowel syndrome and control subjects with painful and non-painful rectal distention. *Gastroenterology* 2000;118:842–848.

Ritchie J. Pain from distension of the pelvic colon by inflating a balloon in the irritable colon syndrome. *Gut* 1973;14:125–132.

Silverman DHS, Munakata JA, Ennes H, et al. Regional cerebral activity in normal and pathological perception of visceral pain. *Gastroenterology* 1997;112:64–72.

Thompson WG, Creed F, Drossman DA, et al. Functional bowel disorders and functional abdominal pain. *Gastroenterol Int* 1992;5:75–91.

Thompson WG, Longstreth GF, Drossman DA, et al. Functional bowel disorders and functional abdominal pain. *Gut* 1999;45(suppl II):43–47.

Whitehead WE, Holtkotter B, Enck P, et al. Tolerance for rectosigmoid distention in irritable bowel syndrome. *Gastroenterology* 1990;98:1187–1192.

Chapter 7. How Is IBS Diagnosed?

Cash BD, Schoenfeld P, Chey WD. The utility of diagnostic tests in irritable bowel syndrome patients: a systematic review. *Am J Gastroenterol* 2002;97:2812–2819.

Chey WD, Olden K, Carter E, et al. Utility of the Rome I and Rome II criteria for irritable bowel syndrome in US women. *Amer J Gastroenterol* 2002;97:2803–2811.

Drossman DA. Irritable bowel syndrome: how far do you go in the workup? *Gastroenterology* 2001;121:1515.

Drossman DA, Corazziari E, Talley NJ, et al. *Rome II. The Functional Gastrointestinal Disorders. Diagnosis, Pathophysiology and Treatment: A Multinational Consensus.* 2nd ed. McLean, Va.: Degnon Associates, 2000.

Kruis W, Thieme CH, Weinzierl M, et al. A diagnostic score for the irritable bowel syndrome: its value in the exclusion of organic disease. *Gastroenterology* 1984;87:1–7.

Manning AP, Thompson WG, Heaton KW, et al. Towards positive diagnosis of the irritable bowel. *Brit Med J* 1978;2:653–654.

Sanders DS, Carter MJ, Hurlstone DP, et al. Association of adult celiac disease with irritable bowel syndrome: a case-control study in patients fulfilling ROME II criteria referred to secondary care. *Lancet* 2001;358:1504–1508.

Smith RC, Greenbaum DS, Vancouver JB, et al. Gender differences in Manning criteria in the irritable bowel syndrome. *Gastroenterology* 1991;100:591–595.

Thompson WG, Creed FH, Drossman DA, et al. Functional bowel disorders and functional abdominal pain. *Gastroenterol Int* 1992;5:75–91.

Vanner SJ, Depew WT, Paterson WG, et al. Predictive value of the Rome criteria for diagnosing the irritable bowel syndrome. *Am J Gastroenterol* 1999;94:2912–2917.

Chapter 9. *IBS and Other Medical Disorders*

Cady R and Dodick DW. Diagnosis and treatment of migraine. *Mayo Clinic Proceedings* 2002;77:255–261.

Goadsby PJ, Lipton RB, and Ferrari MD. Migraine: current understanding and treatment. *N Engl J Med* 2002;346:257–270.

Chapter 13. *Treatment Basics*

Akehurst R, Kaltenthaler E. Treatment of irritable bowel syndrome: a review of randomised controlled trials. *Gut* 2001;48:272–282.

Camilleri M. Review article: clinical evidence to support current therapies of irritable bowel syndrome. *Aliment Pharmacol Ther* 1999;13(suppl 12):48–53.

Jailwala J, Imperiale TF, Kroenke K. Pharmacologic treatment of the irritable bowel syndrome: a systematic review of randomized, controlled trials. *Ann Intern Med* 2000;133:136–147.

Klein KB. Controlled treatment trials in the irritable bowel syndrome. *Gastroenterology* 1988;95:232–241.

Chapter 16. *Treatment Options for IBS with Constipation*

Camilleri M, Kerstens R, Rykx A, Vandeplassche L. A placebo-controlled trial of prucalopride for severe chronic constipation. *N Engl J Med* 2008;358:2344–2354.

Drossman DA, Chey WD, Johanson JF, et al. Clinical trial: lubiprostone in patients with constipation-associated irritable bowel syndrome—results of two randomized, placebo-controlled studies. *Aliment Pharmacol Ther* 2009;29:329–341.

Ford A, Brandt L, Young C, et al. Efficacy of 5-HT3 antagonists and 5-HT4 agonists in irritable bowel syndrome: systematic review and meta-analysis. *Am J Gastroenterol* 2009;104:183–93.

Johanson JF, Morton D, Geenen J, Ueno R. Multicenter, 4-week, double-blind, randomized, placebo-controlled trial of lubiprostone, a locally-acting type-2 chloride channel activator, in patients with chronic constipation. *Am J Gastroenterol* 2008;103:170–177.

Johnston JM, Kurtz CB, Macdougall JE, et al. Linaclotide improves abdominal pain and bowel habits in a phase IIb study of patients with irritable bowel syndrome with constipation. *Gastroenterology* 2010;139:1877–1886.

Jones MP, Talley NJ, Nuyts G, Dubois D. Lack of objective evidence of efficacy of laxatives in chronic constipation. *Dig Dis Sci* 2002;47:2222–2230.

Kellow J, Lee OY, Chang FY, et al. An Asia-Pacific, double blind, placebo controlled, randomized study to evaluate the efficacy, safety, and tolerability of tegaserod in patients with irritable bowel syndrome. *Gut* 2003;52:671–676.

Lacy BE, Cole MS. Constipation in the older adult. *Clin Geriatrics* 2004;12:44–54.

Lacy BE, Loew B, Crowell MD. Prucalopride for chronic constipation. *Drugs Today* 2009;45:843–853.

Lacy BE, Yu S. Tegaserod: a new 5-HT4 agonist. *J Clin Gastroenterol* 2002;34:27–33.

Muller-Lissner S, Fumagalli I, Bardhan KD, et al. Tegaserod, a 5-HT4 receptor partial agonist, relieves symptoms in irritable bowel syndrome patients with abdominal pain, bloating, constipation. *Aliment Pharmacol Ther* 2001;15:1655–1666.

Novick J, Miner P, Krause R, et al. A randomized, double-blind, placebo-controlled trial of tegaserod in female patients suffering from irritable bowel syndrome with constipation. *Aliment Pharmacol Ther* 2002;16:1877–1888.

Nyhlin H, Bang C, Elsborg L, et al. A double-blind, placebo-controlled, randomized study to evaluate the efficacy, safety and tolerability of tegaserod in patients with irritable bowel syndrome. *Scan J Gastroenterol* 2004;39:119–126.

Patel S, Berrada D, Lembo A. Review of tegaserod in the treatment of irritable bowel syndrome. *Expert Opinion Pharmacother* 2004;5:2369–2379.

Chapter 17. Treatment Options for IBS with Diarrhea

Camilleri M, Chey WY, Mayer EA, et al. A randomized controlled clinical trial of the serotonin type 3 receptor antagonist alosetron in women with diarrhea-predominant irritable bowel syndrome. *Arch Int Med* 2001;161:1733–1740.

Cann PA, Read NW, Holdsworth CD, Barends D. Role of loperamide and placebo in management of irritable bowel syndrome. *Dig Dis Sci* 1984;29:239–247.

Coremans G, Clouse RE, Carter F, et al. Cilansetron, a novel 5-HT3 antagonist, demonstrated efficacy in males with irritable bowel syndrome with diarrhea-predominance. *Gastroenterology* 2004;126:A643.

Higgins PDR, Davis KJ, Laine L. The epidemiology of ischemic colitis. *Aliment Pharmacol Ther* 2004;19:729–738.

Lembo T, Wright RA, Bagby B, et al. Alosetron controls bowel urgency and provides global symptom improvement in women with diarrhea-predominant irritable bowel syndrome. *Am J Gastroenterol* 2001;96:2662–2670.

Chapter 18. Medications for Abdominal Pain Associated with IBS

Broekaert D, Vos R, Gevers A, et al. A double-blind, randomized placebo-controlled crossover trial of citalopram, a selective 5-hydroxytryptamine reuptake inhibitor, in irritable bowel syndrome. *Gastroenterology* 2001;120:A641.

Drossman DA, Toner BB, Whitehead WE, et al. Cognitive-behavioral therapy versus education and desipramine versus placebo for moderate to severe functional bowel disorders. *Gastroenterology* 2003;125:19–31.

Lin HC. Small intestinal bacterial overgrowth: a framework for understanding irritable bowel syndrome. *JAMA* 2004;292:852–858.

Masand PS, Gupta S, Schwartz TL, et al. Paroxetine in patients with irritable bowel syndrome: a pilot open-label study. *J Clin Psychiat* 2002;4:12–16.

Mathias JR, Clench MH, Abell TL, et al. Effect of leuprolide acetate in treatment of abdominal pain and nausea in premenopausal women with functional bowel disease. *Dig Dis Sci* 1998;43:1347–1355.

Page JG, Dirnberger GM. Treatment of the irritable bowel syndrome with Bentyl (dicyclomine hydrochloride). *J Clin Gastroenterol* 1981;3:153–156.

Pimentel M, Chow EJ, Lin HC. Eradication of small intestinal bacterial overgrowth reduces symptoms of irritable bowel syndrome. *Am J Gastroenterol* 2000;95:3503–3506.

Pimentel M, Chow EJ, Lin HC. Normalization of lactulose breath testing correlates with symptom improvement in irritable bowel syndrome: a double blind, randomized controlled study. *Am J Gastroenterol* 2003;98:412–419.

Poynard T, Naveau S, Mory B, Chaput JC. Meta-analysis of smooth muscle relaxants in the treatment of irritable bowel syndrome. *Aliment Pharmacol Ther* 1994;8:499–510.

Tabas G, Beaves M, Wang J, et al. Paroxetine to treat irritable bowel syndrome not responding to high-fiber diet: a double-blind, placebo-controlled trial. *Am J Gastroenterol* 2004;99:914–920.

Chapter 19. Treatments for Gas and Bloating

Ringel Y, Williams RE, Kalilani L, Cook SF. Prevalence, characteristics, and impact of bloating symptoms in patients with irritable bowel syndrome. *Clin Gastroenterol Hepatol* 2009;7:68–72.

Chapter 21. Complementary and Alternative Medicine

Bazzocchi G, Gionchetti P, Almerigi PF, et al. Intestinal microflora and oral bacteriotherapy in irritable bowel syndrome. *Dig Liver Dis* 2002;34(suppl):48–53.

Bensoussan A, Talley NJ, Hing M, et al. Treatment of irritable bowel syndrome with Chinese herbal medicine: a randomized controlled trial. *JAMA* 1998;280:1585–1589.

Kim HJ, Camilleri M, McKinzie S, et al. A randomized controlled trial of a probiotic, VSL#3, on gut transit and symptoms in diarrhoea-predominant irritable bowel syndrome. *Aliment Pharmacol Ther* 2003;17:895–904.

Niedzielin K, Kordecki H, Birkenfeld B. A controlled double-blind randomized study on the efficacy of *Lactobacillus plantarum* 299V in patients with irritable bowel syndrome. *Eur J Gastroenterol Hepatol* 2001;13:1143–1147.

Nobaek S, Johansson ML, Molin G, et al. Alternation of intestinal microflora is associated with reduction in abdominal bloating and pain in patients with irritable bowel syndrome. *Am J Gastroenterol* 2000;95:1231–1238.

Pittler MH, Ernst E. Peppermint oil for irritable bowel syndrome: a critical review and meta-analysis. *Am J Gastroenterol* 1998;93:1131–1135.

Rohrbock RBK, Hammer J, Vogelsang H, et al. Acupuncture has a placebo effect on rectal perception but not on distensibility and spatial summation: a study in health and IBS. *Am J Gastroenterol* 2004;99:1990–1997.

Sen S, Mullan MM, Parker TJ, et al. Effect of *Lactobacillus plantarum* 299V on colonic fermentation and symptoms of irritable bowel syndrome. *Dig Dis Sci* 2002;47:2615–2620.

Spanier JF, Howden CW, Jones MP. A systematic review of alternative therapies in the irritable bowel syndrome. *Arch Int Med* 2003;163:265–274.

Yadav SK, Jain AK, Tripathi SN, Gupta JP. Irritable bowel syndrome: therapeutic evaluation of indigenous drugs. *Indian J Med Res* 1989;90:496–503.

Chapter 22. Psychological, Hypnotherapeutic, and Psychiatric Therapies

Fricchione G. Generalized anxiety disorder. *N Eng J Med* 2004;351:675–682.

Gonsalkorale WM, Miller V, Afzal A, Whorwell PJ. Long-term benefits of hypnotherapy for irritable bowel syndrome. *Gut* 2003;52:1623–1629.

Greene B, Blanchard EB. Cognitive therapy for irritable bowel syndrome. *J Consult Clin Psychol* 1994;62:576–582.

Heymann-Monnikes I, Arnold R, Florin I, et al. The combination of medical treatment plus multicomponent behavioral therapy is superior to medical treatment alone in the therapy of irritable bowel syndrome. *Am J Gastroenterol* 2000;95:981–994.

Jackson JL, O'Malley PG, Tomkins G, et al. Treatment of functional gastrointestinal disorders with antidepressant medications: a meta-analysis. *Am J Med* 2000;108:65–72.

Otto MW, Smits JA, Reese HE. Cognitive-behavioral therapy for the treatment of anxiety disorders. *J Clin Psych* 2004;65 (suppl 15):34–41.

Chapter 24. IBS and Children

Crane C, Martin M. Illness-related parenting in mothers with functional gastrointestinal symptoms. *Am J Gastroenterol* 2004;99:694–702.

El-Matary W, Spray C, Sandhu B. Irritable bowel syndrome: the commonest cause of recurrent abdominal pain in children. *Eur J Pediatr* 2004;163:584–588.

Howell S, Talley NJ, Quine S, et al. The irritable bowel syndrome has origins in the childhood socioeconomic environment. *Am J Gastorenterol* 2004;99:1572–1578.

Kanazawa M, Endo Y, Whitehead WE, et al. Patients and nonconsulters with irritable bowel syndrome reporting a parental history of bowel problems have more impaired psychological distress. *Dig Dis Sci* 2004;49:1046–1053.

Lackner JM, Gudleski GD, Blanchard EB. Beyond abuse: the association among parenting style, abdominal pain, and somatization in IBS patients. *Behav Res Ther* 2004;42:41–56.

Levy RL, Whitehead WE, Von Korff MR, Feld AD. Intergenerational transmission of gastrointestinal illness behavior. *Am J Gastroenterol* 2000;95:451–456.

Miele E, Simeone D, Marino A, et al. Functional gastrointestinal disorders in children: an Italian prospective survey. *Pediatrics* 2004;114:73–78.

Index

Page numbers in **bold** refer to figures or tables.